Pediatric Robotic Assisted Surgery

Ciro Esposito • Thomas Blanc
Arnaud Bonnard
Editors

Pediatric Robotic Assisted Surgery

Step-by-step Techniques, Tips & Tricks

Springer

Editors
Ciro Esposito
Pediatric Surgery Department
University of Naples Federico II
Napoli, Napoli, Italy

Thomas Blanc
Department of Paediatric Urology
Paediatric Surgery & Transplantation
Hôpital Necker-Enfants Malades
AP-HP, Université Paris Cité
Paris, France

Arnaud Bonnard
Robert Debre University Children's Hospital
Paris, France

ISBN 978-3-031-99531-6 ISBN 978-3-031-99532-3 (eBook)
https://doi.org/10.1007/978-3-031-99532-3

This Springer imprint is published by the registered company Springer Nature Switzerland AG
The registered company address is: Gewerbestrasse 11, 6330 Cham, Switzerland

To my wife Marina and my children Giovanni and Giorgia, the three most beautiful and precious things I have ever had in my life
To my father, the best pediatric surgeon I've ever met, I thank him for the continuous teaching and for transferring to me his love for children we care for every day.
To my proctor of Robotics and my friend Lorenzo Masieri

Ciro Esposito

To my family
To my colleagues and friends of the Department of Paediatric Urology, Paediatric Surgery & Transplantation at Hôpital Necker-Enfants malades
To the FRUCT (FRench Urology Children Team)

Thomas Blanc

To the children and their parents, we will always try to make the best for them
To my mentor, Pascal de Lagausie…I'm sure you are still observing us and I hope you are proud of what we achieved
To my colleagues and friends, with them I'm sure that the best of care is provided to the children while I'm away of the department
To my family I'm cheering every days

Arnaud Bonnard

Preface

The field of minimally invasive surgery in children has undergone remarkable changes in the last few years and, above all, in the field of robotic surgery.

Robotic surgery has been developed in adult surgery over the last 20 years, but this technology was applied also for pediatric surgery in the last 10 years.

This book of pediatric robotic surgery covers all the fields of pediatric surgery (thoracic, abdominal, urology, oncology, and gynecology).

International experts of pediatric robotic surgery are involved in it, providing current indications to robotic surgery; technical notes are illustrated in detail to show patient position, robotic assessment, and the optimal use of robotic instruments.

This book is addressed to all the specialists involved in robotics, pediatric surgeons, pediatric urologists, urologists, general surgeons but also anesthesiologists, pediatricians, and scrub nurses.

The chapters are arranged in different sections to guide the readers step by step in performing the different procedures thanks also to the images at the end to each chapter.

Nowadays the more common robotic procedure performed in the pediatric population is pyeloplasty but several other urological, gastrointestinal, thoracic, and gynecological procedures can be performed with the robotic system, and all these procedures are accurately described in this book.

This book is intended to provide all the instruments to start a pediatric robotic program in a pediatric surgical unit.

We sincerely hope that upon completion of this text the reader will learn the basic and advanced robotic-assisted surgical techniques to assist them in their pediatric robotic surgery activity. Despite the huge development of robotics in the last few years, the current robotic systems are still not able to replace the surgeon who maintains a key role in the performance of surgical procedure and that above all must decide the surgical indications, the operative setting, and know how to manage surgical complications. The format to this book is designed to be readily accessible, and it will be certainly a must and a real opportunity for the new generation of pediatric surgeons and pediatric urologists.

Napoli, Napoli, Italy — Ciro Esposito
Paris, France — Thomas Blanc
Paris, France — Arnaud Bonnard

Acknowledgments

The editors gratefully acknowledge the contributing authors for their work and for sharing their wisdom for the preparation of their individual chapters.

We express our thanks to Madona Samuel, project coordinator at Springer Nature, the executive editor Donatella Rizza, who provided professional support, without whom this book would never have reached print.

Contents

General

Pediatric Anesthesia in Robotic Surgery

Giuseppe Cortese, Andrea Uriel de Siena, Carola Visani, Immacolata Fontana, Tiziana Rossi, Giuseppina Faccioli, Loredana Grande, Maria Silvia Barone, and Giuseppe Servillo

1 Introduction

Robotic surgery has revolutionized various surgical fields by offering enhanced precision, dexterity, and control, particularly in complex and minimally invasive procedures. In pediatric patients, the application of robotic systems presents unique challenges and opportunities for anesthesiologists. Unlike adult patients, children undergoing robotic surgery require specialized care due to their physiological and anatomical differences, including smaller airways, immature organ systems, and unique pharmacokinetic and pharmacodynamic profiles.

The role of the anesthesiologist in pediatric robotic surgery extends beyond traditional anesthesia delivery. The anesthetic plan must accommodate the surgical requirements of robotic systems, which often involve prolonged insufflation, steep Trendelenburg positions, and restricted access to the patient during the procedure. These factors necessitate meticulous attention to ventilation, hemodynamic stability, and intraoperative monitoring, as well as the possible complications such as pneumoperitoneum-related effects, airway pressure challenges, and the risk of cardiovascular compromise.

Furthermore, the perioperative management of pediatric patients involves careful preoperative assessment, considering comorbidities and developmental considerations that may affect anesthesia delivery. Postoperative care, including pain management, the risk of postsurgical nausea and vomiting (PONV), and the potential for delayed recovery, requires a tailored approach to ensure optimal outcomes.

This chapter explores the anesthetic considerations, strategies, and advancements in pediatric robotic surgery, providing anesthesiologists with a comprehensive framework to manage these complex cases effectively. By understanding the intricacies of pediatric physiology in the context of robotic surgery, anesthesiologists can optimize patient safety and surgical outcomes.

*Giuseppe Cortese, *Andrea Uriel de Siena, Carola Visani, Immacolata Fontana, Catello La Storia, Costanza Tognon, Tiziana Rossi, Giuseppina Faccioli, Loredana Grande, Maria Silvia Barone and Giuseppe Servillo *contributed equally with all other contributors.

G. Cortese (✉) · A. U. de Siena · C. Visani · I. Fontana · T. Rossi · G. Faccioli · L. Grande · M. S. Barone · G. Servillo
Department of Neurosciences, Reproductive and Odontostomatological Sciences, University of Naples, Federico II, Naples, Italy

C. Esposito et al. (eds.), *Pediatric Robotic Assisted Surgery*,
https://doi.org/10.1007/978-3-031-99532-3_1

2 Robotic Surgery

2.1 Introduction to Robotic Surgery

Robotic surgery (RS) is becoming more and more popular, because it gives surgeons a three-dimensional view of the operating field, allows for smaller incisions, and allows for fine motor control of robotic arms. These benefits include decreased blood loss; a decreased risk of damaging neural, vascular, and parenchymal structures; and less pain following surgery. However, it also requires the patient to be positioned in an extreme manner, which may increase the risk of certain side effects, such as atelectasis [1, 2]. RS has also a high cost, and the main problem is the size of the instrument: The difference in size could potentially limit the access of the anesthetist and/or assistance to the patient and cause arm and instrument collision outside the patient. Moreover, the respiratory and cardiovascular balance is significantly altered by pneumoperitoneum, which has to be understood and treated. Considering this background, it is important to understand the anesthesiologist challenges and their management. All the changes during surgery and their consequences are summarized in Table 1.

2.2 Physiological Effect of Robotic Surgery and Anesthesia Consideration

RS affects mainly three systems: respiratory, cardiovascular, and neuroendocrine ones. These three systems are stressed by two main conditions: the pneumoperitoneum and the position of the patient. The pneumoperitoneum involves an augmented abdominal pressure and carbon dioxide (CO_2) levels and hypothermia due to the low

Table 1 Pneumoperitoneum consequences

Target	Intra-abdominal pressure↑	Hypercarbia	Possible consequences
Cerebral	Intracranial pressure↑	Cerebral blood flow↑	Cerebral edema Late awakening
Eye	Ocular pressure↑	–	Retin lesion
Pulmonary system	Diaphragm cranial migration Airway pressure↑ Ventilation/Perfusion mismatch Lung compliance↓ Functional residual capacity↓	Pulmonary arterial pressure↑ Pulmonary vascular resistance↑ Gas embolism Subcutaneous emphysema	Pulmonary hypertensionDesaturation with or without pCO_2↑ Cardiac arrest Airway device displacement
Cardiovascular system	Right atrial pressure↑ Systemic vascular resistance↑ Cardiac output↓ Mean arterial pressure↑ Inferior vena cava or/and aortic compression	Arrhythmia Myocardial depression or/and ischemia Impaired hemoglobin affinity Systemic vascular resistance↓	Mismatch delivery O_2/consumption O_2 Hypertension or hypotension Respiratory acidosis Pulmonary hypertension Myocardial infraction Cardiac arrest
Kidney	Renal blood flow↓ Glomerular filtration rate↓ Oliguria	Renal proton excretion↑	Oliguria Acute kidney injury Renin/aldosterone system activation Bicarbonate loss
Splanchnic	Blood flow↓ Hepatic artery/portal vein blood flow↓ Gut blood flow↓ Risk of gastric regurgitation↑	Hepatic/intestine local tissue acidosis	Hepatic dysfunction Risk of pneumonia due to aspiration Risk of prolonged postoperative ileus

temperature of the gas; on the other side, the deep Trendelenburg or deep anti-Trendelenburg positions heavily affect the hemodynamic response and the pulmonary function.

2.2.1 Respiratory System

During pediatric robotic surgery, the pulmonary effects are a critical concern due to the cephalad displacement of the mediastinum and diaphragm due to the increase of intra-abdominal pressure, leading to a decrease in functional residual capacity and pulmonary compliance [3]. The decreasing of functional residual capacity and pulmonary compliance promotes ventilation-perfusion (V/Q) mismatch and shunting, inducing hypoxia due to mixture of unoxygenated blood with oxygenated one, and increases atelectasis, leading to a reduction of functional residual capacity, which raises peak airway pressures [4]. These challenges are further exacerbated with Trendelenburg position, commonly used in robotic surgery, which induce a cephalic migration of abdominal organs. To counteract the absorption of carbon dioxide (CO_2) from insufflation, minute ventilation (MV) must be increased; the increase of the MV could be reached by increasing tidal volume (TV) or respiratory rate (RR) [5]. It is important to consider that the increasing of TV is associated with the increase of volutrauma and barotrauma, meanwhile the increasing of RR is associated with the increase of mechanical power [6]. The absorption of CO_2, alongside physical compression of the lungs, can induce pulmonary vasoconstriction complicating gas exchange. In obese patients, this is particularly problematic, as the alveolar-arterial oxygen gradient widens in the Trendelenburg position, although insufflation may provide slight relief [7]. Over time, CO_2 absorption tends to plateau at around 1 hour. However, complications such as subcutaneous emphysema and intrabronchial migration of the endotracheal tube (ETT), due to cephalad movement of the carina or increased ETT cuff pressure, can arise. Notably, elevated CO_2 levels can shift the oxyhemoglobin dissociation curve to the right via the Haldane effect, aiding oxygen delivery to tissues and mitigating ischemic damage [8].

2.2.2 Cardiovascular and Neuroendocrine Effects

The physiological alterations given by pneumoperitoneum and patient position have a major influence on the cardiovascular system in pediatric robotic surgery. Inhaling carbon dioxide into the belly causes hypercarbia, which sets off a chain reaction in the neuroendocrine system that results in elevated cortisol, vasopressin, and catecholamine release [9]. Increased systemic vascular resistance, mean arterial pressure, and central venous pressure are the outcomes of this hormone surge. Furthermore, the insufflated abdomen's direct compression of the aorta raises systemic vascular resistance even further.

Pneumoperitoneum-related intrathoracic pressure increases heart filling pressures, but it can also compress the inferior vena cava, lowering preload and venous return. Variations in cardiac output may result from this, and after about 15 minutes of insufflation, early drops in the cardiac index usually return to normal. Moreover, compression of the spleen and liver, among other abdominal organs, might increase intravascular volume and complicate the cardiovascular response; this leads to a decrease in cardiac index of about 13%, especially when the pneumoperitoneum is above 12 mmHg [10].

The placement of the patient is also very important. While reverse, which is prevalent in upper gastrointestinal procedures, can cause venous pooling and lower cardiac output, especially in hypovolemic patients, the Trendelenburg position, which is frequently employed in pelvic surgeries, improves venous return and raises ventricular filling pressures [11]. It is important to consider also the ventricular interdependence phenomenon due to pneumo-cardiac interaction: Post-expiratory end pressure (PEEP) is often set at high level to reduce the atelectasis, and this could increase the pressure in the right chambers with a slide of the interventricular septum to the left and a reduction of left ventricular chamber [9].

Prolonged hypercarbia can cause acidosis, which can impair cardiac contractility and increase susceptibility to arrhythmias and augment the dissociation of hemoglobin, due to a right shift of the curve [12]. Hypercarbia can also cause tachyarrhythmias and bradyarrhythmia through a vagal response. During pediatric robotic surgery, hemodynamic stability must be maintained by controlling these cardiovascular consequences.

2.2.3 Splanchnic Circulation Consequences

Pneumoperitoneum and patient posture have both mechanical and neuroendocrine impacts on splanchnic circulation, which make them a crucial factor to consider while doing pediatric robotic surgery. Insufflation lowers intestinal perfusion and total hepatic blood flow, especially at pressures higher than 15 mmHg. But splanchnic vasodilation, which happens in reaction to hypercarbia during the surgery, frequently cancels out this reduction [13]. Therefore, in most situations, the total effect on splanchnic circulation is not clinically significant. Even yet, renal perfusion may be lower and so will urine production as a result of parenchymal compression. In order to minimize these consequences and sustain renal function, it is advised to keep insufflation pressures below 15 mmHg.

2.3 Fluid Balance

The decrease of renal blood flow induces a similar response of hypovolemic state: plasma renin and aldosterone level improvement lead to the increase of peripheral vascular resistance [14]. Moreover, decreased renal plasma flow and glomerular filtration pressure may result in reduced urine output, but these changes are generally well compensated in healthy patients, with no evidence of long-term renal impairment. Three regimens are possible in fluid administration: liberal, restricted, and a new approach called targeted directed therapy (GDT). A recent network metanalysis conducted on adult patient undergoing nonvascular abdominal surgery concluded that GDT is linked to a better outcome for wounds complications and postoperative anastomotic leak, lung, and cardiovascular complications: Indeed, restricted regimen could cause more hypotensive events, but liberal one improves lung complications and can worsen the intraoperative cerebral edema [15]. The 4-2-1 rule multiplied by the hours of fasting could be applied.

2.4 Temperature

Exposure of the peritoneal cavity to large volumes of cold, non-humidified CO_2 can contribute to hypothermia. The cardiovascular system and coagulation may be affected by hypothermia during prolonged surgeries, especially in neonates. Moreover, hypothermia moves the dissociation curve of hemoglobin to the left, increasing its affinity to oxygen but reducing the supply of the peripheral tissue, worsening the hypothermia-induced peripheral acidosis [12].

2.5 Intracranial Pressure

Cerebral blood flow and intracranial pressure may increase. A study in adults undergoing laparoscopy showed that significant changes in cerebral oxygenation are uncommon and similar trends were observed in pediatric populations during laparoscopic surgery. Furthermore, hypercarbia raises intracranial pressure (ICP) and cerebral blood flow, which calls for close observation, particularly in those with comorbid cerebrovascular diseases [16]. This raise of ICP could lead to cerebral edema, which could justify a delay in awakening at the end of the surgery. The Trendelenburg posture, which is frequently used in robotic surgery, might make things more difficult by raising intraocular pressure, which can last for up to an hour after procedure. Therefore, sustaining systemic and splanchnic perfusion in pediatric patients requires careful intraoperative regulation of insufflation pressures and carbon dioxide levels.

2.6 Peritoneal Morphology

Carbon dioxide has both local and systemic effects. Studies on rats have shown that CO_2 reacts with peritoneal fluid, reducing peritoneal pH and creating an acidic environment that limits inflammation. The degree of intra-abdominal pressure and the type of insufflation gas affect the extent of inflammation [17]. Low pressure with CO_2 causes fewer peritoneal changes compared to high pressure or air insufflation. Increased inflammatory cells, such as eosinophils, mast cells, and lymphocytes, have been observed, though no clinical significance has been identified.

2.7 Intestinal Function

RS is associated with faster postoperative recovery compared to open surgery, including quicker return of bowel function, early removal of devices, improved mobilization, and better pain control. A minimally invasive approach also reduces the inflammatory response and the incidence of postoperative wound infections, facilitating faster recovery [14]. Preoperative education, patient optimization, intraoperative management of surgical stress, multimodal analgesia, early mobilization, and early oral nutrition have all contributed to improved outcomes [13].

3 Preoperative Evaluation

The preoperative phase is a crucial phase where it is possible to get to know the patient, to decide the best anesthesia strategy, to explain the strategy and solve children's and parents' doubt, and to acquire the informed consent, considering, if possible, children's will.

3.1 Assessment and Investigation

For the safe administration of anesthesia and to foresee potential complications arising from the special physiological and anatomical challenges that pediatric patients undergoing robotic surgery present, a preoperative evaluation is crucial. Given the complexity of robotic-assisted surgery (RAS), selecting the right patient is essential. This is especially true for children under the age of 1 year or weighing under 10 kg, as these patients may have anatomical space limitations or robotic instrumentation limitations that make the procedure more challenging. There is no agreement on standardized selection criteria for pediatric RAS, despite the fact that robotic surgeries have been carried out on patients as small as 7 kg [18].

Preanesthetic assessment entails a comprehensive assessment to detect any comorbidities that may affect the patient's physiological response to pneumoperitoneum and other intraoperative challenges, particularly in the respiratory, cardiovascular, and nervous systems. Pneumoperitoneum, for instance, can alter hemodynamics, so congenital abnormalities, especially those affecting the cardiovascular system, should be carefully evaluated. According to available data, even in children with congenital heart disease, intra-abdominal pressures (IAP) of 8 to 12 mmHg are generally well tolerated; however, close observation is necessary for those with more severe conditions [19].

The evaluation of potential risk factors, such as elevated intraocular pressure and central venous pressure during steep Trendelenburg positioning that may affect intracranial pressure or vision, should also be a part of the preoperative phase. Nonetheless, research indicates that individuals without underlying ocular or brain disorders typically manage these pressures quite well. While certain conditions like glaucoma or high intracranial pressure need to be considered, using RAS is not always prohibited by them.

A thorough physical examination and a thorough anamnesis are required to evaluate the patient's general health, medication use, allergies, and level of hydration. To address any abnormalities, preoperative investigations such as electrocardiograms (recommended to be 6 month old at the latest) and laboratory tests (especially in high risk surgery) should be scheduled well in advance. During this phase, it is important to investigate any possible hereditary illness and ask parents or pediatric patient if abnormal blood loss after a wound or a dentary loss/extraction was found. Indeed, there are some studies that underline that laboratory exams cannot identify all coagulation disfunctions [20]. It is important to investigate a possible pregnancy in female patients in childbearing age.

All fasting guidelines, including those pertaining to the consumption of infant formula and breast milk, should be adhered to. Bowel preparation is recommended occasionally to increase intraoperative working space, particularly for gastrointestinal procedures. The fasting timing recommended are as follows:

- 2 hours from clear liquids (water, fruit juice without pulp, clear tea, black coffee)
- 4 hours from breast milk
- 6 hours from nonhuman milk and light meal (toast with water)

3.2 Informed Consent

Informed consent is the most important step for election surgery. It is important to involve the children considering his/her intellective and psychological growth stage according to his/her age. Informed consent is acquired by the parents or legal tutor. It is important to refer to the local law and protocols about informed consent for underaged patient.

4 Anesthesia Management

Anesthesia management is the most challenging part for the anesthesiologist due to a difficult access to the patient and the physiological changes inducted by RS and pneumoperitoneum.

4.1 Premedication and Patient Preparation

The first step is to prepare all the equipment. The SOAPME acronym is a valid approach to ensure that the operative room is ready to accept the patient:

- S (suction): Size-appropriate suction catheters.
- O (oxygen): Adequate O_2 supply and ventilator.
- A (airway): Size-appropriate airway equipment (facial masks, laryngoscope blades, endotracheal and rhino-tracheal tubes, stylet, any devices for difficult airway management).
- P (pharmacy): All basic drugs needed to support any phase of anesthesia.
- M (monitors): Pulse oximeter, ECG, noninvasive pressure, capnography, and stethoscope are always required; defibrillator periodically checked.
- E (equipment): Any special equipment or drugs for a particular case.

Premedication for pediatric patients receiving RS should be customized to the patient's anxiety level and general physical state, using the same guidelines as other surgical procedures. A good premedication is important to reduce the possibility of a psychological trauma [21]. One of the frequently prescribed drugs is midazolam, which is taken orally 30 minutes prior to the induction of anesthesia at a dose of 0.5 mg/kg. Alternative delivery methods like rectal (0.5 mg/kg), sublingual (0.3 mg/kg), or nasal (0.3 mg/kg) can be taken into consideration if oral administration is not practical [18]. In the last years, intranasal dexmedetomidine demonstrated a safe profile with a good efficacy [22]. Furthermore, premedication may be combined with anticholinergic medications like atropine or glycopyrrolate to lessen airway secretions and avoid reflex bradycardia brought on by abdominal insufflation, even if in the routine a prior use is not more diffused due to their side effects [23].

In order to guarantee surgical access and patient safety during robotic procedures, the placement of the patient on the operating table is essential. The anesthesiologist must have access to the patient for monitoring and intervention, and the position must allow for the best possible visibility of the surgical field. Adequate padding is used at pressure points, such as the face, elbows, and heels, to prevent complications like nerve compression injuries or pressure ulcers [24]. The patient's arms are usually positioned alongside the body, with at least one arm kept accessible for monitoring intravenous access; anti-decubitus aids and eye protection are also applied. Maintaining stability while on the table is very important, particularly when performing robotic surgery and requiring steep Trendelenburg positions. To stop patients from moving during the procedure, use straps that secure the patient without obstructing access and anti-slip mattresses [24].

Vascular access is crucial, because the robot's docking may make it more difficult to access the patient afterward. In situations where blood loss is anticipated, two intravenous lines are preferred but at least one is needed. To prevent pneumoperitoneum from limiting the administration of fluids and medications, venous access should ideally be positioned above the diaphragm. During this phase, it is possible to induce the patient with sevoflurane gas to acquire a vascular access if the premedication was not successful or the patient is not collaborative [18]. Patients who require frequent blood sampling or who are more likely to experience complications may be candidates for central venous access or arterial lines. In order to improve visibility of the surgical field and lower the risk of gastric injury during the procedure, it is also recommended a nasogastric tube to be positioned correctly. Furthermore, bladder catheterization is advised for managing fluids and keeping track of urine output [18].

4.2 Airway Management and Intraoperative Phase

The airway management could be a challenge for the anesthesiologist. The main problems are the difficult access to the head during surgery, pneumoperitoneum that increases the risk of airway device displacement, and difficult airway management of the children. The use of laryngeal mask is not recommended, especially if the surgery lasts some time, due to the high risk of displacement of the device with difficulty in replacing it. Endotracheal intubation (ETI) with a cuffed tube is generally preferred for improved airway protection and controlled ventilation, especially in younger children, non-cuffed tube could be used in patient aged less than 8 years old [18]. A protocol of rapid series induction should be considered in kids with excessive threat of regurgitation and pulmonary aspiration.

The primary goals of anesthesia during pediatric robotic surgery are to keep the optimal conditions for the surgery while managing physiological alterations caused by pneumoperitoneum and patient position [17]. General anesthesia with neuromuscular blockade, endotracheal intubation, and positive pressure ventilation is typically used. Standard monitoring includes continuous ECG, noninvasive blood pressure, pulse oximetry, capnography, and temperature control, though capnography may not accurately reflect arterial CO_2 levels in infants due to a variable gradient between arterial and end-tidal CO_2. Induction of anesthesia may be intravenous or inhalational, depending on the patient's age and tolerance for intravenous catheter placement. Intravenous induction, commonly with propofol, is preferred in older children due to its rapid onset, reduced risk of bronchospasm, and antiemetic properties. Inhalational induction is an option for younger children, though desflurane is generally avoided due to its potential to cause airway irritation and laryngospasm. Rapid sequence induction may be necessary for patients at high risk of aspiration, often combined with the use of H2-receptor antagonists like ranitidine [18].

Ventilation strategies during robotic surgery must be carefully managed to prevent lung injury. Pressure-controlled ventilation with low tidal volumes (6–7 mL/kg) is recommended to reduce the risk of barotrauma; an augment of about 30% of respiratory rate could be used to maintain the normocarbia, with a target of end-tidal CO_2 of 35–40 mmHg. Positive end-expiratory pressure (PEEP) of at least 5 cm H_2O should be applied to prevent atelectasis, especially in the Trendelenburg position, even if the PEEP guided by driving pressure (DP, less than 12 mmHg) or calculated on pressure/volume curve (on the lower inflection point) are the most recommended [9]. In cases of hypoxia, alveolar recruitment maneuvers (RMs) should be performed cautiously to minimize lung trauma, adjusting FiO_2 based on oxygen saturation or arterial oxygenation; RMs via PEEP should be preferred [11].

Pneumoperitoneum-induced hemodynamic changes are generally well tolerated in healthy pediatric patients; euvolemia is carefully maintained. Fluid management aims to preserve extracellular volume with an isotonic polyelectrolyte solution (10 ml/kg/h) buffered possibly, and additional boluses may be administered to maintain hemodynamic stability [18]. Close monitoring of vital signs, acid-base balance, and urinary output is necessary to ensure stability during surgery. The infusion should be administered with syringe pump and not by normal via.

In pediatric patients, hypothermia is a significant concern due to prolonged exposure to cold insufflation gases and surgical duration. Therefore, it is critical to monitor and maintain body temperature using warming devices, heated intravenous fluids, and a warm operating room environment. The hypothermia could be reduced by a low rate of gas insufflation (2 L/min) [18].

Neuromuscular blockade is maintained throughout the procedure to ensure muscle relaxation and stabilization of insufflation pressure. Peripheral nerve stimulation is used to monitor the depth of blockade, and using sugammadex if possible a complete reversal of neuromuscular agents is essential to avoid postoperative respiratory complications. For pain management, a multimodal approach combining systemic analgesics and regional anesthesia is recommended to control both incisional and visceral pain [18].

Antibiotic prophylaxis is recommended for pediatric RS in cases of clean-contaminated procedures, clean surgeries involving prosthetic implants, or when infection could lead to severe consequences. However, it is generally not required for clean surgeries. The decision to use prophylaxis should consider factors such as the ASA score, wound classification, and the procedure's duration. For pelvic, abdominal, or thoracic RS classified as clean-contaminated, perioperative prophylaxis should follow local antimicrobial guidelines, with intravenous antibiotics administered 30–60 minutes before incision and additional doses considered if the surgery exceeds the drug's half-life or involves significant blood loss. Postoperative antibiotics are only continued for 24 hours in high-risk cases [18].

4.3 Postoperative Management and Complications

Postoperative care for pediatric patients following robotic surgery requires careful monitoring and a structured approach to pain management, prevention of complications, and recovery. While drains are generally not used in pediatric RS, they may be necessary in some cases, such as abdominal or thoracic procedures, due to unforeseen surgical events. When drains are used, their placement should be minimized to reduce the risk of infection and other complications [18].

Effective postoperative analgesia is crucial and should begin immediately upon anesthesia emergence. Multimodal pain management, including a combination of opioids, NSAIDs, paracetamol, and regional anesthesia, is highly recommended to minimize discomfort and optimize recovery. Intravenous administration of fentanyl (1–2 mcg/kg), paracetamol (15 mg/kg), morphine (0.1 mg/kg), and ketorolac IV (0.5 mg/kg) is common in managing postoperative pain [25]. For ongoing pain relief, paracetamol can be administered at regular intervals, either intravenously or orally. Rescue analgesia, such as tramadol, may be used if necessary. Additionally, transversus abdominis plane (TAP) blocks are increasingly used as a valid and effective method for postoperative pain control in lower abdominal surgeries [18]. This regional technique offers long-lasting relief while reducing the need for systemic opioids, thus minimizing the risk of respiratory depression.

Postoperative nausea and vomiting (PONV) are a frequent complications, particularly in laparoscopic procedures, with an incidence rate of about 39% in pediatric patients [26]. A multimodal approach to PONV prevention is essential and should include preoperative risk evaluation, adequate IV fluid hydration, opioid-sparing pain management, and antiemetic prophylaxis. Dexamethasone is superior to ondansetron in preventing postoperative nausea 4–6 hours after surgery, though both are equally effective in preventing vomiting within the first 24 hours. The use of a prophylactic antiemetic protocol and a postoperative vomiting in children (POVOC) score are recommended to manage PONV effectively [26]. Figure 1 reports the main steps in evaluation and treatment of PONV.

Thromboprophylaxis is generally unnecessary in pediatric patients due to the low incidence of venous thromboembolism (approximately 0.2%). However, risk assessment should be conducted for each patient, and perioperative thromboprophylaxis is advised for those with confirmed thromboembolic risk factors or when prolonged immobilization is expected. Thromboprophylaxis should begin immediately after surgery and continue for 48–72 hours, with reevaluation of the patient's risk profile afterward [27]. Table 2 reports the risk factors, meanwhile Fig. 2 shows an algorithm for thromboprophylaxis management.

Lastly, the anesthesiologist must be prepared to manage potential postoperative complications. These include hemodynamic instability, respiratory complications such as hypoxia or hypercarbia, and the rare but serious risk of gas embolism. Monitoring for subcutaneous emphysema, capnothorax, and capnomediastinum is critical, especially in cases of unexplained increases in airway pressure or hypoxemia. Prompt intervention with hyperventilation, PEEP optimization, and, in severe cases, abdominal desufflation may be necessary to resolve these complications [29]. Carbon dioxide embolism in a large vein or artery is a rare but potentially life-threatening complication. It typically presents as cardiovascular collapse, with a sudden drop in end-tidal CO_2, oxygen saturation, blood pressure, and the onset of various arrhythmias. In severe cases, it can be

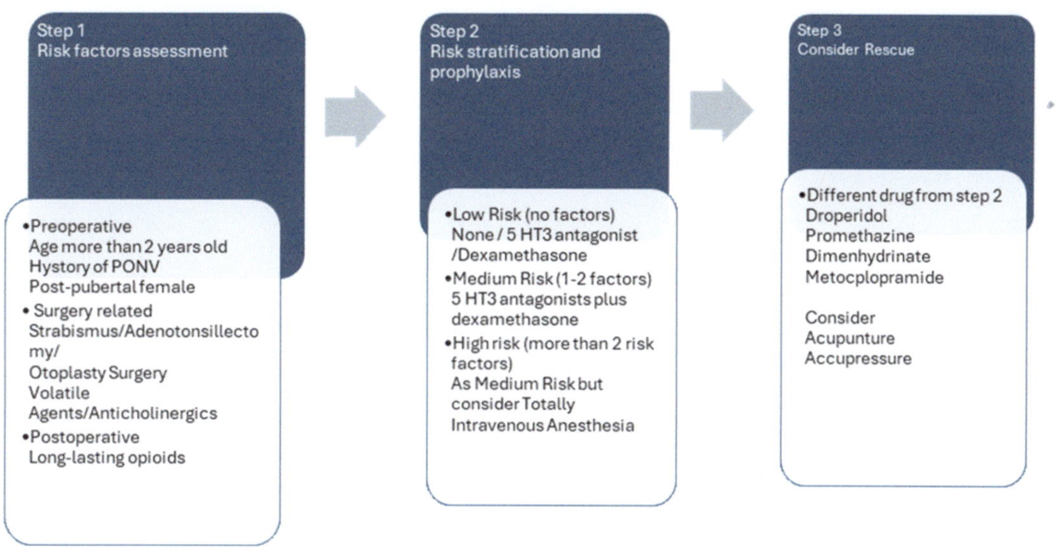

Fig. 1 PONV assessment and treatment

Table 2 Bleeding and thrombosis risk factors according to APAGBI guidelines [28]

	Bleeding risk	Thrombosis risk
Patient related	Acquired bleeding disorder Untreated inherited bleeding disorder Use of anticoagulants Thrombocytopenia Uncontrolled hypertension >230/120 mmHg	Central venous catheter Active cancer or cancer treatment Dehydration Thrombophilia Obesity Significant medical condition Personal history or first-degree relative aged less than 40 years old with an history of venous thromboembolism Estrogen therapy Pregnancy or < 6 weeks after the partum
Admission related	Neurosurgery or eye surgery Neuraxial anesthesia or lumbar puncture within 12 hours Active bleeding	Reduced mobility Severe trauma Severe burns Spinal cord injury with paralysis Total surgical procedure >90 minutes (>60 minutes if pelvic or lower limb surgery) Critical care patient

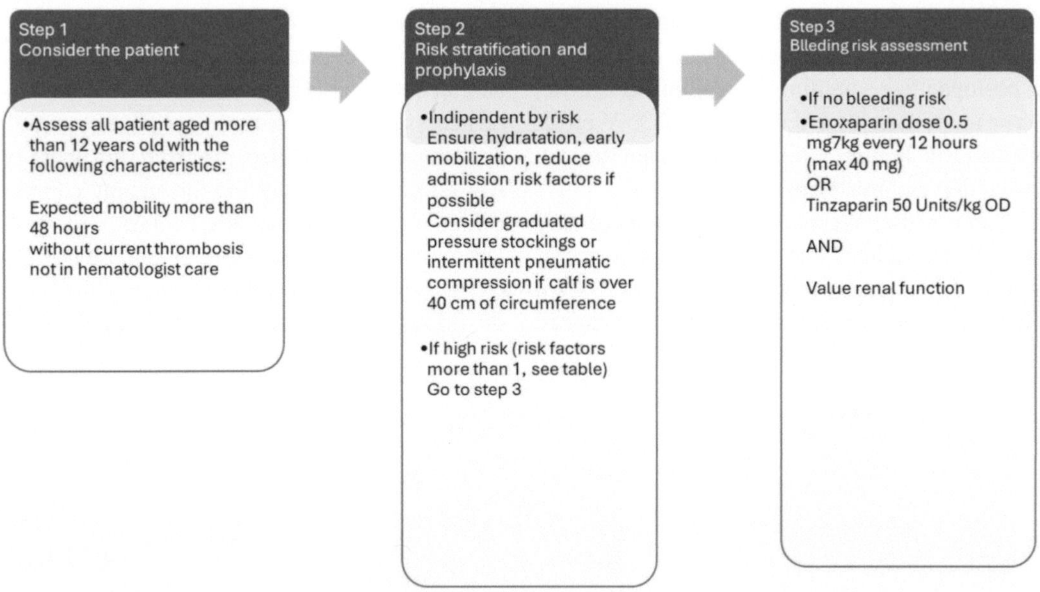

Fig. 2 Algorithm for postoperative thromboprophylaxis

fatal, depending on the size of the embolus [30]. Critical interventions include aspirating the gas through a central venous catheter, positioning the patient in Durant's position, and performing cardiopulmonary resuscitation (CPR).

5 Discussion

Pediatric anesthesia for robotic surgery presents a unique set of challenges that require careful planning, meticulous intraoperative management, and close postoperative monitoring. As RS becomes more prevalent in pediatric populations, anesthesiologists must be fully aware of the physiological alterations induced by pneumoperitoneum, patient positioning, and the use of minimally invasive techniques. The balance between the benefits of robotic surgery—such as reduced recovery time, smaller incisions, and less postoperative pain—and the complexities of maintaining respiratory, cardiovascular, and splanchnic stability, forms the core of anesthetic management.

The impact of patient positioning, particularly in steep Trendelenburg or reverse Trendelenburg, on respiratory and cardiovascular systems cannot be overstated. Careful ventilation strategies, including the use of pressure-controlled modes, positive end-expiratory pressure (PEEP), and cautious application of recruitment maneuvers, are essential to prevent barotrauma, atelectasis, and hypercarbia. Hemodynamic monitoring and fluid management are equally important, as pneumoperitoneum induces changes in preload, afterload, and cardiac output, necessitating vigilant control of intraoperative fluid balance and close monitoring of cardiovascular parameters.

The postoperative phase focuses on effective pain management, prevention of nausea and vomiting, and early detection of complications such as gas embolism or respiratory distress. Multimodal analgesia, incorporating systemic opioids, NSAIDs, and regional blocks like the transversus abdominis plane (TAP) block, ensures better pain control while minimizing opioid-related side effects such as respiratory depression. Prophylactic antiemetic protocols are vital to prevent the high incidence of postoperative nausea and vomiting (PONV) associated with laparoscopic surgeries, with dexamethasone and ondansetron being key agents in these strategies.

Thromboprophylaxis is generally not required in pediatric patients without specific risk factors for venous thromboembolism. However, in cases where prolonged immobilization or other risks are present, early intervention with thromboprophylaxis is warranted.

In conclusion, the anesthetic management of pediatric patients undergoing robotic surgery requires a tailored approach that considers the unique physiological demands of this patient population. Through a combination of advanced monitoring techniques, protective ventilation strategies, multimodal analgesia, and a proactive approach to managing potential complications, anesthesiologists can optimize surgical outcomes and ensure the safety and well-being of their young patients.

References

1. Luca F, Valvo M, Ghezzi TL, Zuccaro M, Cenciarelli S, Trovato C, Sonzogni A, Biffi R. Impact of robotic surgery on sexual and urinary functions after fully robotic nerve-sparing total mesorectal excision for rectal cancer. Ann Surg. 2013;257:672–8. https://doi.org/10.1097/SLA.0b013e318269d03b.
2. Baukloh J-K, Perez D, Reeh M, Biebl M, Izbicki JR, Pratschke J, Aigner F. Lower gastrointestinal surgery: robotic surgery versus laparoscopic procedures. Visc Med. 2018;34:16–22. https://doi.org/10.1159/000486008.
3. Gokdemir BN, Cekmen N. Laparoscopic surgery and anesthesia. JARSS. 2023;31:173–87. https://doi.org/10.54875/jarss.2023.63496.
4. Meininger D, Westphal K, Bremerich DH, Runkel H, Probst M, Zwissler B, Byhahn C. Effects of posture and prolonged pneumoperitoneum on hemodynamic parameters during laparoscopy. World J Surg. 2008;32:1400–5. https://doi.org/10.1007/s00268-007-9424-5.
5. Vieillard-Baron A, Prin S, Augarde R, Desfonds P, Page B, Beauchet A, Jardin F. Increasing respiratory rate to improve CO2 clearance during mechanical ventilation is not a panacea in acute respiratory failure. Crit Care Med. 2002;30:1407–12. https://doi.org/10.1097/00003246-200207000-00001.
6. Paudel R, Trinkle CA, Waters CM, Robinson LE, Cassity E, Sturgill JL, Broaddus R, Morris PE. Mechanical power: a new concept in mechanical ventilation. Am J Med Sci. 2021;362:537–45. https://doi.org/10.1016/j.amjms.2021.09.004.
7. Atkinson TM, Giraud GD, Togioka BM, Jones DB, Cigarroa JE. Cardiovascular and ventilatory consequences of laparoscopic surgery. Circulation. 2017;135:700–10. https://doi.org/10.1161/CIRCULATIONAHA.116.023262.
8. Haldane Effect - an Overview | ScienceDirect Topics. Available online: https://www.sciencedirect.com/topics/medicine-and-dentistry/haldane-effect. Accessed on 18 Sept 2024.
9. Buonanno P, Marra A, Iacovazzo C, Vargas M, Coviello A, Squillacioti F, Nappi S, de Siena AU, Servillo G. Impact of ventilation strategies on pul-

monary and cardiovascular complications in patients undergoing general anaesthesia for elective surgery: a systematic review and meta-analysis. Br J Anaesth. 2023; https://doi.org/10.1016/j.bja.2023.09.011.
10. Ortega AE, Peters JH, Incarbone R, Estrada L, Ehsan A, Kwan Y, Spencer CJ, Moore-Jeffries E, Kuchta K, Nicoloff JT. A prospective randomized comparison of the metabolic and stress hormonal responses of laparoscopic and open cholecystectomy. J Am Coll Surg. 1996;183:249–56.
11. Buonanno P, Marra A, Iacovazzo C, Merola R, De Siena AU, Servillo G, Vargas M. Electric impedance tomography and protective mechanical ventilation in elective robotic-assisted laparoscopy surgery with steep trendelenburg position: a randomized controlled study. Sci Rep. 2023;13:2753. https://doi.org/10.1038/s41598-023-29860-x.
12. Oxygen-Haemoglobin Dissociation Curve - an overview | ScienceDirect Topics. Available online: https://www.sciencedirect.com/topics/medicine-and-dentistry/oxygen-haemoglobin-dissociation-curve. Accessed on 19 Sept 2024.
13. Hatipoglu S, Akbulut S, Hatipoglu F, Abdullayev R. Effect of laparoscopic abdominal surgery on splanchnic circulation: historical developments. World J Gastroenterol. 2014;20:18165–76. https://doi.org/10.3748/wjg.v20.i48.18165.
14. Rist M, Hemmerling TM, Rauh R, Siebzehnrübl E, Jacobi KE. Influence of pneumoperitoneum and patient positioning on preload and splanchnic blood volume in laparoscopic surgery of the lower abdomen. J Clin Anesth. 2001;13:244–9. https://doi.org/10.1016/s0952-8180(01)00242-2.
15. Yang TX, Tan AY, Leung WH, Chong D, Chow YF. Restricted versus liberal versus goal-directed fluid therapy for non-vascular abdominal surgery: a network meta-analysis and systematic review. Cureus. 15:e38238. https://doi.org/10.7759/cureus.38238.
16. Effects of hypocapnia and hypercapnia on splanchnic circulation and hepatic function in the Beagle - PubMed Available online: https://pubmed.ncbi.nlm.nih.gov/2504078/. Accessed on 18 Sept 2024.
17. Esposito C, Escolino M, Farina A, Cerulo M, Cortese G, Caprio MG, De Pascale T, Settimi A. The role of bowel preparation to optimize working space in laparoscopic inguinal hernia repair in infants. J Pediatr Surg. 2014;49:1536–7. https://doi.org/10.1016/j.jpedsurg.2014.05.013.
18. Tesoro S, Gamba P, Bertozzi M, Borgogni R, Caramelli F, Cobellis G, Cortese G, Esposito C, Gargano T, Garra R, et al. Pediatric robotic surgery: issues in management—expert consensus from the Italian Society of Pediatric and Neonatal Anesthesia and Intensive Care (SARNePI) and the Italian Society of Pediatric Surgery (SICP). Surg Endosc. 2022;36:7877–97. https://doi.org/10.1007/s00464-022-09577-0.
19. Gillory LA, Megison ML, Harmon CM, Chen MK, Anderson S, Chong AJ, Chaignaud BE, Beierle EA. Laparoscopic surgery in children with congenital heart disease. J Pediatr Surg. 2012;47:1084–8. https://doi.org/10.1016/j.jpedsurg.2012.03.008.
20. Halimeh S, Rott H, Kappert G, Siebert M. Is a standardized preoperative questionnaire a good tool to detected coagulation disorders in children. Blood. 2013;122:4786. https://doi.org/10.1182/blood.V122.21.4786.4786.
21. Dave NM. Premedication and induction of anaesthesia in paediatric patients. Indian J Anaesth. 2019;63:713–20. https://doi.org/10.4103/ija.IJA_491_19.
22. Peng K, Wu S, Ji F, Li J. Premedication with dexmedetomidine in pediatric patients: a systematic review and meta-analysis. Clinics (Sao Paulo). 2014;69:777–86. https://doi.org/10.6061/clinics/2014(11)12.
23. Boriosi JP, Lasarev MR, Peters ME, Ferrazzano P, Hollman GA. Anticholinergics and serious adverse events in pediatric procedural sedation: a report of the pediatric sedation research consortiums. Paediatr Anaesth. 2022;32:665–72. https://doi.org/10.1111/pan.14403.
24. Chang C, Steinberg Z, Shah A, Gundeti MS. Patient positioning and port placement for robot-assisted surgery. J Endourol. 2014;28:631–8. https://doi.org/10.1089/end.2013.0733.
25. Bannister CF, Brosius KK, Wulkan M. The effect of insufflation pressure on pulmonary mechanics in infants during laparoscopic surgical procedures. Paediatr Anaesth. 2003;13:785–9. https://doi.org/10.1046/j.1460-9592.2003.01149.x.
26. Ames WA, Machovec K. An update on the management of PONV in a pediatric patient. Best Pract Res Clin Anaesthesiol. 2020;34:749–58. https://doi.org/10.1016/j.bpa.2020.05.007.
27. Aceto P, Antonelli Incalzi R, Bettelli G, Carron M, Chiumiento F, Corcione A, Crucitti A, Maggi S, Montorsi M, Pace MC, et al. Perioperative Management of Elderly Patients (PriME): recommendations from an Italian intersociety consensus. Aging Clin Exp Res. 2020;32:1647–73. https://doi.org/10.1007/s40520-020-01624-x.
28. Dunn T, Misra L. Intraoperative capnothorax during robotic diaphragmatic endometriosis excision. Case Rep Anesthesiol. 2022;2022:5935312. https://doi.org/10.1155/2022/5935312.
29. d'Arcy JL, Coffey S, Loudon MA, Kennedy A, Pearson-Stuttard J, Birks J, Frangou E, Farmer AJ, Mant D, Wilson J, et al. Large-scale community echocardiographic screening reveals a major burden of undiagnosed valvular heart disease in older people: the OxVALVE population cohort study. Eur Heart J. 2016;37:3515–22. https://doi.org/10.1093/eurheartj/ehw229.
30. Park EY, Kwon JY, Kim KJ. Carbon dioxide embolism during laparoscopic surgery. Yonsei Med J. 2012;53(3):459–66. https://doi.org/10.3349/ymj.2012.53.3.459. PMID: 22476987; PMCID: PMC3343430.

Training in Robotic Surgery

Maria Escolino, Annalisa Chiodi, Claudia Di Mento, Leonardo Continisio, and Ciro Esposito

1 Introduction

The introduction of robotic systems into the medical field has fundamentally revolutioned the landscape of surgery, representing one of the most significant technological breakthroughs in modern healthcare. The advent of robotic-assisted surgery allows for unprecedented levels of precision, dexterity, and control, offering surgeons the ability to perform intricate procedures that would be exceedingly difficult, if not impossible, to execute manually. These systems have transformed several key surgical disciplines, including urology, gynecology, and cardiothoracic surgery, but their impact is perhaps most visible in general surgery, where the potential for reduced patient recovery times and minimally invasive approaches has reshaped patient outcomes [1]. Since its inception, robotic surgery has evolved to become a key tool in the surgeon's armamentarium, particularly with the da Vinci Surgical System, which remains the market leader in robotic-assisted technologies.

Robotic surgery offers several advantages over traditional open and laparoscopic approaches. Not only it facilitates higher precision in complex surgical procedures, but it also significantly improves ergonomics for the surgeon, reducing fatigue and strain. These innovations contribute to fewer intraoperative complications and faster patient recovery times, making it a preferred method for many complex surgeries. Over the last 10 years, robotic surgery has been increasingly adopted also in pediatric patients, especially in complex reconstructive procedures such as pyeloplasty or lower urinary tract reconstruction, which benefit from the enhanced dexterity that robotic instruments provide [1].

However, with these advancements come new challenges, particularly in the realm of surgical training. Unlike traditional open surgery, where surgeons rely heavily on tactile feedback, robotic surgery requires a different set of skills, including enhanced hand-eye coordination, depth perception, and a mastery of the robotic interface. As a result, the training required to proficiently use robotic systems is more complex and longer than traditional surgical training programs [2]. Furthermore, the cost of acquiring, maintaining, and training on robotic systems is significant, leading to disparities in access to robotic surgery training, particularly in less well-funded

M. Escolino (✉) · A. Chiodi · C. Di Mento · C. Esposito
Pediatric Surgery Unit, University of Naples Federico II, Naples, Italy
e-mail: maria.escolino@unina.it; annalisa.chiodi@unina.it; claudia.dimento@unina.it; ciroespo@unina.it

L. Continisio
CEINGE Advanced Biotechnology Center, Naples, Italy
e-mail: leonardo.continisio01@universitadipavia.it

C. Esposito et al. (eds.), *Pediatric Robotic Assisted Surgery*,
https://doi.org/10.1007/978-3-031-99532-3_2

healthcare systems. This chapter aims to explore the current status of robotic training and related challenges, the methodologies developed to address them, and the technological advancements that continue to shape the field of robotic surgery.

2 Technological Advancements in Robotic Surgery

The technological evolution of robotic surgery systems has been characterized by rapid innovation and continuous refinement. The da Vinci Surgical System, which remains the most widely used robotic surgery platform today, offers numerous advantages over earlier forms of laparoscopic surgery. These include articulated instruments with multiple degrees of freedom, high-definition 3D visualization, and intuitive controls that translate the surgeon's movements into precise micro-movements of the surgical instruments. These capabilities are particularly advantageous in surgeries that require delicate tissue manipulation, such as pyeloplasty or lower urinary tract reconstruction, where precision is paramount [1].

In recent years, new advancements have pushed the boundaries of what is possible in robotic surgery. One of the most significant developments has been the integration of artificial intelligence (AI) into robotic systems. AI has the potential to revolutionize robotic surgery by enabling systems to learn from vast datasets of previous surgeries. These AI-driven systems can provide real-time guidance, assisting surgeons with decision-making by suggesting optimal techniques or identifying potential complications. For example, AI can analyze preoperative data and intraoperative images to recommend the best course of action for individual patients, thereby improving both efficiency and outcomes. However, AI integration requires extensive retraining of surgeons to effectively interpret and act upon these AI-generated insights [3].

Another emerging technology in robotic surgery is augmented reality (AR), which has the potential to significantly enhance the surgeon's ability to visualize critical anatomical structures during surgery. AR systems can overlay real-time, patient-specific anatomical data onto the surgeon's field of view, providing enhanced context and enabling more precise surgical interventions. This technology is particularly useful in procedures involving complex anatomy or when visibility is limited due to patient-specific factors, such as scar tissue from previous surgeries. For example, in liver surgery, AR can help surgeons visualize blood vessels or tumor margins that are not visible to the naked eye, thereby reducing the risk of accidental injury [4].

3 Challenges in Robotic Surgery Training

Training in robotic surgery presents a unique set of challenges compared to traditional surgical training. Robotic surgery demands a different skill set, including enhanced hand-eye coordination, proficiency with the robotic console, and a deep understanding of the system's capabilities and limitations. Unlike traditional surgery, where tactile feedback is a key component of the surgeon's skillset, robotic surgery requires the surgeon to rely almost entirely on visual feedback provided by the high-definition 3D cameras within the system. This shift from tactile to visual feedback can be disorienting for many surgeons, especially those trained in conventional methods, and requires extensive retraining [5].

One of the most significant challenges in robotic surgery training is the steep learning curve associated with mastering robotic systems. Research has shown that many surgeons need dozens, if not hundreds, of cases to become fully proficient with robotic systems. This prolonged learning period is due in part to the complexity of the robotic interface, which requires surgeons to operate in a completely different manner than they would during traditional open or laparoscopic surgery. Mastering the hand-eye coordination necessary to operate the robotic arms effectively is a major hurdle, as is developing the cognitive ability to control the robotic instruments in a way that mirrors their natural hand movements [6].

Another significant barrier to training is the financial burden associated with acquiring and maintaining robotic systems. Robotic surgery systems are among the most expensive medical technologies currently in use, with individual systems costing millions of dollars. In addition to the initial purchase price, hospitals must also invest in regular maintenance, software updates, and the training of personnel. These financial costs can be prohibitive for smaller institutions, limiting access to robotic surgery training and creating disparities in the availability of robotic surgery between well-funded hospitals and those with fewer resources [7].

Moreover, the limited availability of experienced mentors and proctors poses a further challenge. Robotic surgery is still a relatively new field, and the number of experienced surgeons who are capable of training others is limited. This is particularly problematic in regions where access to robotic surgery is less widespread, leading to bottlenecks in training and delays in the adoption of robotic surgery by new surgeons. The shortage of mentors also exacerbates the learning curve, as surgeons must often rely on self-directed learning or simulation-based training without the benefit of real-time feedback from experienced robotic surgeons [8].

4 Training Methodologies in Robotic Surgery

To address the challenges associated with robotic surgery training, a variety of training methodologies have been developed, each designed to provide surgeons with the skills and knowledge necessary to operate robotic systems safely and effectively. These methodologies include simulation-based training, dry lab exercises, wet lab practice, fellowships, and proctorships.

4.1 Simulation-Based Training

Simulation-based training has emerged as a cornerstone of robotic surgery education. In simulation-based training, surgeons practice their skills in a virtual environment that replicates the conditions of real surgeries without the risks associated with operating on live patients. Virtual reality (VR) refers to technology that enables users to interact with three-dimensional, deformable computerized environments in real time, using their natural senses and abilities. VR surgical training is becoming increasingly accessible and immersive, allowing trainees to hone essential skills through repetitive practice in a controlled setting, which results in shorter operative times, fewer complications, and better patient outcomes. Currently, there are four commercially available VR simulation platforms for surgical training, all validated and proven effective in developing robotic surgery skills. These include the Robotic Surgery System (Simulated Surgical Systems, USA), the dV-Trainer (Mimic, USA), the da Vinci Skills Simulator (Intuitive Surgical, USA), and the recently launched RobotiX Mentor (3D Systems, USA). These simulators provide high-fidelity, 3D representations of the surgical environment, allowing trainees to practice suturing, cutting, and tissue manipulation in a safe and controlled setting.

Furthermore, VR simulators provide performance metrics that allow trainees to track their progress and receive feedback on their performance [9]. However, the degree of immersion can vary, and the experience may sometimes feel artificial.

Simulation-based training offers several key advantages over traditional methods [9]. First, it allows trainees to practice procedures repeatedly, helping them to build the muscle memory and cognitive skills required for robotic surgery. Second, it provides a risk-free environment where mistakes can be made and corrected without consequence, fostering a learning environment where surgeons can refine their techniques without the pressure of operating on a live patient. Finally, simulators can be customized to replicate specific surgical scenarios, providing a tailored learning experience that meets the needs of individual trainees.

4.2 Dry Lab and Wet Lab Training

In addition to simulation, dry labs and wet labs offer valuable hands-on experience for surgeons in training. Dry lab simulation utilizes synthetic models with robotic consoles to develop specific skills like grasping, suturing, placement, cutting, and camera control. These exercises help surgeons develop the motor skills, spatial awareness, and familiarity with robotic instruments necessary for successful surgery. It's a cost-effective method for training basic psychomotor abilities and ensures consistent training across different locations. However, it offers the least surgical realism compared to other simulation methods, leading to diminishing returns for skill improvement. Additionally, its assessment capabilities are limited, typically focusing on basic metrics such as time taken to complete tasks or error prevention [10].

Wet lab simulation uses organic tissue to create a more realistic environment for developing skills in tissue handling and understanding tissue responses to instruments and diathermy. This method provides sensory feedback that can be applied in real surgeries. Wet lab models include synthetic and cadaveric models from humans and animals. While cadavers offer the highest level of realism, they are costly and lack physiological responses such as vascular injuries and tissue hemostasis. Animal models, on the other hand, provide more realistic physiological responses but face challenges related to anatomical differences, ethical concerns, sample preparation, and cost. Live porcine and ovine models have been used to simulate bleeding, which increases trainee confidence and leads to greater participation in robotic surgery training. However, all these models are limited by their high cost and limited availability. This type of training is essential for helping surgeons understand the nuances of tissue interaction, such as how to manage intraoperative complications and how to handle delicate tissues during surgery. Although wet labs are costly and raise ethical concerns, they remain an invaluable component of comprehensive robotic surgery training programs [11].

4.3 Basic and Advanced Courses

Basic courses focus on basic skills, while advanced courses explore more specialized technical abilities and procedural techniques. This distinction is important, because the objective of each type of training influences the approach and, consequently, the evaluation method. Beginners in robotic surgery typically start with virtual or dry lab training, whereas more experienced robotic surgeons often train in wet labs using animal tissue models. The goal of basic training is to familiarize trainees with the robotic surgery system, including its controls, interface, camera, and robot docking while helping them develop initial technical skills (Fig. 1). On the other hand, advanced training aims to refine existing skills and apply them to high-fidelity models before transitioning to real-world practice.

4.4 Fellowships and Proctorships

For surgeons who have completed their residency training, fellowship or mini-fellowship programs provide an opportunity for advanced, specialized training in robotic surgery. Fellowships typically last 1 to 2 years and offer surgeons the chance to work alongside experienced robotic surgeons in a clinical setting. These programs combine hands-on surgical experience with simulation-based training and theoretical education, ensuring that fellows develop a deep understanding of robotic surgery techniques and principles. Fellows also gain experience in case selection, preoperative planning, and postoperative care, all of which are essential for independent practice [12].

Proctorships provide another form of mentorship, in which experienced robotic surgeons guide trainees through live surgeries. Proctorships allow trainees to receive real-time feedback and guidance from skilled mentors during actual sur-

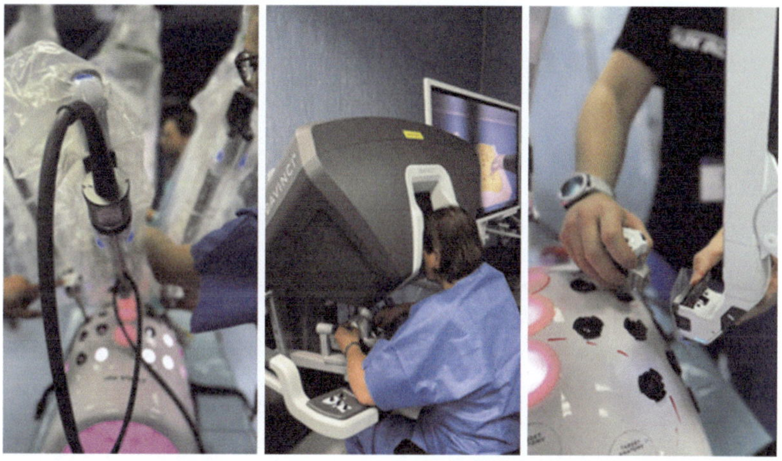

Fig. 1 Robotic basic course in the dry-lab setting

gical procedures. This hands-on learning experience is crucial for bridging the gap between simulation training and live patient surgeries. However, the effectiveness of proctorships is dependent on the quality of the mentorship, and the availability of experienced proctors can be a limiting factor, particularly in regions where robotic surgery is less common [8]. The duration of proctoring needed will also vary by individual surgeon, and critical self-assessment and reflection is essential during the training period.

5 Proposition of Robotic Surgical Training Curriculum

The robotic curriculum for surgical training, as highlighted in several studies, is structured to provide a comprehensive and progressive learning experience that integrates different training modalities [5, 13, 14]. This training curriculum aims to equip surgeons with the necessary skills to proficiently use advanced robotic systems, meeting the growing demand for minimally invasive procedures across various fields like general, urological, and thoracoabdominal surgery.

The curriculum is initially developed based on expert opinions or a Delphi consensus. Next, a pilot validation is conducted by breaking down the surgery into key steps and assessing the complexity of each. Steps with similar levels of complexity are then organized into modules, independent of their order in the actual surgical procedure. Safety is assessed by comparing clinical outcomes to the standard of care. Lastly, the effectiveness of the curriculum is evaluated by considering the total number of steps and modules the trainee has attempted and successfully completed. This curriculum typically follows a multistage approach, beginning with pre-console training, which focuses on developing fundamental skills, such as camera control, instrument manipulation, and spatial awareness. Trainees also learn to navigate robotic platforms like da Vinci, Versius, Hugo RAS, and RobotiX Mentor, mastering the console and understanding docking procedure. Simulation plays a pivotal role, incorporating both virtual reality (VR) training and dry/wet lab simulations. VR simulators, such as the SimNow and dV-Trainer, allow trainees to practice repeatedly in a risk-free environment, improving technical skills like suturing, tissue manipulation, and precision in robotic movements. These simulations not only enhance proficiency but also reduce mental workload, preparing trainees for real-life surgical scenarios. Wet lab models using animal tissue further enhance sensory and tissue-handling skills, bridging the gap between simulation and live surgery. The curriculum is often based on proficiency-based progression (PBP), where surgeons advance through increasingly complex tasks, using objective metrics to assess performance. Tools like the Global Evaluative Assessment of Robotic Skills (GEARS) and Robotic Objective Structured Assessments of

Technical Skills (R-OSATS) help evaluate competency in critical areas such as bimanual dexterity, depth perception, and efficiency [5]. The ERUS Robotic Curriculum is a prime example, integrating evidence-based practices with a focus on moving trainees from novice to expert levels through deliberate practice [14]. Future efforts should be directed to design a training curriculum specific for pediatric surgeons, considering the peculiarities of this surgical specialty and its applications.

6 Financial Implications of Robotic Surgery Training

The financial implications of adopting robotic surgery systems are considerable, and the costs associated with training surgeons in their use add a significant burden on healthcare institutions. The acquisition of a robotic surgery system can cost anywhere from $one million to $2.5 million, depending on the model and the number of instruments included. In addition to the initial purchase price, hospitals must also factor in the costs of maintenance, software updates, and the disposable instruments used during surgeries, which can add hundreds of thousands of dollars to the overall cost each year.

Moreover, the training programs required to bring surgeons up to proficiency with robotic systems are expensive as well. Simulation platforms, wet lab facilities, and the salaries of trainers and proctors all contribute to the cost of training. Smaller hospitals, particularly those in rural or less affluent areas, often struggle to afford these costs, which can create disparities in access to robotic surgery. Hospitals that are unable to afford these systems may find themselves falling behind in the adoption of new technologies, ultimately affecting patient care. As robotic surgery continues to expand and new technologies such as AI and AR are integrated into these systems, the costs associated with training are likely to increase further [15].

To offset these costs, many institutions are turning to partnerships with medical device companies or seeking government grants to help fund their robotic surgery programs. In some cases, larger hospitals may share their robotic systems and training resources with smaller hospitals, allowing more surgeons access to this advanced training. However, these solutions are not always feasible, and the financial burden remains a significant barrier to widespread adoption of robotic surgery [5].

7 Current and Future Trends in Robotic Surgery Training

The field of robotic surgery training is evolving rapidly, driven by advances in technology and the increasing demand for robotic surgery expertise. One of the most significant trends is the growing use of simulation-based training, which continues to become more sophisticated. Recent advancements in VR and haptic feedback have made it possible for simulators to offer highly realistic and immersive training experiences. Haptic feedback, which mimics the sensation of touch, allows surgeons to feel the resistance and texture of tissues as they practice, providing a level of realism that was previously unattainable. This enhancement is particularly valuable in training for procedures where tactile feedback is critical, such as tissue dissection or suturing [10, 11].

The integration of AI and AR into robotic surgery systems is also expected to play an increasingly important role in training. AI-driven systems have the potential to provide real-time feedback on a surgeon's performance, identifying mistakes and offering suggestions for improvement. Similarly, AR can enhance training by overlaying anatomical models onto the trainee's field of view, allowing them to practice complex procedures with greater accuracy and context. These technologies are still in the early stages of adoption but are likely to become more widespread as they prove their value in improving training outcomes [3].

Another trend in robotic surgery training is the increased emphasis on remote learning. With advancements in telemonitoring and teleproctoring technologies, experienced robotic surgeons can now mentor trainees from remote locations. This flexibility allows for broader access to high-quality training, particularly in regions where there are few experienced robotic surgeons available. Telemonitoring also enables real-time feedback during live surgeries, providing trainees with the support they need while performing complex procedures.

Looking to the future, it is likely that training programs will continue to evolve to keep pace with the rapid developments in robotic surgery technology. As robotic systems become more advanced and more widely adopted, the demand for highly trained robotic surgeons will continue to grow. Training programs must therefore continue to adapt, incorporating new technologies and methodologies to ensure that surgeons are well-prepared for the challenges of robotic surgery [12].

8 Ethical and Practical Considerations

While the benefits of robotic surgery are clear, there are also ethical and practical considerations that must be addressed in both the adoption of these systems and the training of surgeons. One of the primary concerns is the cost of robotic surgery and the potential for this technology to exacerbate inequalities in health care. As previously mentioned, the high cost of robotic systems and the training required to use them can create disparities in access to care, with wealthier hospitals and patients benefiting from the latest technologies while others are left behind.

Another ethical consideration is the use of animal models in training. While wet labs provide an invaluable training environment for surgeons, they also raise ethical questions about the use of animals in medical education. Many institutions are exploring alternatives to wet lab training, such as high-fidelity simulators that can replicate the feel and behavior of live tissues without the need for animal models. However, these alternatives are not yet as effective as wet labs in providing the tactile feedback necessary for certain procedures [11].

Finally, as AI becomes more integrated into robotic systems, there are concerns about the role of human decision-making in surgery. While AI has the potential to greatly enhance surgical outcomes, there is also a risk that surgeons may become overly reliant on these systems, leading to a loss of critical thinking skills. Training programs must therefore strike a balance between leveraging the benefits of AI and ensuring that surgeons maintain their ability to make independent, informed decisions during surgery.

9 Conclusion

The integration of robotic systems into surgery has transformed the field by offering unprecedented precision and control while improving patient outcomes. However, these advancements come with significant challenges, particularly in training. The complexity of robotic surgery, the steep learning curve, and the high cost of training programs present significant barriers to widespread adoption. Nevertheless, using simulation-based training, dry and wet labs, fellowships, and proctorships, surgeons can develop the skills necessary to perform robotic surgeries safely and effectively.

As technology continues to evolve, particularly with the integration of AI and AR, the future of robotic surgery training looks promising. These advancements will likely make training more accessible, more effective, and more tailored to the individual needs of surgeons. Major challenges include the high cost of equipment and limited access to experts, but technologies like remote mentoring and augmented reality can help lower costs and bridge geographical gaps. These emerging technologies provide real-time feedback and immersive environments, ultimately leading to better patient outcomes.

References

1. Spinoit AF, Nguyen H, Subramaniam R. Role of robotics in children: a brave new world! Eur Urol Focus. 2017;3(2–3):172–80. https://doi.org/10.1016/j.euf.2017.08.011.
2. Liss MA, McDougall EM. Robotic surgical simulation. Cancer J. 2013;19(2):124–9. https://doi.org/10.1097/PPO.0b013e3182885d79.
3. Howard KK, Makki H, Novotny NM, Mi M, Nguyen N. Value of robotic surgery simulation for training surgical residents and attendings: a systematic review protocol. BMJ Open. 2022;12(6):e059439. https://doi.org/10.1136/bmjopen-2021-059439.
4. Costello DM, Huntington I, Burke G, Farrugia B, O'Connor AJ, Costello AJ, Thomas BC, Dundee P, Ghazi A, Corcoran N. A review of simulation training and new 3D computer-generated synthetic organs for robotic surgery education. J Robot Surg. 2022;16(4):749–63. https://doi.org/10.1007/s11701-021-01302-8.
5. Sinha A, West A, Vasdev N, Sooriakumaran P, Rane A, Dasgupta P, McKirdy M. Current practises and the future of robotic surgical training. Surgeon. 2023;21(5):314–22. https://doi.org/10.1016/j.surge.2023.02.006.
6. Gonçalves MR, Mück B, Faure JP, Topart P, Sousa MC. RoboticSurgery4all: are discovery courses important for robotic surgery skills acquisition? J Robot Surg. 2024;18(1):322. https://doi.org/10.1007/s11701-024-02077-4.
7. O'Kelly F, Farhat WA, Koyle MA. Cost, training and simulation models for robotic-assisted surgery in pediatric urology. World J Urol. 2020;38(8):1875–82. https://doi.org/10.1007/s00345-019-02822-7.
8. Ben-Or S, Nifong LW, Chitwood WR Jr. Robotic surgical training. Cancer J. 2013;19(2):120–3. https://doi.org/10.1097/PPO.0b013e3182894887.
9. Bric JD, Lumbard DC, Frelich MJ, Gould JC. Current state of virtual reality simulation in robotic surgery training: a review. Surg Endosc. 2016;30(6):2169–78. https://doi.org/10.1007/s00464-015-4517-y.
10. Raison N, Gavazzi A, Abe T, Ahmed K, Dasgupta P. Virtually competent: a comparative analysis of virtual reality and dry-lab robotic simulation training. J Endourol. 2020;34(3):379–84. https://doi.org/10.1089/end.2019.0541.
11. Raison N, Poulsen J, Abe T, Aydin A, Ahmed K, Dasgupta P. An evaluation of live porcine simulation training for robotic surgery. J Robot Surg. 2021;15(3):429–34. https://doi.org/10.1007/s11701-020-01113-3.
12. Azadi S, Green IC, Arnold A, Truong M, Potts J, Martino MA. Robotic surgery: the impact of simulation and other innovative platforms on performance and training. J Minim Invasive Gynecol. 2021;28(3):490–5. https://doi.org/10.1016/j.jmig.2020.12.001.
13. Seeliger B, Pavone M, Schröder W, Krüger CM, Bruns CJ, Scambia G, Mutter D, Marescaux J, Fuchs HF. Skill progress during a dedicated societal robotic surgery training curriculum including several robotic surgery platforms. Surg Endosc. 2024;38(9):5405–12. https://doi.org/10.1007/s00464-024-11128-8.
14. Basile G, Gallioli A, Diana P, Gallagher A, Larcher A, Graefen M, Harke N, Traxer O, Tilki D, Van Der Poel H, Emiliani E, Angerri O, Wagner C, Montorsi F, Wiklund P, Somani B, Buffi N, Mottrie A, Liatsikos E, Breda A. Current standards for training in robot-assisted surgery and endourology: a systematic review. Eur Urol. 2024;86(2):130–45. https://doi.org/10.1016/j.eururo.2024.04.008.
15. Rahimi AM, Uluç E, Hardon SF, Bonjer HJ, van der Peet DL, Daams F. Training in robotic-assisted surgery: a systematic review of training modalities and objective and subjective assessment methods. Surg Endosc. 2024;38(7):3547–55. https://doi.org/10.1007/s00464-024-10915-7.

Robotic-Assisted Surgery and Artificial Intelligence in Pediatric Surgery

Stefano Pomati and Sara Lazzaretti

1 The Gold Standard of Minimally Invasive Surgery and Robotics

Minimally invasive surgery (MIS), including laparoscopic procedures pioneered in the 1980s and 1990s, has become a prominent approach for many surgical specialties. Today, the laparoscopic approach is considered the gold standard for some surgical procedures across many specialties.

Laparoscopic surgery is a minimally invasive technique that employs specialized instruments inserted through small incisions to perform surgical procedures. Compared to traditional open surgery, this approach results in reduced tissue trauma. Notably beneficial for pediatric patients, laparoscopy often leads to decreased postoperative pain, faster recovery, and improved cosmetic outcomes due to smaller incisions [1, 2].

Over the past few decades, MIS has been embraced by both adult and pediatric surgeons, and many have also adopted robotic surgical methods for the benefits of increased precision and dexterity. Since the first soft-tissue robotic surgery was performed over 20 years ago, more than 12 million robotic-assisted surgeries (RAS) have been performed worldwide.

S. Pomati (✉) · S. Lazzaretti
Asensus Surgical Inc, Research Triangle, NC, USA
e-mail: spomati@asensus.com; slazzaretti@asensus.com

While RAS benefits are recognized across a variety of surgical specialties, the limited availability of smaller-diameter robotic instruments has inhibited the use of RAS by pediatric surgeons. In fact, the lack of 3 mm and 5 mm instruments, which are widely used in pediatric surgery, has meant that traditional robotic solutions have overlooked the unique needs and importance of preserving MIS benefits for the pediatric population. The lack of appropriately sized robotic instruments could force pediatric surgeons to compromise on Halsted's Principles, which emphasize minimal tension and gentle handling of tissues during surgery. Consequently, many pediatric patients have not been able to benefit fully from RAS advancements. This gap highlights the need for the development and availability of smaller robotic instruments to ensure that children can receive the same high standards of care and the added benefits of RAS as adults.

2 History of Robotic-Assisted Surgery in Surgery

Robotic-assisted surgery has a fascinating history marked by technological advancements and medical milestones.

The integration of machines in surgical procedures began between the 1950s and 1970s, driven by advancements in computer technology and early mechanical systems. Initially, surgical

C. Esposito et al. (eds.), *Pediatric Robotic Assisted Surgery*,
https://doi.org/10.1007/978-3-031-99532-3_3

robots were employed for tasks requiring precision, such as the positioning of needles for biopsies. In 1985, the *PUMA 560*, an industrial robotic arm, was utilized for a neurosurgical biopsy, marking one of the earliest documented instances of robotic-assisted surgery.

In 1988, the *PROBOT*, developed at Imperial College London, successfully performed prostate surgery, demonstrating the potential of robotic systems for precise interventions in urology. By the 1990s, rapid advancements in robotic-assisted surgery ensued. The *ROBODOC* system, introduced in 1992, was specifically designed for orthopedic surgeries such as hip replacements, enhancing the accuracy of bone cuts and the fit of implants. In 1994, Intuitive Surgical was founded, later developing the *Da Vinci Surgical System*, which has since become one of the most prominent robotic surgery platforms worldwide.

The Da Vinci Surgical System received FDA approval in 2000, revolutionizing minimally invasive surgery by offering enhanced precision, flexibility, and control for surgeons. In 2001, the *ZEUS Robotic Surgical System* enabled the historic transatlantic "Lindbergh Operation," where a surgeon in New York performed surgery on a patient in France, demonstrating the feasibility of remote surgery [3].

The 2010s marked continued innovation in robotic surgery. In 2011, the release of the Da Vinci Si model introduced improved 3D-HD vision and enhanced ergonomics. In 2013, the *Senhance Surgical System* by TransEnterix (now Asensus Surgical) received CE Mark approval, bringing haptic feedback and eye-tracking camera control to robotic surgery. By 2017, both the Da Vinci X and da Vinci Xi systems were launched, while the Senhance Surgical System received FDA approval, further advancing the field.

The 2020s have seen ongoing progress in robotic-assisted surgery, with the integration of artificial intelligence, machine learning, and enhanced robotic dexterity. New systems, including the *Versius* by CMR Surgical and the *HUGO* by Medtronic, have entered the market, fostering competition and innovation in the field of robotic surgery.

Robotic systems are now used in a wide range of procedures, including general surgery, gynecology, cardiothoracic surgery, and more. Future trends indicate greater automation and improved robotic control, enhanced imaging technologies for better visualization, augmented reality (AR) and virtual reality (VR) integration for surgical planning and training, and AI-driven decision support to assist surgeons during procedures.

3 Robotics in Pediatric Surgery

3.1 State of the Art

The use of robotic-assisted surgery (RAS) in pediatric surgery has evolved significantly over the past two decades. While adult surgical specialties, such as urology, gynecology, and general surgery, have widely adopted RAS, its application in pediatrics remains relatively limited due to some challenges. However, advances in robotic systems and miniaturized instrumentation are gradually overcoming these barriers, allowing pediatric surgeons to explore the benefits of RAS with improved dexterity, precision, and ergonomics [4].

Da Vinci Surgical System by Intuitive Surgical remains the most widely used robotic platform in pediatric surgery. Its three-dimensional high-definition (3D-HD) visualization, tremor filtration, and wristed instrumentation provide significant advantages over conventional laparoscopy. However, it does not offer 3 mm and 5 mm wristed instrument sizes or force feedback for all the instruments, and considerable space is required for docking the robotic arms in small pediatric patients [5]. Despite these constraints, the Da Vinci system has been successfully used in pediatric patients in all the specialties, demonstrating in pediatric urology reduced complication rates and shorter hospital stays compared to conventional laparoscopic approaches [6, 7].

To address some of the limitations of the Da Vinci system, newer robotic platforms have emerged, including the Senhance Surgical System by Asensus Surgical, the Versius by CMR Surgical, and the HUGO RAS by Medtronic.

The Senhance system offers haptic feedback and eye-tracking camera control. It uses 3 mm and 5 mm instruments, which may be more suitable for pediatric applications. Additionally, the open-console design provides a more natural ergonomic position for surgeons, which could reduce fatigue during prolonged pediatric procedures [8].

The Versius system by CMR is another recent innovation that is gaining attention in pediatric surgery. Its modular and compact design allows greater flexibility in small operating rooms, the use of 6.8 mm wristed instruments, and the open console are some examples.

Furthermore, the HUGO RAS platform by Medtronic incorporates AI-driven analytics and cloud connectivity, potentially enhancing surgical planning and postoperative performance assessments.

Overall, the state of the art in pediatric robotic surgery is rapidly advancing, with novel systems addressing long-standing challenges.

4 Advantages and Limitations of Robotic-Assisted Surgery in Pediatrics

Robotic-assisted surgery (RAS) has introduced significant advantages in pediatric surgery, particularly in terms of precision, dexterity, and minimally invasive approaches. However, several limitations still restrict its widespread adoption. Understanding these benefits and drawbacks is essential for optimizing the use of RAS in pediatric procedures and guiding future advancements in surgical robotics.

4.1 Advantages of Robotic-Assisted Surgery in Pediatrics

One of the main advantages of RAS is enhanced *surgical precision and dexterity*. The robotic system provides *tremor elimination* and *motion scaling*, allowing more refined movements than human hands can achieve. These attributes may benefit pediatric surgery, where delicate and small anatomical structures require extreme precision to minimize trauma and ensure optimal surgical outcomes. Studies have demonstrated that robotic systems enable superior suturing capabilities and more refined dissection, reducing complications in complex pediatric cases such as pyeloplasty and fundoplication [9].

Another major benefit of RAS is *improved ergonomics for the surgeon*. Unlike conventional laparoscopy, which requires the surgeon to maintain uncomfortable postures for extended periods, robotic platforms offer a seated console with easy hand controls. This setup reduces surgeon fatigue, thereby potentially enhancing performance and reducing intraoperative errors [10].

RAS also offers *three-dimensional high-definition (3D-HD) vision*, which improves depth perception during surgery. Traditional laparoscopic procedures rely on two-dimensional imaging, which can make intricate maneuvers more challenging. The enhanced visualization provided by robotic platforms could improve spatial awareness and accuracy [11].

4.2 Limitations of Robotic-Assisted Surgery in Pediatrics

Despite its advantages, RAS presents several challenges, particularly for pediatric patients. One of the primary limitations is *the size of the robotic instruments and of the systems*. Many robotic platforms were originally designed for adult surgery, and the absence of appropriately scaled instruments has made pediatric applications difficult. The lack of *3 mm and 5 mm instruments* has limited the feasibility of RAS in smaller children [12].

Another major concern is *the high cost of robotic surgery*. RAS is significantly more expensive than conventional laparoscopy due to high initial investment costs, disposable instrument expenses, and maintenance fees. Many pediatric surgical centers, especially in developing regions, face financial barriers to acquiring robotic systems, which limit accessibility and widespread adoption [13].

Additionally, *the learning curve for robotic surgery remains steep*, particularly for pediatric surgeons who may not have extensive exposure to robotic systems during training. The transition from traditional laparoscopic techniques to robotic-assisted surgery requires specialized training and credentialing, which can pose logistical challenges for hospitals implementing RAS programs [14].

4.3 Overcoming the Limitations of Current Robotic-Assisted Surgery Systems in Pediatrics

The limitations of robotic-assisted surgery (RAS) in pediatric surgery—such, as discussed, as the lack of appropriately sized instruments, the absence of haptic feedback, steep learning curves, and high costs—have hindered its widespread adoption. However, several robotic systems now incorporate features that mitigate these challenges. For instance, the Senhance Surgical System, developed by Asensus Surgical, and the Versius, developed by CMR, have been designed to address some of these challenges while preserving the benefits of robotic-assisted procedures. Let's now see how these new technologies are overcoming the current limitations of RAS in pediatric surgery.

4.3.1 Miniaturized Instruments for Pediatric Surgery

One of the primary challenges in applying RAS to pediatric patients has been the *lack of appropriately sized instruments*. Many traditional robotic platforms, such as the Da Vinci Surgical System, utilize 8 mm instruments, which may be too large for small pediatric patients. The Senhance system directly addresses this limitation by providing *3 mm and 5 mm instruments*. The Versius system provides *6.8 mm instruments*. The availability of these smaller-diameter instruments is believed to enable surgeons to perform delicate procedures while minimizing trauma to developing tissues, thereby preserving the key principles of minimally invasive surgery [15].

4.3.2 Open-Console Design and Surgeon Ergonomics

The traditional closed-console design of many robotic systems limits surgeon's visibility of the operating room and requires an adjustment period for hand-eye coordination. New RAS systems, in contrast, feature an *open-console design*, allowing surgeons to maintain direct communication with the surgical team. This configuration enhances *situational awareness and teamwork*, which is particularly advantageous in complex surgeries that require coordinated effort among multiple specialists. Additionally, the open-console system's ergonomic design, with an optimized seated position and Senhance, with eye-tracking camera control, *is believed to reduce surgeon fatigue and strain*.

4.3.3 Shorter Learning Curve and Greater Procedural Adaptability

Another major barrier to the widespread adoption of RAS in pediatric surgery is *the steep learning curve* associated with traditional robotic systems. The transition from laparoscopy to robotics often requires extensive training, leading to prolonged procedure times and increased costs in the early phases of implementation. The Senhance system, for example, helps mitigate this issue by offering *laparoscopic-like instrument control*, which may allow surgeons already skilled in laparoscopic techniques to transition more smoothly to robotic surgery.

Furthermore, new RAS systems in the market support *multi-quadrant surgery*, meaning the robotic arms can be repositioned without redocking, which is a limitation in some traditional robotic systems. This feature may be particularly useful in pediatric surgeries where delicate tissue handling and precise movements across different anatomical sites are required.

4.3.4 Cost Considerations and Increased Accessibility

One of the most significant obstacles to RAS adoption in pediatric surgery has been *the high cost of robotic platforms*, including the purchase price, maintenance fees, and disposable instrument expenses. New systems in the market aim to make robotic-assisted surgery more accessible by *reducing per-procedure costs* through reusable instruments, which can significantly lower operating expenses over time. Reusable tools help alleviate financial constraints and increase cost-effectiveness, making RAS a more viable option for pediatric surgical centers with limited budgets.

5 Artificial Intelligence in Surgery

Artificial intelligence (AI) is revolutionizing the field of surgery by enhancing decision-making, improving precision, and facilitating automation. AI applications in surgery range from preoperative planning and intraoperative navigation to postoperative monitoring and surgical education. Through machine learning algorithms, deep learning, and data-driven analytics, AI offers the promise of enabling more precise diagnoses, predicting surgical outcomes, and assisting surgeons in optimizing techniques [16].

One of AI's primary roles in surgery is *image analysis and surgical navigation*. AI-driven imaging techniques assist surgeons by providing enhanced visualization of anatomical structures and pathology, allowing for more accurate surgical planning. Advanced algorithms can segment organs, detect anomalies, and guide robotic systems during complex procedures. In particular, AI-assisted radiology and pathology analysis have become instrumental in some cancer surgeries, where AI can detect malignancies with an accuracy comparable to that of expert radiologists [17].

Another significant contribution of AI is in *robotic-assisted surgery*. Conventional robotic systems, such as the Da Vinci platform, enhance a surgeon's dexterity and precision. However, with AI integration, surgical robots can learn from vast datasets, adapt to individual patient anatomy, and even provide real-time intraoperative recommendations based on predictive analytics [18]. AI-powered robotic platforms are moving toward semiautonomous and even fully autonomous surgical procedures, where machines assist with routine tasks while surgeons focus on complex decision-making.

AI is also transforming *surgical training and education*. By analyzing vast amounts of surgical performance data, AI can assess a surgeon's technique, identify errors, and provide personalized feedback. AI-driven virtual reality (VR) and augmented reality (AR) simulators are being developed to enhance skill acquisition for trainees, enabling realistic surgical practice in a risk-free environment. These AI-based education platforms are expected to revolutionize how surgeons are trained, ensuring a higher level of competency before they enter the operating room.

Another emerging field in AI-assisted surgery is *predictive analytics and patient outcome forecasting*. AI models analyze patient data, including medical history, genetic markers, and real-time physiological responses, to predict complications and personalize treatment strategies. If trained on this information, AI can suggest optimal surgical approaches, anticipate adverse events, and guide postoperative care, reducing the risk of complications and readmissions [19].

Despite its promise, AI in surgery presents several challenges. *Ethical and legal concerns* and questions about safety and privacy continue to be evaluated and addressed. Surgeons must also contend with *AI's limitations in adaptability and decision-making*, as current AI systems still lack the intuition, experience, and contextual judgment of human surgeons [20]. Nevertheless, as AI technology continues to evolve, its integration into surgical practice is expected to enhance patient outcomes, streamline workflows, and push the boundaries of modern surgery.

6 Artificial Intelligence Applications in Pediatric Surgery

Artificial intelligence (AI) is making significant strides in pediatric surgery, offering solutions to some of the unique challenges associated with operating on children. AI has been applied in various stages of pediatric surgical care, from preoperative assessment and intraoperative guidance to postoperative monitoring and outcome prediction. While the field is still evolving, emerging research highlights AI's potential in improving surgical precision, enhancing decision-making, and facilitating minimally invasive techniques [20].

One of the most promising applications of AI in pediatric surgery is *image-based diagnosis and preoperative planning*. AI-driven imaging technologies, such as deep learning-based segmentation of organs and pathology detection, have been used to enhance preoperative visualization. By integrating AI with radiological imaging techniques like MRI and CT scans, pediatric surgeons can obtain more accurate, high-resolution 3D reconstructions of anatomical structures, which are particularly beneficial in complex congenital anomalies and tumor resections [21].

AI is also meant to enhance *robotic-assisted surgery in pediatric patients*, improving surgical precision and overcoming some limitations of traditional robotic platforms [22]. AI-enhanced procedures could assist surgeons with *real-time intraoperative decision support*, particularly in delicate pediatric procedures that require meticulous tissue handling.

In addition, AI is being used for *predictive analytics and perioperative risk assessment*. By analyzing large datasets of pediatric surgical outcomes, AI models can predict the likelihood of complications, guide anesthetic management, and personalize surgical approaches [23].

Another emerging application is *the use of artificial intelligence for surgical training and skill assessment*. AI-powered surgical simulators and virtual reality-based training platforms analyze a surgeon's movements, provide real-time feedback, and assess surgical proficiency. These innovations are expected to play a crucial role in training the next generation of pediatric surgeons.

Despite these advancements, challenges remain in the widespread adoption of AI in pediatric surgery, mostly limited by the scarcity of pediatric-specific data, which renders it necessary to compromise with training on adult data for pediatric applications [24].

7 Open Challenges and Future Directions of RAS and AI in Pediatric Surgery

Despite the significant progress in robotic-assisted surgery (RAS) and artificial intelligence (AI) applications in pediatric surgery, several challenges remain that must be addressed to facilitate broader adoption and optimization. One of the most pressing issues is the lack of appropriately scaled robotic instruments for pediatric patients, which only few commercial applications, like the Senhance and the Versius, currently cover. While advancements in miniaturized instruments are ongoing, many current robotic platforms still lack the flexibility required for smaller anatomical structures, limiting their usability in neonates and infants.

Cost remains a substantial barrier in pediatric robotic surgery, given the significant initial investment required for acquiring robotic systems, as well as ongoing expenses related to maintenance, pediatric-specific disposable instruments, and specialized surgeon training. These financial burdens particularly restrict adoption in lower-resource pediatric centers. Furthermore, dedicated training and credentialing programs should be available to ensure the proficiency of pediatric robotic surgical teams.

From an AI standpoint, the availability and standardization of pediatric surgical data represent significant challenges. Pediatric surgical cases are inherently less frequent than adult procedures, making it difficult to collect the extensive datasets required for training accurate and generalizable AI models. Ethical considerations surrounding AI integration in pediatric settings—such as safeguarding patient data privacy, maintaining algorithm transparency, and ensuring appropriate surgeon oversight—are critical for gaining acceptance from both clinicians and regulatory bodies. Additionally, AI-based decision support tools specifically designed for pediatric patients must undergo rigorous validation processes to guarantee reliability and minimize biases that could adversely affect clinical outcomes for children.

Addressing these barriers will require sustained collaboration among pediatric surgeons, engineers, data scientists, and regulatory agencies. Future research must prioritize the development of cost-effective robotic platforms tailored to pediatric care, refinement of AI-driven clinical decision support systems specific to pediatric needs, and the establishment of standardized pediatric datasets to enhance AI training and validation. Overcoming these challenges will be essential for fully leveraging the transformative potential of AI-powered robotics in pediatric surgery.

8 Conclusions

The integration of robotic-assisted surgery and artificial intelligence is transforming pediatric surgery by enhancing precision, reducing invasiveness, and improving patient outcomes. While robotic platforms have been widely adopted in adult surgery, their application in pediatrics has been constrained by factors such as instrument size, cost, and the need for specialized training. Advances in miniaturized robotic systems, AI-driven decision support, and real-time surgical guidance are progressively overcoming these barriers, making RAS more accessible and beneficial for pediatric patients.

AI is further optimizing surgical workflows, from preoperative planning to intraoperative guidance and postoperative monitoring. The introduction of AI-enhanced imaging, predictive analytics, and automated skill assessment tools is shaping the future of pediatric surgical practice, ensuring greater accuracy, efficiency, and patient safety.

However, the full integration of RAS and AI into pediatric surgery still requires addressing technical, financial, and ethical challenges. As research and technological advancements continue, interdisciplinary collaboration will be essential to refine these systems, expand accessibility, and improve pediatric surgical outcomes. The future of pediatric surgery will increasingly rely on robotics and AI, paving the way for more precise, efficient, and safer surgical interventions tailored to the unique needs of young patients.

Disclosure of Interest *The authors of this chapter are both employed by Asensus Surgical. This chapter represents our best efforts to provide a thorough, unbiased, and well-researched overview of the topic of Robotics and AI in Pediatrics, based on the information available to us at the time of writing.*

While our professional affiliations may have influenced our perspectives and access to specific data, we have strived to present information in a manner that is both comprehensive and impartial. We have made an effort to ensure that all information reported in this chapter is accurate, up-to-date, and free from undue bias.

Any conclusions or opinions expressed herein reflect our individual analyses and interpretations and not necessarily those of Asensus Surgical or any of its affiliates. We have disclosed all relevant data and insights available to us, with the intention of contributing to a balanced and insightful discussion of the subject matter.

References

1. Ponsky TA, Rothenberg SS, Petersen K, et al. Minimally invasive surgery in children. Pediatr Clin N Am. 2009;56(2):407–28.
2. Holcomb GW, Murphy JP, Ostlie DJ. Ashcraft's pediatric surgery. 6th ed. Elsevier; 2014.
3. Lanfranco AR, Castellanos AE, Desai JP, Meyers WC. Robotic surgery: a current perspective. Ann Surg. 2004;239(1):14–21.
4. O'Brien LP, Hannan E, Antao B, Peirce C. Pediatric robotic surgery: a narrative review. J Robot Surg. 2023;17:1171–9.
5. Navarrete-Arellano M. Robotic-assisted minimally invasive surgery in children. In: Latest developments in medical robotics systems. IntechOpen; 2021.
6. Silay MS, Spinoit AF, Undre S, et al. Global minimally invasive pyeloplasty study in children: results from the Pediatric Urology Expert Group of the European Association of Urology Young Academic Urologists working party. J Pediatr Urol. 2016;12(4):229.e1–7.
7. Song SH, Lee C, Jung J, et al. A comparative study of pediatric open pyeloplasty, laparoscopy-assisted extracorporeal pyeloplasty, and robot-assisted laparoscopic pyeloplasty. PLoS One. 2017;12:e0175026.
8. Puentes MC, Rojnica M, Sims T, Jones R, Bianco FM, Lobe E. Senhance robotic platform in pediatrics: early US experience. Children. 2023;10(2):178.
9. Cundy TP, Shetty K, Clark J, Chang TP, Sriskandarajah K, Gattas NE, et al. The first decade of robotic surgery in children. J Pediatr Surg. 2013;48:858–65.

10. Pérez-Salazar MJ, Caballero D, Sánchez-Margallo JA, Sánchez-Margallo F. Comparative study of ergonomics in conventional and robotic-assisted laparoscopic surgery. Sensors. 2024;24(12):3840.
11. Zwimpfer TA, Wismer C, Fellmann-Fischer B, Geiger J, Schötzau A, Heinzelmann-Schwarz V. Comparison of 2D 4K vs. 3D HD laparoscopic imaging systems using a pelvitrainer model: a randomized controlled study. Updat Surg. 2021;74(7)
12. Al-Bassam A. Robotic-assisted surgery in children: advantages and limitations. J Robot Surg. 2010;4(1):19–22.
13. Iacob ER, Iacob R, Ghenciu LA, Popoiu T-A, Stoicescu ER, Popoiu CM. Small scale, high precision: robotic surgery in neonatal and pediatric patients—A narrative review. Children. 2024;11(3):270.
14. Maizlin I, Shroyer CM, Yu DC, Martin AC, Chen K, Russell T. Survey on robot-assisted surgical techniques utilization in US pediatric surgery fellowships. J Laparoendosc Adv Surg Tech. 2017;27(2):191–6.
15. Bergholz R, Botden S, Verweij J, Tytgat S, Van Gemert W, Boettcher M, Ehlert H, Reinshagen K, Gidaro S. Evaluation of a new robotic-assisted laparoscopic surgical system for procedures in small cavities. J Robot Surg. 2020;14(1):191–7.
16. Tsai AY, Carter SR, Greene AC. Artificial intelligence in pediatric surgery. Semin Pediatr Surg. 2024;33(1):151390.
17. Tarassoli DS, Bahramiazar DF. Advancements in image-guided navigation for surgical procedures. J Med Res Surg. 2023;4(5):86–91.
18. Abbasi N, Hussain HK. Integration of artificial intelligence and smart technology: AI-driven robotics in surgery precision and efficiency. JAIGS. 2024;5(1):381–92.
19. Alowais SA, Alghamdi SS, Alsuhebany N, Alqahtani T, Alshaya AI, Almohareb SN, Aldairem A, Alrashed M, Bin Saleh K, Badreldin HA, Al Yami MS, Al Harbi S, Albekairy AM. Revolutionizing healthcare: the role of artificial intelligence in clinical practice. BMC Med Educ. 2023;23(1):689.
20. Guni A, Ahmad T, Smith JP. Artificial intelligence in surgery: the future is now. Eur Surg Res. 2024;65(1):22–39.
21. Chowdhury AT, Salam A, Naznine M, Abdalla D, Erdman L, Chowdhury MEH, Abbas TO. Artificial intelligence tools in pediatric urology: a comprehensive review of recent advances. Diagnostics. 2024;14(18):2059.
22. Alex Joseph AF, Sathik Raja M, Basha VAA, Muthukumaran D, Gowthami V. Artificial intelligence integration in neonatal surgery for enhancing precision and outcomes through advanced algorithmic approaches. J Neonatal Surg. 2025;14(4S):61–71.
23. Dundaru-Bandi D, Antel R, Ingelmo PM. Advances in pediatric perioperative care using artificial intelligence. Curr Opin Anaesthesiol. 2024;37(3):251–8.
24. Rollan-Martinez-Herrera M, Díaz AA, Estépar RSJ, Sanchez-Ferrero GV, Ross JC, Nardelli P. CNNs trained with adult data are useful in pediatrics: a pneumonia classification example. PLoS One. 2024;19(7):e0306703.

Gastrointestinal

Robotic-Assisted Surgery for Esophageal Atresia with Trachea-Esophageal Fistula

Laurent Fourcade, Pauline Lopez, Antoine Bedu, Laure Ponthier, and Quentin Ballouhey

1 Introduction

Esophageal atresia (EA) is a life-threatening condition in newborn infants, because it makes oral feeding impossible and may lead to respiratory distress due to pulmonary inhalation. It is generally diagnosed at birth by checking the permeability of the esophagus with a gastric tube. Several types of EA have been described [1]. In type III EA, stenosis of the esophagus is associated with an ectopic connection of the lower part of the esophagus to the trachea. Until recently, thoracotomy [2] was the only way to cure atresias of this type, but then, several years ago, a thoracoscopic method was proposed [3, 4]. Each of these methods has advantages but also drawbacks [5].

Robot-assisted surgical procedures are now a proposed surgery in children. Several authors published pediatric uses of robotic procedures, mainly uronephrologic and abdominal interventions [6]. Thus, the development of these techniques has opened up new possibilities for the treatment of EA. However, these robotic procedures require fine-tuning for use in such small patients. We report here the use of a robotic approach, together with a thoracoscopic approach, to correct type III esophageal atresia.

2 Patient Positioning and Planning

We described here the case of a newborn girl, with a birth weight of 3.570 g, measuring 51 cm in length and with an Apgar score of 5-6-9-10, born in a maternity ward close to our university hospital. She was transferred to our surgical team 4 hours after birth. Respiration was normal and remained so without support until anesthesia. Saliva overflow into the lungs was prevented by maintaining the infant in a partly upright position and by continuous aspiration of the upper esophageal pouch with a Replogle® tube. The delivery had occurred at 41 weeks of gestation, with no evident problems and no prenatal diagnosis of atresia. The surgical intervention took place 36 hours after birth (H36).

Type III esophageal atresia (EA with distal tracheoesophageal fistula) was diagnosed upon feeding tube arrest. The requested chest X-ray showed that the feeding tube stopped and was bent in the esophagus and that the stomach contained a large amount of air (Fig. 1b). No other

L. Fourcade (✉) · P. Lopez · Q. Ballouhey
Pediatric Surgery Unit, University of Limoges, Limoges, France
e-mail: laurent.fourcade@unilim.fr; quentin.ballouhey@chu-limoges.fr

A. Bedu · L. Ponthier
Department of Neonatology, University of Limoges, Limoges, France
e-mail: antoine.bedu@chu-limoges.fr; laure.ponthier@chu-limoges.fr

C. Esposito et al. (eds.), *Pediatric Robotic Assisted Surgery*,
https://doi.org/10.1007/978-3-031-99532-3_4

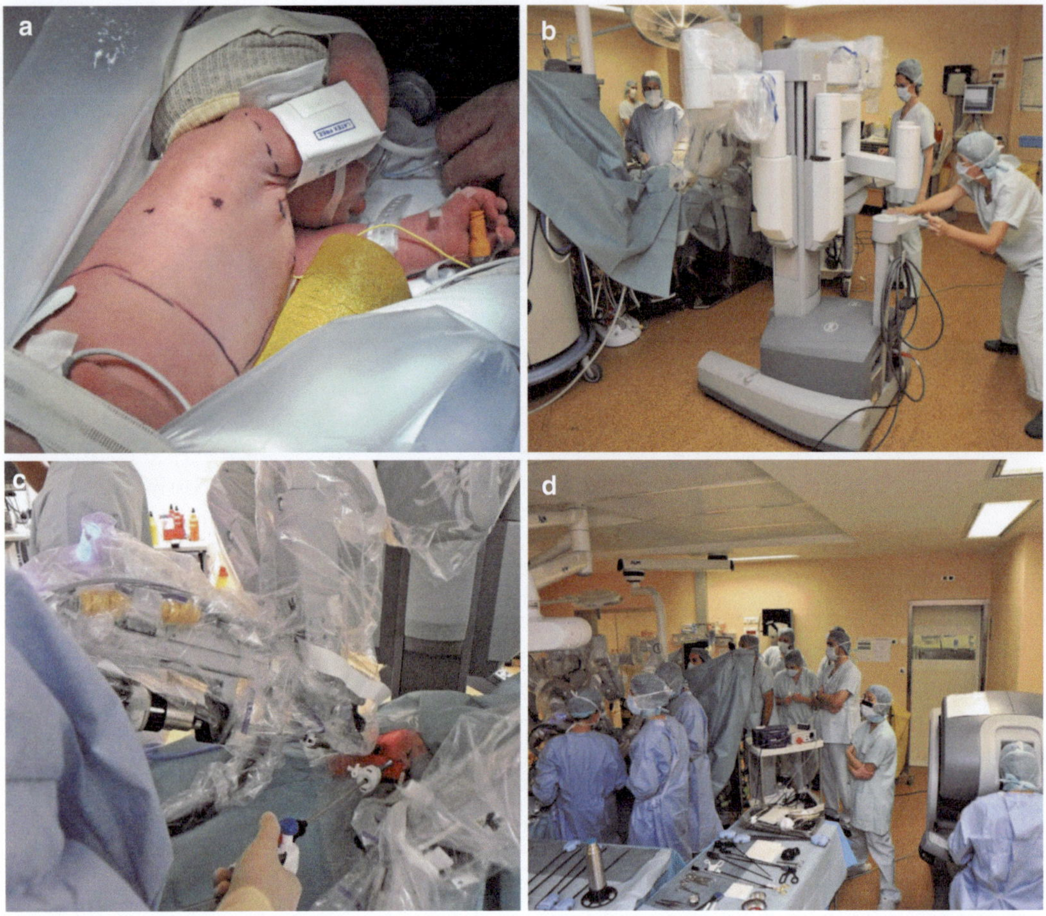

Fig. 1 (**a**) Positioning of the baby, (**b**) Robot positioning, (**c**) Ports positioning, (**d**) Overall view of the operative room

anatomical abnormality was detected. Informed consent was obtained from both parents for the intervention.

2.1 Anesthesia and Positioning of the Patient

Anesthesia was induced after the insertion of a tracheal tube (no. 3). As recommended by many anesthesiologists [7], we adopted a ventilation strategy aiming to limit pressure peaks: Spontaneous ventilation with inspiratory support was maintained before intubation, and the neonate was placed under pressure-controlled ventilation after intubation. Ventilator settings were adjusted to yield an arterial oxygen saturation of between 90% and 98%, an airway pressure of less than 18 cm H_2O and an end-tidal P_{CO2} (ETPCO2) exceeding 45 mm Hg. Selective ventilation was not required.

The patient was placed on the operating table in a lateral, slightly prone position. A urinary catheter was also implanted (Fig. 1a).

3 Incision and Ports Placement

The robot used for this intervention was a Da Vinci surgical system (Intuitive Surgical Inc., Sunnyvale, CA). This Da Vinci system has four robotic arms, but we used only three of these arms during the procedure. Three ports were used to dock the robot: an 8-mm port for the three-dimensional camera and two 8-mm ports for the instruments used—cautery hooks, grasping forceps, and microneedle forceps. An accessory 5-mm nonrobotic port was also used for suction and sutures.

The localization of the robotic ports is a crucial step in the procedure. It was adapted from previously described localizations [8] and was as follows: One port was below the tip of the right scapula (camera), one was on the anterior axillary line (anterior port for instruments), and the remaining port was on the posterior axillary line (posterior port for instruments), all these ports being located in the fifth intercostal space (Fig. 1c).

The first port to be installed was the camera port, as this facilitated the installation of the other two ports under visual guidance. The accessory port was located between the anterior and the middle port in the sixth intercostal space. It is essential to insert these ports less deeply into the body of the infant than is generally the case in adults to allow sufficient space for the manipulation of instruments in this very limited space.

4 Robot Positioning

The robot was placed to the right of the patient (Fig. 1b). The anesthesia team members were at the head of the patient slightly to the left side of the patient's head in order to leave room for the robot. The bedside assistant and the scrub nurse were on the left, close to the patient, and the main surgeon (right part of the picture) was sitting at the console, 3 meters away from the patient (Fig. 1d). Once the ports were fully operational, the robot was connected to the ports (docking procedure), and the digital display (console) was switched on. The main surgeon then went to the console and the joysticks controlling the movements of the instruments. The second surgeon (bedside assistant) and the scrub nurse remained close to the patient to manipulate the instruments and the ports in a sterile manner.

4.1 Insufflation

Carbon dioxide gas was insufflated into the body through the robotic ports, at a flow rate of 0.1 L/min, with maintenance at a positive pressure between 2 and 4 mm Hg throughout the intervention, to ensure that there was sufficient space to manipulate the instruments comfortably.

5 Procedure Steps

The intervention can be schematically split into three phases: (i) identification and ligation of the TEF, (ii) dissection of the upper pouch of the esophagus, and (iii) one-layer end-to-end anastomosis of the upper and lower parts of the esophagus.

The TEF was identified by locating the azygos vein and observing the inflation of the TEF by ventilation. The azygos vein was dissected, coagulated, and cut (Fig. 2a). The TEF was then carefully dissected, transfixed, and sutured with nonabsorbable 5/0 Ticron® (3 stitches) and cut below the stitches (Fig. 2b). The lower end of the esophagus was left free for the last step (anastomosis). During this phase, great care was taken to avoid damage to the vagus nerve, with the aid of the three-dimensional images supplied by the camera.

The upper part of the esophagus was identified in the operative field by gently mobilizing the Replogle® tube inserted into the esophagus by the anesthesiologist. The blind end was grasped with atraumatic forceps and mobilized (dissected) until the two ends of the esophagus were close enough to be ligated without tension (Fig. 2c).

The blind end was then progressively cut open, and three stitches (Polysorb 5/0®) were made to join the posterior walls of the two ends of the esophagus. The feeding tube was then inserted further into the lower part of the esophagus. This action was carried out for two reasons:

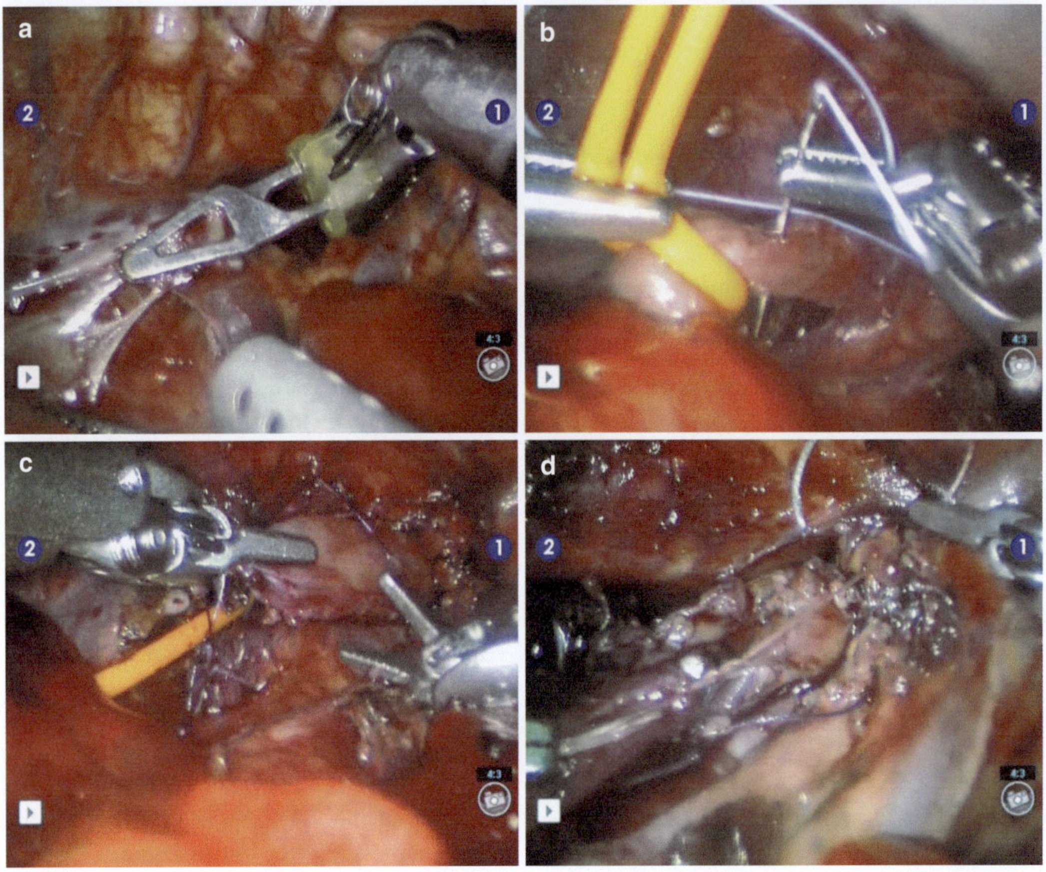

Fig. 2 Perioperative view of the main operative steps (**a**) Azygos vein coagulation (**b**) Closure of the tracheaesophageal atresia fistula using stitches—the needle holder is used completely folded, thanks to the double wrist and then is not too much space consuming (**c**) Dissection of the upper part of the esophagus (**d**) View of the anastomosis

to facilitate the completion of anastomosis and provide a transanastomotic feeding tube for the patient [9]. The ligation was then completed by four additional stitches on the lateral and anterior sides of the esophagus (Fig. 2d).

A chest tube was introduced via the accessory port hole and was left close to the anastomosis (it was left in place for the next 5 days). The instruments were then removed, the robot was undocked, and the port holes were closed in two layers, with 5/0 Monocryl®.

The intervention (from patient positioning to skin closure) took 4 hours. The installation of the ports and robot docking took 45 min. The surgeon spent 2 1/2 hours at the robotic console.

6 Postoperative Period

The respiratory tube can be removed 24 hour after the surgical intervention.

A feeding tube (10-French) is inserted from day 0 to day 10. Thereafter, the status of the esophagus was checked with an upper GI tract series, and a thinner feeding tube was inserted from day 10 to day 18. Enteral feeding with maternal breast milk is allowed 72 hour after surgery (8 × 5 ml). Oral feeding with enriched mother's milk was started 10 days after surgery and was fully operational (6 × 120 ml) on day 18, making it possible to remove the thinner enteral feeding tube. During this period, parenteral feeding was carried out with an umbilical vein catheter from day 1 to day 3 and a percutaneously inserted central venous catheter from day 3 to day 13.

The chest drain can be removed 5 days after surgery. An upper GI tract series was performed 10 days after surgery and showed the esophagus to be continuous, with no leakage of the contrast agent. Due to the novelty of this procedure, the patient was kept in hospital for longer than was strictly necessary. The patient was discharged from hospital 1 month after surgery. The patient weighed 3570 g at birth, 3200 g 36 hour later, and 3975 g on discharge from hospital.

7 Tips and Tricks

Neonatal robotic surgery is every pediatric surgeon's dream. However, as the equipment is still totally dedicated to adults, it is necessary to adapt existing equipment to the constraints of pediatrics. While in abdominal surgery, working space can be increased by insufflation, this is not possible in thoracoscopic surgery.

Nevertheless, thanks to the mobility of the instruments and the double articulation, better vision and absence of tremors, it is possible to have a thoracoscopic robotic approach.

Of course, this is not the place to start and experience of urological or digestive surgery on children weighing 10–15 kg would seem to be essential [10].

In our experience, it has not been possible to perform this procedure on children weighing less than 3 kg, which is the norm. Indeed, the 8-mm diameter of the ports made it impossible to mobilize the instruments without the child also moving. It should also be noted that in the case described here, the patient developed a scoliotic attitude outside any VACTERL, probably due to a lesion of the rib periosteum.

Some authors, in order to benefit from the robotic approach, delay surgery to obtain a higher weight for robot use. This seems to me to be questionable, given the pulmonary complications of such a delay [11].

Communication with anesthetists is another essential key point. They are at a distance from the infant but need to be able to react very quickly. We had a case of displacement of the intubation tube in the eso-tracheal fistula and only experience and access to the trachea enabled us to understand and solve the problem.

8 Conclusions

The robotic approach to esophageal cancer is still rare, with very few publications [12].

The learning curve for the thoracoscopic approach to esophageal atresia remains long, despite the benefits of simulation, and democratization remains slow despite all these advantages [13]. It is certain that the robotic approach, once instruments dedicated to pediatrics have been developed, will enable the majority of esophageal atresia to be operated on thoracoscopically, even by nonexperts.

The robot-assisted method described here provides clear three-dimensional images of the operative field, allows high-quality anastomosis, and can easily be taught to other surgeons, and it results in a good esthetic appearance. It is still too early to tell whether this method is less painful than thoracotomy, but we would expect pain levels to be similar to those for thoracoscopy. Thus, we believe the robotic procedure described here combines the advantages of the two reference methods—thoracotomy and thoracoscopy—without having any of their main drawbacks. We therefore strongly believe this robotic method will allow skipping the thoracoscopic intervention and will soon be used by many pediatric surgery teams.

References

1. Spitz L. Oesophageal atresia. Orphanet J Rare Dis. 2007;2:24.
2. Burford JM, Dassinger MS, Copeland DR, Keller JE, Smith SD. Repair of esophageal atresia with tracheo-esophageal fistula via thoracotomy: a contemporary series. Am J Surg. 2011;202(2):203–6.
3. Rothenberg SS. Thoracoscopic repair of esophageal atresia and tracheo-esophageal fistula. Semin Pediatr Surg. 2005;14(1):2–7.
4. Allal H, Kalfa N, Lopez M, et al. Benefits of the thoracoscopic approach for short- or long-gap esophageal atresia. J Laparoendosc Adv Surg Tech A. 2005;15(6):673–7.
5. Szavay PO, Zundel S, Blumenstock G, et al. Perioperative outcome of patients with esophageal atresia and tracheo-esophageal fistula undergoing open versus thoracoscopic surgery. J Laparoendosc Adv Surg Tech A. 2011;21(5):439–43.
6. de Lambert G, Fourcade L, Centi J, et al. How to successfully implement a robotic pediatric surgery program: lessons learned after 96 procedures. Surg Endosc. 2013;27(6):2137–44.
7. Alabbad SI, Shaw K, Puligandla PS, Carranza R, Bernard C, Laberge JM. The pitfalls of endotracheal intubation beyond the fistula in babies with type C esophageal atresia. Semin Pediatr Surg. 2009;18(2):116–8.
8. van der Zee DC, Bax KNMA. Thoracoscopic treatment of esophageal atresia with distal fistula and of tracheomalacia. Semin Pediatr Surg. 2007;16(4):224–30.
9. Alabbad SI, Ryckman J, Puligandla PS, Shaw K, Nguyen LT, Laberge J-M. Use of transanastomotic feeding tubes during esophageal atresia repair. J Pediatr Surg. 2009;44(5):902–5.
10. Ballouhey Q, Villemagne T, Cros J, Vacquerie V, Bérenguer D, Braik K, et al. Assessment of paediatric thoracic robotic surgery. Interact Cardiovasc Thorac Surg. 2015;20:300–3.
11. Zhang M, Huang J, Jin Z, Zhang X, Zhou Y, Chi S, et al. Comparison of robotic versus thoracoscopic repair for congenital esophageal atresia: a propensity score matching analysis. Int J Surg févr. 2024;110(2):891–901.
12. Li S, Cao G, Zhou R, Zhang X, Zhou Y, Tang S, tao. Feasible techniques in robotic thoracoscopic repair of congenital esophageal atresia: case report and literature review. Surg Case Rep déc. 2021;7(1):142.
13. Zee DC, Tytgat SHAJ, Zwaveling S, Herwaarden MYA, Vieira-Travassos D. Learning curve of thoracoscopic repair of esophageal atresia. World J Surg. 2012;36(9):2093–7.

Robotic Gastric Fundoplication for GER

Lacher Martin, Gabriel Goetz, Richard Wagner, Richard Gnatzy, Lena Bode, Peter Zimmermann, and Jan Gosemann

1 Introduction

Laparoscopic surgery has become the "gold standard" for treating gastroesophageal reflux disease (GERD) in children. This minimally invasive approach is especially critical for neurologically impaired children who suffer from symptomatic GERD and require anti-reflux surgery. The indications for laparoscopic fundoplication mirror those for the traditional open approach, with the choice between complete (Nissen) or partial (Thal, Toupet) wraps left to the surgeon's discretion. The debate over which type of wrap is superior continues, but current literature suggests that the type of wrap is not the primary factor influencing outcomes.

Regardless of the surgical technique employed, three essential steps are fundamental to all fundoplications [1, 2].

1. Creation of intra-abdominal length of the distal esophagus.
2. Narrowing of the diaphragmatic hiatus.
3. Fixation of the fundus against or around the distal esophagus, with or without additional stitches to the diaphragm.

L. Martin (✉) · G. Goetz · R. Wagner · R. Gnatzy · L. Bode · P. Zimmermann · J. Gosemann
University of Leipzig, Department of Pediatric Surgery, Leipzig, Germany
e-mail: martin.lacher@medizin.uni-leipzig.de

Robot-assisted anti-reflux surgery (ARS) has also been explored through randomized clinical trials and subsequent meta-analyses [3, 4]. These studies indicate that while robot-assisted ARS results in longer operating times, it does not demonstrate superiority over conventional laparoscopic approaches. However, these studies are often limited by small sample sizes, heterogeneity, short-term follow-up, and a lack of focus on the differences between complete and partial fundoplication [5].

Studies in pediatric cohorts show that robot-assisted laparoscopic fundoplication is safe and effective. However, it is still not widely adopted for children [6].

The aim of this chapter is to provide a comprehensive, step-by-step guide to performing robot-assisted complete and partial fundoplication in pediatric surgery.

2 Patient Positioning and Planning

The North American Society for Pediatric Gastroenterology, Hepatology, and Nutrition (NASPGHAN) and the European Society for Pediatric Gastroenterology, Hepatology, and Nutrition (ESPGHAN) recommend conducting a detailed history and physical examination in children presenting with typical GERD symptoms. If alarm signs are present or if medical treatment

C. Esposito et al. (eds.), *Pediatric Robotic Assisted Surgery*,
https://doi.org/10.1007/978-3-031-99532-3_5

fails, further diagnostic steps are warranted, including esophagogastroscopy with biopsies to diagnose or rule out complications of GERD or other conditions such as eosinophilic esophagitis, infections, and Crohn's disease. A contrast study of the upper GI tract is useful for detecting anatomical abnormalities like hiatal hernia, gastric outlet obstruction, or malrotation. Additionally, 24-hour impedance pH monitoring measures acid and nonacid reflux episodes, providing a comprehensive assessment of GERD [7].

Preoperative preparation should include administering an enema to enhance intra-abdominal visualization by sufficiently emptying the colon. Robotic-assisted fundoplication is performed under general anesthesia with endotracheal intubation [8]. The stomach is decompressed using a nasogastric tube, which is then removed, and a large esophageal bougie, approximately the size of the patient's thumb, is inserted. If available, perioperative epidural anesthesia may be administered by a dedicated pain service.

Positioning is critical for optimal surgical outcomes. For infants, a supine frog-leg positioning is recommended. Older children should be positioned supine with legs on abductable leg holders. The hip should be placed over the bending point of the table to allow hyperextension just above the hip, facilitating a better range of movement for the instruments. Positioning on a beanbag ensures easy, firm, and safe positioning (Fig. 1).

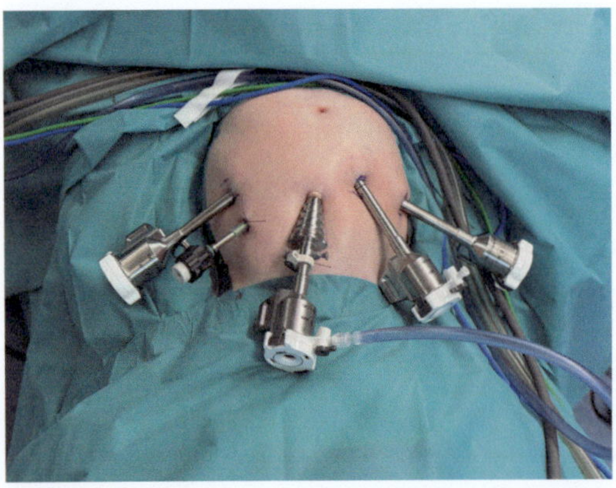

Fig. 1 Port placement

3 Incision and Port Placement

This section outlines the operative steps using the Da Vinci Xi surgical robot.

An infraumbilical incision is made using scissors, followed by a purse-string placement of a Polyglactin 0 suture. An 8-mm trocar with a Hasson cone is introduced through the mini-laparotomy. The purse-string suture is then tightened and secured to the Hasson cone on both sides, ensuring an airtight and firm fixation of the first trocar.

The capnoperitoneum is insufflated using a pressure of 6–8 mmHg and a flow rate of 4–6 L/min, depending on the age of the child. For liver retraction, either a Nathanson retractor can be used via a subxiphoid incision or an 8 mm Da Vinci instrument can perform this function.

When using four 8-mm trocars, they should be placed in a horizontal or semicircular fashion, with a minimum distance of four fingers between each trocar (Fig. 1). Additionally, a 3-mm or 5-mm assistant port may be utilized for the later retraction of the stomach.

This systematic approach to incision and port placement ensures optimal access and visualization during robotic-assisted fundoplication, enhancing the precision and safety of the procedure.

4 Robot Positioning

The final step in the setup involves docking the surgical robot. The robot can approach from either the patient's left or right side. In our operating room configuration, docking is performed from the patient's left side. This method is straightforward and consistently reproducible (see accompanying video for demonstration) (Fig. 2).

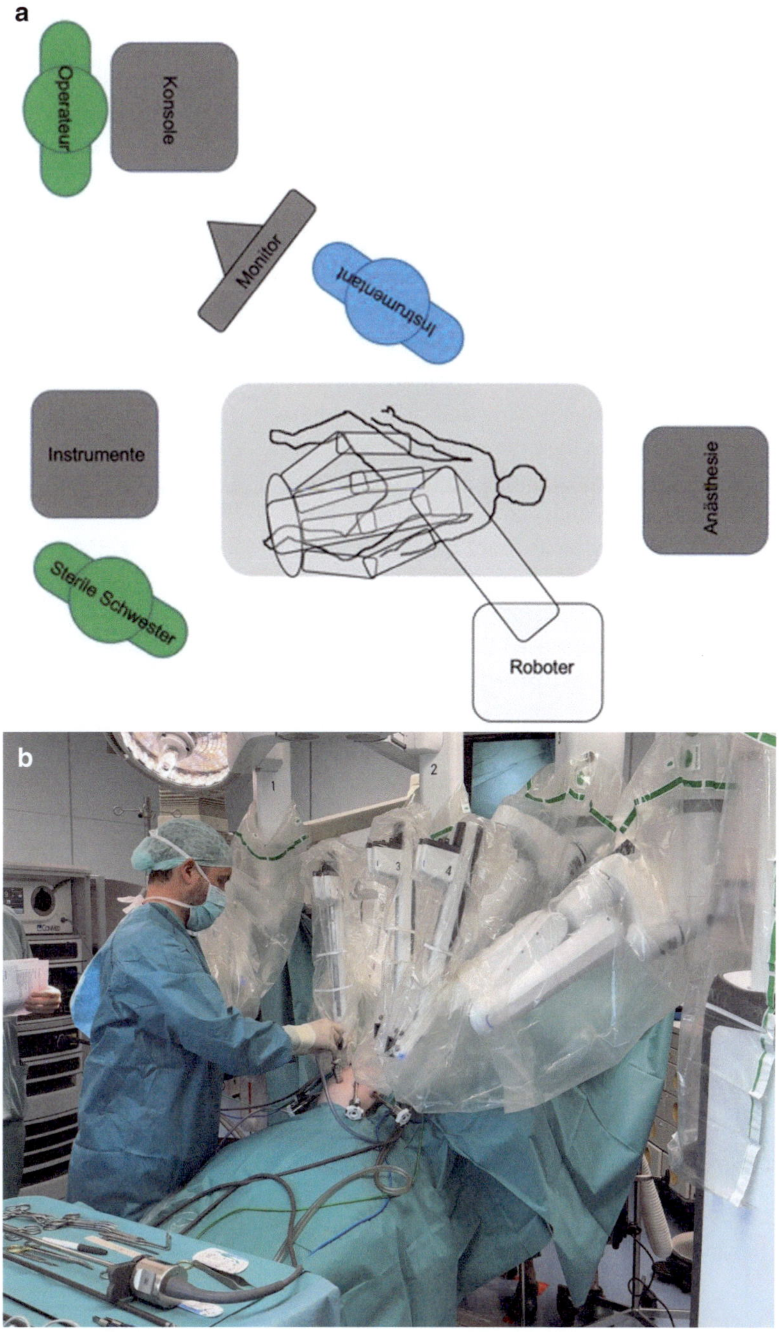

Fig. 2 Robot position diagram (**a**) and picture (**b**)

5 Procedure Steps

5.1 Liver Retraction and Initial Exposure

An 8-mm Da Vinci atraumatic grasper, such as a Cadiere or fenestrated bipolar forceps, is used for liver retraction. An atraumatic grasper is inserted via the 3-mm or 5-mm umbilical assistant trocar to apply traction on the distal esophagus and fundus. This maneuver ensures adequate exposure of the hepatogastric and phrenoesophageal ligaments. The hepatogastric and phrenoesophageal ligaments are then divided using Maryland bipolar forceps or monopolar scissors. Care must be taken to avoid injury to the anterior or posterior vagus nerve or an aberrant left hepatic artery.

5.2 Dissection and Creation of Retroesophageal Space

The right crus is identified, and a retroesophageal space is created by approaching from the patient's right side using blunt dissection (Fig. 3). Before proceeding to the patient's left side (left crus), the short gastric vessels are divided to prevent traction on the spleen while mobilizing the fundus. A window is created behind the esophagus, a vessel loop is placed around the esophagus for retraction, and it is secured using a 5-mm locking clip. Dissection of the posterior wall and the hiatus is then completed (Fig. 4), allowing the distal esophagus to be brought into the abdominal cavity.

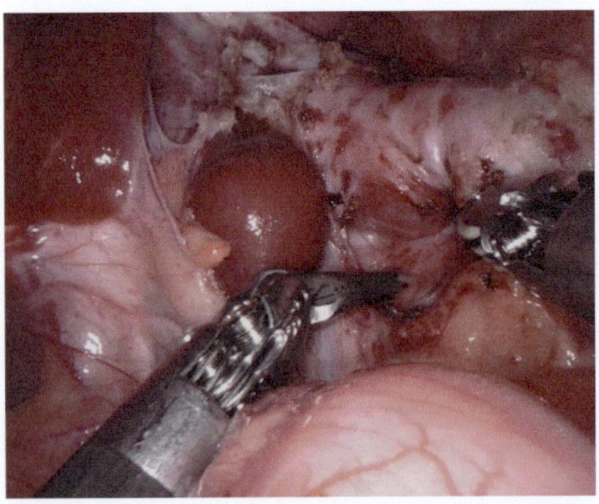

Fig. 3 Identification of the right crus is identified, and a retroesophageal space is created by approaching from the patient's right side using blunt dissection

5.3 Narrowing of the Hiatus

The second step in every anti-reflux procedure involves narrowing the hiatus (Fig. 5). These sutures are placed from the patient's right side

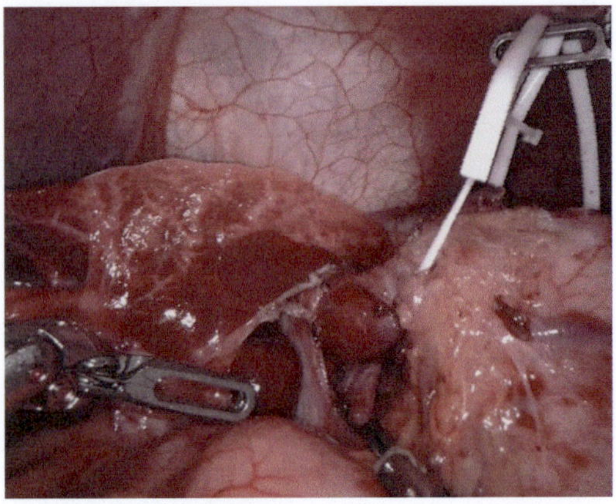

Fig. 4 A window is created behind the esophagus, a vessel loop is placed round the esophagus for retraction, and it is secured using a 5-mm locking clip. Dissection of the posterior wall and the hiatus is then completed

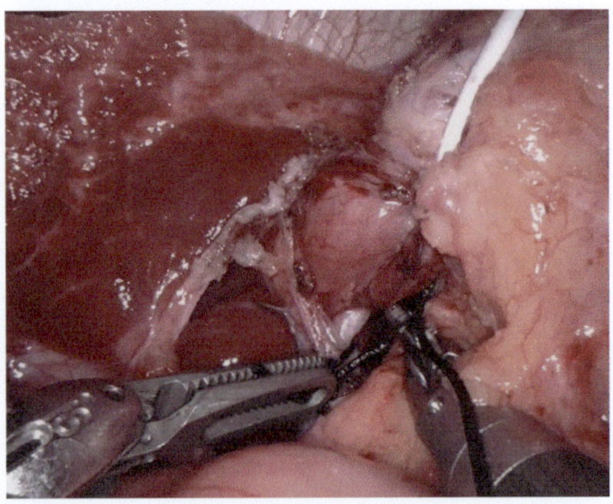

Fig. 5 Narrowing of the hiatus. Stiches are performed from the right to the left side, using either silk or polyester suture. The uppermost suture may include the posterior esophageal wall. During the plastic reconstruction of the hiatus, the esophageal bougie is placed into the stomach to avoid narrowing of the esophagus

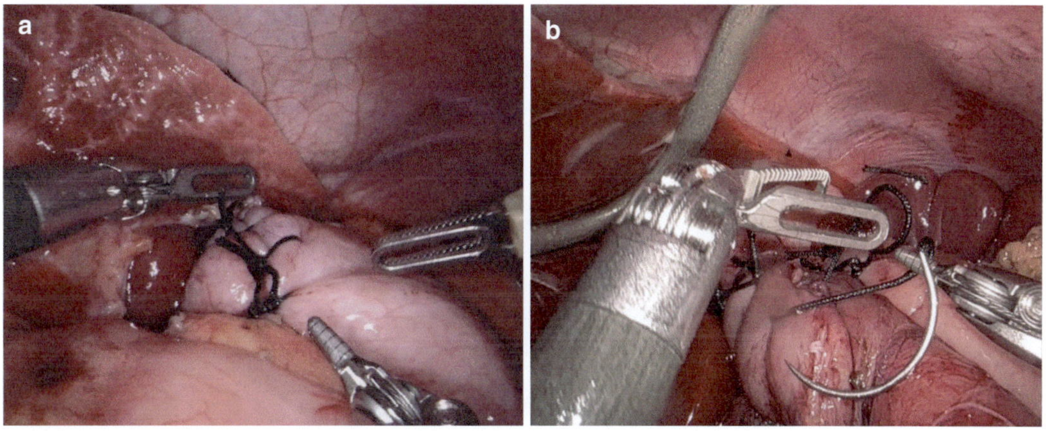

Fig. 6 (**a**) Nissen fundoplication (**b**) Toupet fundoplication

using silk or polyester suture (0). The uppermost suture may include the posterior esophageal wall to secure the intra-abdominal position of the distal esophagus. During hiatus reconstruction, the esophageal bougie is left in place to prevent esophageal narrowing, and it is removed afterward.

5.4 Nissen Fundoplication

The fundus of the stomach is passed behind the esophagus, and a shoeshine maneuver is performed to confirm sufficient mobilization and ensure the stomach is not twisted. A fundoplication is created by placing three to four stitches of nonabsorbable material at approximately 1-cm intervals using silk or polyester. The first (most cranial) suture should incorporate a small piece of the anterior esophagus to prevent wrap migration. The wrap should be about 2–3 cm in length (Fig. 6a). The right side of the wrap can also be secured to the right crus.

5.5 Toupet Fundoplication

Following the shoeshine maneuver, the wrap is brought around the retro-cardial window to sit comfortably without tension. A frame stitch (syn: locking stitch) can temporarily stabilize the distal end of the wrap. Three nonabsorbable sutures are placed to approximate the fundus with the right esophagus, with the uppermost suture also including the right diaphragmatic pillar. The same procedure is performed on the left side with two additional sutures to approximate the wrap with the left esophagus, completing the 270-degree wrap (Fig. 6b).

5.6 Closure

After completing the procedure, the instruments are removed, and the abdomen is allowed to desufflate. The 8-mm incisions are closed using polyglactin 4/0 sutures under direct vision, followed by skin glue. Finally, the purse-string suture in the infraumbilical position is closed, followed by the application of skin glue.

6 Postoperative Period

Immediately after surgery, the patient is permitted to start oral feeds, including milk or formula. No food restrictions or special diets are necessary. The child can be discharged home once full enteral feeds are well tolerated. Postoperative complications may include retching, dysphagia, and recurrent GERD. Monitoring and addressing these complications promptly are essential for ensuring a smooth recovery and optimal outcomes.

7 Tips and Tricks

Pearls/Tips and Tricks

1. *Preoperative Preparation*: Administer an enema to empty the colon and enhance intra-abdominal visualization.
2. *Liver Retraction*: Effective liver retraction is crucial for optimal exposure of the operative field. If the colon is dilated and air-filled, puncture it at the linea alba to aspirate the air.
3. *Stomach Maneuvering*: The instrument inserted via the umbilical trocar is consistently used to maneuver the stomach and assist in exposing the operative field.
4. *Esophageal Bougie*: Use an esophageal bougie of appropriate size to prevent esophageal narrowing.
5. *Hemostasis*: The Maryland bipolar forceps facilitate operating similar to open surgery with minimal bleeding.
6. *Esophageal Retraction*: Placing a vessel loop around the esophagus for retraction aids in the dissection of the posterior esophagus and the placement of hiatus-narrowing sutures.

Pitfalls and Ways to Avoid Them

1. *Nerve Injury*: Avoid injury to the anterior or posterior vagus nerve.
2. *Liver Bleeding*: In very young infants, the liver can bleed easily, complicating visualization.
3. *Splenic Injury*: Be cautious when dividing the short gastric vessels to avoid injuring the splenic capsule, especially at the upper pole, which can cause bleeding and obstruct visualization.
4. *Anatomic Variants*: Be aware of anatomical variants such as an aberrant left hepatic artery.
5. *Wrap Suturing*: Ensure that a significant amount of tissue is included when suturing the wrap to prevent disruption.
6. *Recurrence Prevention*: Poorly placed, loose knots can lead to recurrence. Utilize sliding knots to achieve tight and firm knots.

8 Discussion

Robotic-assisted gastric fundoplication represents a significant advancement in the surgical treatment of gastroesophageal reflux disease (GERD) in pediatric patients. This chapter outlines the comprehensive approach to performing this procedure using the Da Vinci Xi surgical robot, emphasizing the systematic steps required to achieve optimal outcomes.

Robotic-assisted surgery offers several advantages over conventional laparoscopic techniques, including enhanced precision, improved visualization, and greater dexterity. These benefits are particularly valuable in pediatric surgery, where the anatomical structures are smaller and more delicate. However, it is crucial to recognize that while robotic-assisted fundoplication demonstrates technical superiority in certain aspects, clinical outcomes such as operating time and complication rates have not consistently shown significant improvements over traditional laparoscopic approaches. This underscores the importance of surgeon expertise and careful patient selection in determining the most appropriate surgical modality.

A key aspect of robotic-assisted fundoplication is the meticulous preoperative preparation and positioning, which are critical for ensuring adequate exposure and maneuverability during the procedure. The detailed steps outlined in this chapter, including incision and port placement, liver retraction, and the creation of a retroesophageal space, provide a clear framework for surgeons to follow. The use of an esophageal bougie and careful suturing techniques are emphasized to prevent complications such as esophageal narrowing and wrap migration.

Regarding the learning curve Binet et al. showed that after 20 procedures, the mean operative time significantly decreased, and there were no conversions to open surgery, with only 4.7% of patients requiring revision surgery [9].

Postoperative care is straightforward, with patients typically able to resume oral feeding immediately after surgery. Monitoring for complications such as retching, dysphagia, and recurrent GERD is essential for a smooth recovery.

Robotic-assisted gastric fundoplication is a valuable technique in the surgical management of pediatric GERD, offering enhanced precision and control. While the procedure is associated with longer operating times compared to conventional laparoscopy, its ability to provide a minimally invasive solution with potentially reduced post-operative discomfort and quicker recovery times makes it an attractive option. Continued advancements in robotic technology and further research into long-term outcomes will help to solidify the role of robotic-assisted surgery in pediatric gastroesophageal reflux disease.

In summary, this chapter provides a detailed guide for performing robotic-assisted gastric fundoplication, highlighting the critical steps and considerations to achieve successful surgical outcomes. By adhering to these principles, surgeons can effectively utilize robotic technology to improve the quality of care for pediatric patients with GERD.

References

1. Gosemann JH, Martynov I, Lacher M. Laparoscopic Thal fundoplication. In: Video Atlas of Pediatric Endosurgery (VAPE). Springer International Publishing (Verlag); 2021.
2. Tan YW, Martynov I, Lacher M, Saxena AK. Laparoscopic Toupet Fundoplication. In: Video Atlas of Pediatric Endosurgery (VAPE). Springer International Publishing (Verlag); 2021. 978-3-030-58042-1 (ISBN).
3. Falkenback D, Lehane CW, Lord RV. Robot-assisted oesophageal and gastric surgery for benign disease: antireflux operations and Heller's myotomy. ANZ J Surg. 2015;85(3):113–20.
4. Wang Z, Zheng Q, Jin Z. Meta-analysis of robot-assisted versus conventional laparoscopic Nissen fundoplication for gastro-oesophageal reflux disease. ANZ J Surg. 2012;82(3):112–7.
5. Jensen JS, Antonsen HK, Durup J. Two years of experience with robot-assisted anti-reflux surgery: a retrospective cohort study. Int J Surg. 2017;39:260–6.
6. Navarrete Arellano M, Garibay GF. Robot-assisted laparoscopic and thoracoscopic surgery: prospective series of 186 pediatric surgeries. Front Pediatr. 2019;7:200.
7. Rosen R, Vandenplas Y, Singendonk M, Cabana M, DiLorenzo C, Gottrand F, et al. Pediatric Gastroesophageal Reflux Clinical Practice Guidelines: joint recommendations of the North American Society for Pediatric Gastroenterology, Hepatology, and Nutrition and the European Society for Pediatric Gastroenterology, Hepatology, and Nutrition. J Pediatr Gastroenterol Nutr. 2018;66:516–54.
8. McNeely JK, Farber NE, Rusy LM, Hoffman GM. Epidural analgesia improves outcome following pediatric fundoplication. A retrospective analysis. Reg Anesth. 1997;22:16–23.
9. Binet A, Fourcade L, Amar S, Alzahrani K, Cook AR, Braïk K, Cros J, Longis B, Villemagne T, Lardy H, Ballouhey Q. Robot-assisted laparoscopic fundoplications in pediatric surgery: experience review. Eur J Pediatr Surg. 2019;29(2):173–8.

Robotic Heller's Cardiomyotomy

Naved Alizai and Melania Matcovici

1 Introduction

Robotic-assisted Heller's cardiomyotomy for paediatric achalasia cardia represents an advanced surgical technique that has gained attention due to its potential benefits over conventional laparoscopic methods. Achalasia cardia is a rare oesophageal motility disorder that requires a surgical approach with effective relief of dysphagia and minimal complications. Heller's cardiomyotomy, traditionally performed laparoscopically, has seen advancements through robotic assistance, offering enhanced precision and reduced risk of mucosal tears [1–4]. Recent studies have begun to compare these methods, highlighting the advantages of robotics in this procedure [1, 5, 6]. When compared to laparoscopy, robotic approach seems to have lower intraoperative blood loss, shorter surgery time and shorter length of stay [1, 7].

We describe our technique of robotic-assisted Heller's cardiomyotomy in children. There are multiple reports of successful outcomes of varying degrees, following dilatation of lower oesophagus. This chapter does not intend to discuss other techniques.

2 Patient Positioning and Set-Up

Theatre room is set up as pictured in Fig. 1. The anaesthetic machine and the drip stand should be positioned away on the right to avoid clash with the arms of the robot.

Patient is positioned supine, with a slight reverse Trendelenburg position to allow gravity retraction of abdominal contents away from the surgical field. Following the induction of anaesthesia, a large size nasogastric tube and urinary bladder catheter are inserted.

N. Alizai (✉) · M. Matcovici
Department of Paediatric Surgery, Leeds Children's Hospital, Leeds, UK
e-mail: naved.alizai@nhs.net

C. Esposito et al. (eds.), *Pediatric Robotic Assisted Surgery*,
https://doi.org/10.1007/978-3-031-99532-3_6

Fig. 1 Theatre set-up

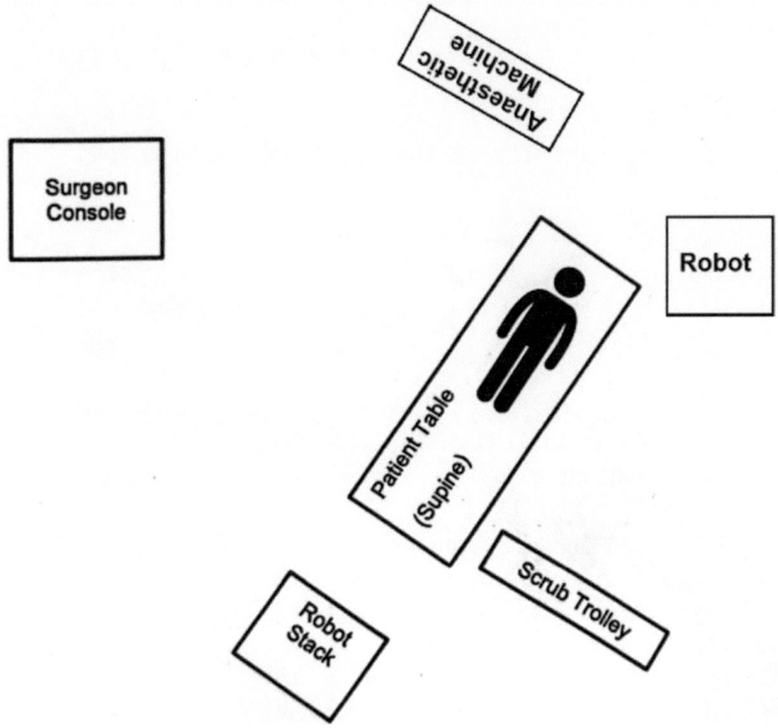

3 Port Placements

The camera port is inserted using a Hasson/open technique via a curved infra-umbilical incision for an 8-mm port. This incision is given just inside the inferior fold of the umbilicus. Such incisions provide a superior long-term cosmetic outcome. Two 8-mm robotic working ports are placed under direct vision in the right and left upper quadrants. A 5-mm accessory port is positioned in the left lower quadrant for assistance with tissue retraction, suction or irrigation (Fig. 2). A Nathanson retractor is introduced through a subxiphoid incision to elevate the liver and improve access to the oesophageal hiatus. While operating in centres where Nathanson is not available, the senior author has used various other means to elevate the left lobe of the liver. A stitch through the liver close to the anterior edge of the left lobe, slinging the falciform with a hanging stitch and stitching the anterior part of the Crura to the abdominal wall are all effective techniques.

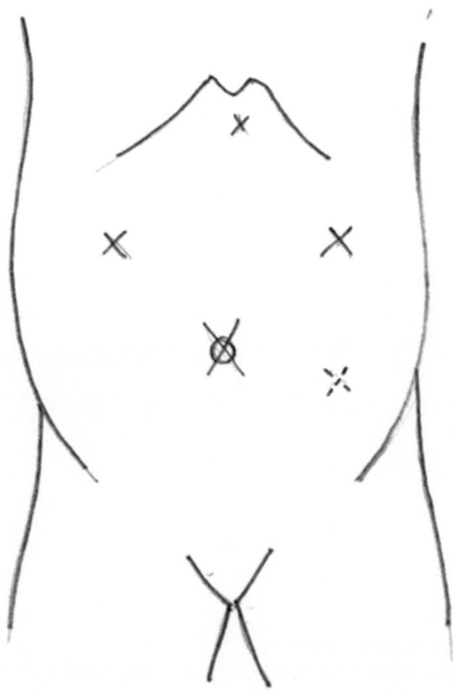

Fig. 2 Port positions

4 Robot Settings

We use three arms of the four-arm da Vinci® Robot X System (Intuitive Surgical, Sunnyvale, CA, USA). We recommend pressure settings between 8 and 12 mmHg with a flow rate of 2 to 4 litres per minute, as almost all patients are of an older age group.

The robot is brought over the left shoulder of the patient with the laser pointer in line with the telescope, which should be looking at the hiatus.

The instruments used are the following:

(i) Cadiere grasping forceps
(ii) Bipolar forceps and/or a monopolar hook
(iii) Suture cut needle holder
(iv) 5 mm laparoscopic Maryland and suction

5 Procedure Steps

The procedure begins with the division of the phreno-oesophageal membrane and dissection to expose the oesophagus circumferentially (Fig. 3), just the way one would approach for a fundoplication. This dissection can be done with a monopolar hook or bipolar forceps, by picking, burning and spreading the attachments. An umbilical tape (around 8 cm long) can be used to pass around the oesophagus, as a sling for retraction. It is needless to say that care needs to be taken to protect the posterior vagus nerve.

The myotomy is performed in the midline of the oesophagus, using bipolar forceps, by creating a window with diathermy and then spreading the oesophageal muscle fibres with forceps to expose the mucosa. It helps and is safer to place the convex surface of the bipolar forceps on the mucosa while spreading (Fig. 3). Robotic precision is advantageous in this step, significantly reducing the risk of mucosal perforation [4].

There is a clear transition with a change of muscle fibre direction, where the oesophagus joins the stomach. It is not unusual to find additional fibres crossing the oesophageal mucosa, especially where the oesophagus joins the stomach. Although the bipolar forceps can be turned back to face the telescope and perform dissection on the stomach, it is easier to create another window in the muscle fibres of the stomach and work in cranial direction to cut the muscle fibres and expose the gastric mucosa (Fig. 4). Care should be taken, and all muscle fibres crossing the mucosa should be divided.

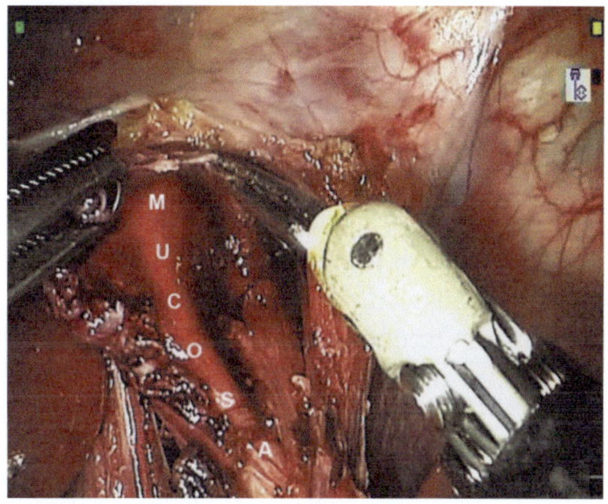

Fig. 3 Oesophageal myotomy

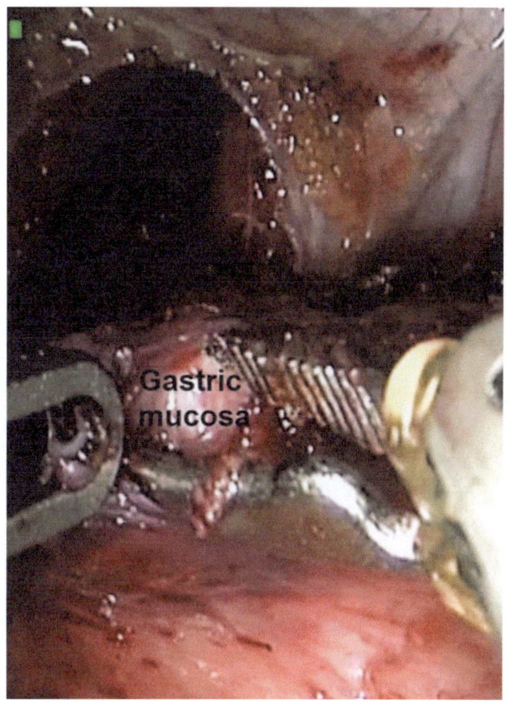

Fig. 4 Gastric end myotomy

The author aims for a total mucosal exposure of 7 cm, 5 cm on the oesophagus and 2 cm on the stomach.

The above dissection can also be performed with a monopolar hook. In author's experience, hook is useful in picking the gastric fibres and makes that part of the procedure easier than bipolar forceps dissection. The oesophageal dissection can also be done with the hook.

Mucosal perforation is a known complication of myotomy. The perforation usually happens when a surgeon mistakes mucosa for muscle fibres and is usually visible, when it happens. If there is no suggestion of a perforation visually, the anaesthetist is asked to inject air in the stomach through the nasogastric tube, and the mucosa should be seen to bulge. If a perforation does occur, the mucosa should be sutured with absorbable monofilament to reduce the risk of braided suture cutting the mucosa. Authors suggest covering the perforation with an anterior fundoplication. The patient should also be given broad-spectrum antibiotics, and gastric feeds should be delayed by couple of days, and patient should stay on soft diet for few days. The authors do not use antibiotics, if there is no perforation.

There is controversy regarding the need of a fundoplication following Heller's cardiomyotomy. Whether to offer a fundoplication or not is outside the remit of this chapter. Author prefers an anterior fundoplication, where the fundus is stitched to both edges of the myotomy and the top of the fundus to the crura (Fig. 5). In author's opinion, such a wrap will protect the mucosa, will keep the muscle edges apart and widely open and will also stop the omentum from getting stuck to the raw area on the mucosa and muscle edges. The length of the wrap is assessed using grasping forceps and by bringing the fundus of the stomach across to the right crura. If necessary, short gastric vessels are taken down using bipolar diathermy to allow adequate mobilisation. Non-absorbable 2–0 braided sutures are used to fix the wrap in place to the crura and to the myotomy layers (Fig. 6).

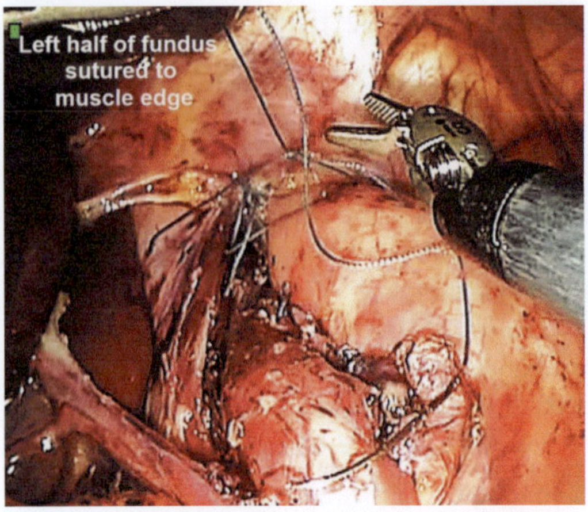

Fig. 5 Left half of anterior fundoplication in place

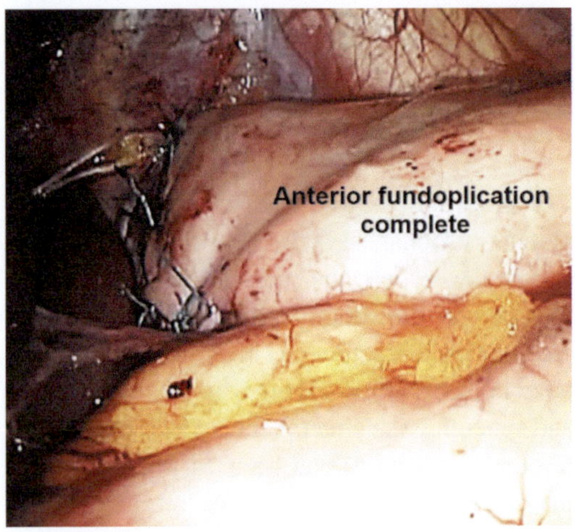

Fig. 6 Completed anterior fundoplication

6 Postoperative Management

Postoperative management includes careful monitoring of vital signs, pain management and early mobilization. The nasogastric tube is typically removed within the first 24 to 48 hours post-surgery. We do not routinely perform a contrast swallow study unless there is suspicion of a leak. Patients are gradually transitioned to a liquid diet and then to soft foods as tolerated. Regular follow-up is essential to monitor for any recurrence of symptoms and ensure adequate oesophageal function.

7 Tips and Tricks

- Preoperative imaging and manometry are essential for precise diagnosis and surgical planning.
- Careful port placement and patient positioning can significantly improve the ease and safety of the procedure.
- Utilizing robotic system's enhanced visualization and dexterity can aid in performing a precise myotomy, minimizing the risk of mucosal tears.

8 Conclusion

Robot-assisted Heller's Cardiomyotomy in children offers a minimally invasive alternative with significant potential benefits over traditional laparoscopic techniques, including enhanced precision and reduced risk of complications.

References

1. Delgado-Miguel C, Amarnath RP, Camps JI. Robotic-assisted vs. laparoscopic Heller's myotomy for achalasia in children. J Pediatr Surg. 2024;59(6):1072–6. https://doi.org/10.1016/j.jpedsurg.2023.11.003. Epub 2023 Nov 10.
2. Ferrero PA, Blanc T, Binet A, Arnaud A, Abbo O, Vatta F, Bonnard A, Spampinato G, Lardy H, Fourcade L, Ballouhey Q. The potential and the limitations of esophageal robotic surgery in children. Eur J Pediatr Surg. 2022;32(2):170–6. https://doi.org/10.1055/s-0040-1721770. Epub 2020 Dec 30.
3. Knight CG, Lorincz A, Gidell KM, Lelli J, Klein MD, Langenburg SE. Computer-assisted robot-enhanced laparoscopic fundoplication in children. J Pediatr Surg. 2004;39(6):864–6; discussion 864-6. https://doi.org/10.1016/j.jpedsurg.2004.02.022.
4. Ballouhey Q, Dib N, Binet A, Carcauzon-Couvrat V, Clermidi P, Longis B, Lardy H, Languepin J, Cros J, Fourcade L. How robotic-assisted surgery can decrease the risk of mucosal tear during Heller myotomy procedure? J Robot Surg. 2017;11(2):255–8. https://doi.org/10.1007/s11701-016-0658-9. Epub 2016 Nov 7.
5. Najmaldin A, Antao B. Early experience of tele-robotic surgery in children. Int J Med Robot. 2007;3(3):199–202. https://doi.org/10.1002/rcs.150.
6. Klein MD, Langenburg SE, Kabeer M, Lorincz A, Knight CG. Pediatric robotic surgery: lessons from a clinical experience. J Laparoendosc Adv Surg Tech A. 2007;17(2):265–71. https://doi.org/10.1089/lap.2006.0034.
7. Chaer RA, Jacobsen G, Elli F, Harris J, Goldstein A, Horgan S. Robotic-assisted laparoscopic pediatric Heller's cardiomyotomy: initial case report. J Laparoendosc Adv Surg Tech A. 2004;14(5):270–3. https://doi.org/10.1089/lap.2004.14.270.

Robotic Cholecystectomy

Arnaud Bonnard and Louise Montalva

1 Introduction

Patients with sickle cell disease (SCD) are prone to multiple complications throughout their lives, including those related to the formation of gallstones. Indeed, these patients are particularly at risk of developing events such as hepatic colic, cholecystitis, or angiocholitis during the course of their disease. Preventing the occurrence of these complications has become a central objective in the management of these patients, and for several years now, the benefit of prophylactic cholecystectomy in case of asymptomatic gallstones has been widely demonstrated. While the superiority of the laparoscopic approach over the open approach is now evident, there is limited data on robotic-assisted cholecystectomies in patients with sickle cell disease. Children with SCD need rigorous monitoring, enabling early detection of biliary complications and preventing morbidity and mortality associated with these complications [1]. These patients are indeed a particularly high-risk population for developing complications related to chronic hemolysis [2, 3].

To date, there is only one study comparing the outcomes of laparoscopic and robot-assisted cholecystectomy in the pediatric population [4]. In this study by Kulaylat et al., the authors demonstrated that the main differences were significantly longer operative duration and higher cost in the robotic group. Single port has been used and reported with the objective of offering a better cosmetic result in teenagers [5].

2 Patient Positioning and Planning

The position is the one described for the use of the SLIP trocars placement.

The patient is positioned using the French position, in a supine position, with the legs spread out and toward the ground. A pad is positioned under the tips of the scapula, at the base of the chest, in order to elevate the thoracic base (Fig. 1). Bladder emptiness is ensured before the procedure, by placing a urinary catheter that can be left in place during surgery, but taken out at the end of the procedure.

A. Bonnard (✉) · L. Montalva
Department of Pediatric Surgery, Robert Debré Children's University hospital and UMR1141 Inserm, Paris Cité University, Paris, France
e-mail: arnaud.bonnard@aphp.fr; louise.montalva@aphp.fr

C. Esposito et al. (eds.), *Pediatric Robotic Assisted Surgery*,
https://doi.org/10.1007/978-3-031-99532-3_7

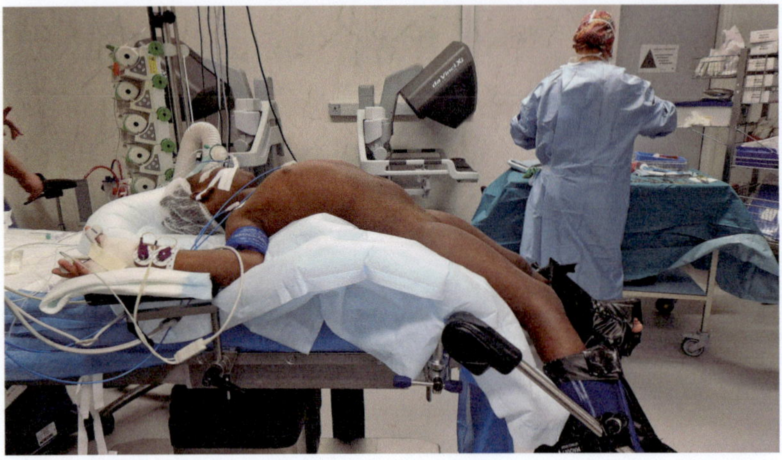

Fig. 1 Patient positioning

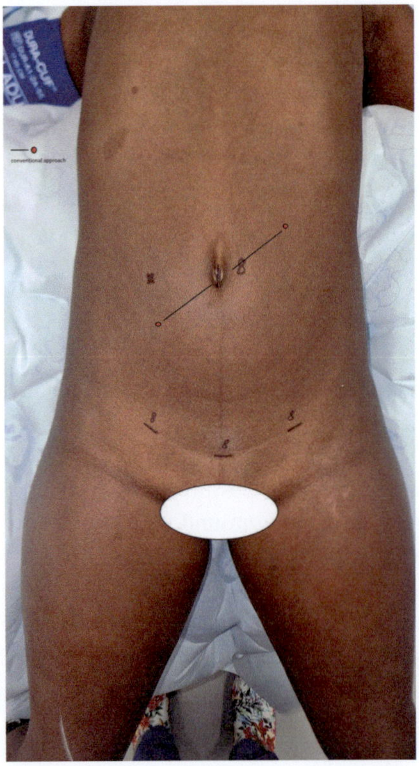

Fig. 2 Trocars placement

3 Incision and Port Placement

The ports are placed in the Pfannenstiel line under direct vision (Fig. 2).

- The first port in inserted through the umbilicus, to have a vision on the pelvic area.
- The second port is then inserted on the midline, in the Pfannenstiel line paying attention to avoiding injury to the bladder.
- The third and the fourth port are inserted on the same line, on the left and on the right side, separated from 4 to 6 cm. The camera is then placed using the port inserted on the midline and the umbilicus closed.
- Recently, we did it keeping the camera in the umbilicus (Xi platform) avoiding the need of a third incision in the Pfannenstiel line.

To expose the Calot triangle and to retract the gallbladder, either a stay stitch in the gallbladder or an extra 3 mm or 2 mm port can be used, placed in the xyphoid area or in the right flank.

The instruments used can be the monopolar scissor or the hook or even monopolar spatula. A bipolar fenestrated forceps can expose the elements you have to dissect. To control the cystic artery and duct, clips can be used but increase the cost of the procedure. Knotting using absorbable suture (vicryl 2/0 or 3/0) is a safe alternative and a good training for the residents and young trainees.

4 Robot Positioning

Using the Xi system, the placement of the robot and the boomer doesn't matter. It can be placed on the right or on the left side of the patient, with robotic settings on superior quadrant. It could be convenient to place an extra monitor for the assistant. Before starting the procedure, conflicts between the robotic arms should be solved and/or anticipated.

5 Procedure Steps

The anatomy of the Calot triangle should be perfectly known, with the liver above, the cystic duct under, and the common bile duct (CBD) medially. Many anatomic variations have been described and do not need to be known perfectly, but knowing the existence of these variations can avoid some catastrophic complications. Recently, indocyanine green has been found to provide an excellent real-time visualization of the extrahepatic biliary tree allowing a faster and safer dissection and minimizing the risk of bile duct injuries [6].

Different steps need to be followed to decrease the operative time and avoid any intraoperative complications:

1. Division and dissection of the Calot triangle: This is done opening the peritoneum in front and in the back of the Calot triangle. The cystic duct is usually the first structure to be individualized.
2. Once the peritoneum has been opened and the cystic duct visualized, a window needs to be created to complete the dissection of the cystic duct. In this window, usually you will find the cystic artery that needs to be divided using only the monopolar cautery or the bipolar forceps. A knot can also be used. Error traps have been published recently and can be summarized as follows [7]:
   - The first trap is the failure to recognize an aberrant posterior right hepatic duct in the operative field. The ICG can help in this situation.
   - The second trap: With significant inflammation, the hepatocystic triangle can be obliterated, and the common hepatic duct (CHD) is adherent to the gallbladder, appearing as part of the gallbladder wall. In this setting, the common bile duct (CBD) is mistaken for the cystic duct.
   - The third trap: In case of important inflammation, a top-down dissection can be used. The gallbladder is densely adherent to the cystic plate. A discernible plane between the back of the gallbladder and the CHD is difficult to identify, which can lead to transection of the CHD.
   - The fourth error trap is the parallel union of the cystic duct with the CBD. Therefore, during dissection of the cystic duct, the CBD or CHD can be misidentified as the cystic duct.
3. After the artery has been controlled, you will have to control the cystic duct. At this moment, the ICG can be useful to visualize how long is it and what is his connection with the CBD. The cystic duct is controlled using a knot and sectioned.
4. Retrograde cholecystectomy: using the monopolar cautery and starting from the gallbladder neck. Care should be taken to avoid pushing the dissection into the liver. This step can be difficult, especially if the patient has a previous history of cholecystitis (Figs. 3, 4, 5 and 6).

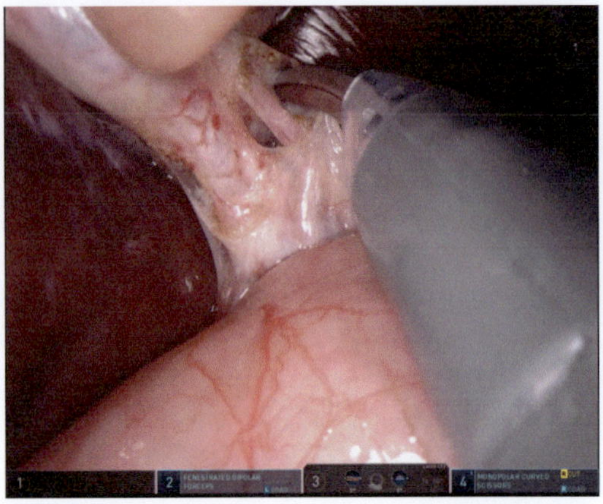

Fig. 3 Dissection of the cystic duct and cystic artery

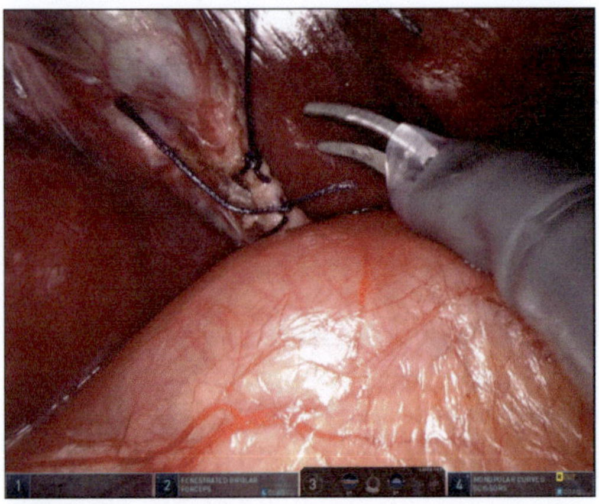

Fig. 4 Control of the cystic duct and section

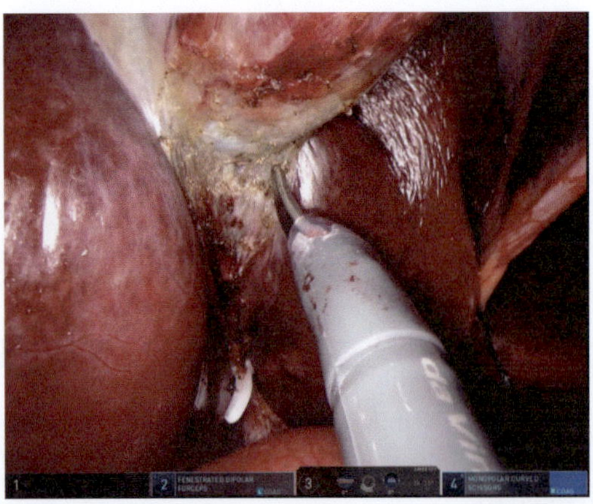

Fig. 5 Dissection of the cystic plate from the gallbladder neck

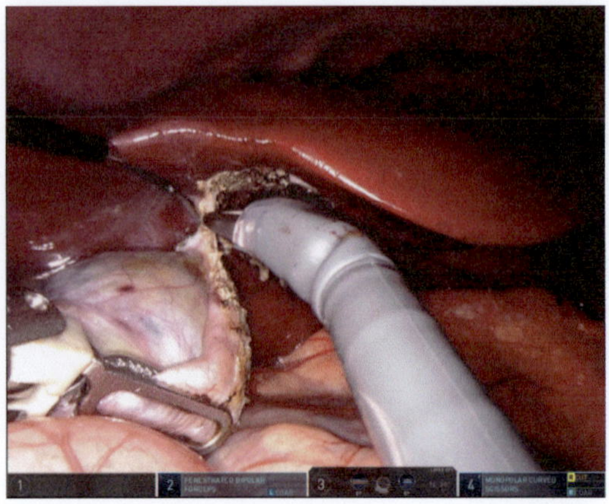

Fig. 6 End of the dissection

6 Postoperative Period

Overall complication rate has been reported to be around 1%. The incidence of bile duct injury remains between 0.2% and 0.4%, even for experienced surgeons. Complications include bleeding from the cystic artery, and rarely a CBD injury resulting in stenosis requiring a Roux-and-Y jejunal loop to replace it. Robotic-assisted cholecystectomy can be safely performed as a day-case surgery for non-Sickle cell disease patient.

7 Tips and Tricks

In case of important inflammation, an anterograde dissection of the gallbladder (top-down technique) can be performed allowing to pediculate the gallbladder on the cystic duct. This is a safer way to manage the dissection of the cystic plate trying to minimize the risk to injure the CBD. The ICG is probably of a great help in these difficult cases.

8 Discussion and Conclusion

Robotic cholecystectomy is a procedure that can be performed using a robotic approach with a suprapubic placement of the trocars. This approach offers a precise dissection of the pedicle, good ergonomic conditions, and a postoperative course similar to the laparoscopic approach. Rules of dissection need to be respected to avoid any complications. Indocyanine green could be the standard of care using a robotic approach.

References

1. Allali S, de Montalembert M, Brousse V, Heilbronner C, Taylor M, Brice J, et al. Hepatobiliary complications in children with sickle cell disease: a retrospective review of medical records from 616 patients. J Clin Med. 2019;8(9):1481.
2. Bender MA, Carlberg K. Sickle cell disease. In: Adam MP, Feldman J, Mirzaa GM, Pagon RA, Wallace SE, Bean LJ, et al., editors. GeneReviews® [Internet]. Seattle: University of Washington; 1993. [cité 23 nov 2023]. http://www.ncbi.nlm.nih.gov/books/NBK1377/.
3. Silva IV, Reis AF, Palaré MJ, Ferrão A, Rodrigues T, Morais A. Sickle cell disease in children: chronic complications and search of predictive factors for adverse outcomes. Eur J Haematol févr. 2015;94(2):157–61.
4. Kulaylat AN, Richards H, Yada K, Coyle D, Shelby R, Onwuka AJ, Aldrink JH, Diefenbach KA, Michalsky MP. Comparative analysis of robotic-assisted versus laparoscopic cholecystectomy in pediatric patients. J Pediatr Surg. 2021;56(10):1876–80.
5. Klazura G, Graf A, Sims T, Rojnica M, Koo N, Lobe TE. Assessment of the da Vinci Single Port robotic platform on cholecystectomy in adolescents. J Laparoendosc Adv Surg Tech A. 2022;32(4):438–41.
6. Esposito C, Settimi A, Cerulo M, Escolino M. Efficacy of indocyanine green (ICG) fluorescent cholangiography to improve intra-operative visualization during laparoscopic cholecystectomy in pediatric patients: a comparative study between ICG-guided fluorescence and standard technique. Surg Endosc. 2022;36(6):4369–75.
7. Seshadri A, Peitzman AB. The difficult cholecystectomy: what you need to know. J Trauma Acute Care Surg. 2024;97(3):325–36.

Robotic-Assisted Excision of Choledochal Cyst and Hepaticojejunostomy in Children

Donatella Di Fabrizio, Naved K. Alizai, and Azad S. Najmaldin

1 Introduction

In children, choledochal cyst is a relatively common congenital malformation of the biliary tract. It presents as a dilation of the common bile duct with or without an intrahepatic bile duct involvement [1]. A timely appropriate management minimizes the risks of the early and late complications, including cholestasis, recurrent pancreatitis, cyst perforation, malignancy, cirrhosis and liver failure. The treatment of choice is cyst excision, cholecystectomy and Roux-en-Y hepaticojejunostomy which traditionally has been performed as an open procedure. In 1995, the first report of laparoscopic choledochal cyst resection appeared in literature [2]. Since, increasing numbers of surgeons, particularly those from high-volume centres, have adopted laparoscopy as the method of choice [3, 4], more recently, robotic-assisted laparoscopic technique has gained some popularity with the first report being published in 2006 [5].

The authors' dedicated minimal access and robotic surgery centre introduced laparoscopic and robotic -assisted approaches in the management of choledochal cyst in 2007 and 2009, respectively [6]. This chapter describes aspects of robotic technique.

D. Di Fabrizio · N. K. Alizai · A. S. Najmaldin (✉)
Department of Paediatric Surgery, Leeds Children's Hospital, Leeds Teaching Hospitals, Leeds, UK

2 Patient Preparation, Position and Set-up

The theatre set-up is similar for all upper abdominal procedures. The operating table may have to be moved and adjusted to suit the theatre environment and optimize safe surgical and anaesthetic access. Extra padding helps retain patient body heat and minimize the risk of pressure sore that can occur during long procedures. As for all conventional and robotic-assisted laparoscopy in infants and small children, the use of a small operating table prevents arms/instruments collision with table. Alternatively, small patients are raised off standard tables by an extra several centimetres thick block of soft mattress. The patient is positioned supine with a slight head up tilt (reverse Trendelenburg). A nasogastric tube and urinary bladder catheter are inserted. Prophylactic intravenous antibiotics are administered to cover the perioperative period.

The anaesthetic team is located at the head of the patient, slightly to the left side, and the slave cart above the right shoulder (old models) or right side of the patient (new models). The main screen is placed further down on the right-hand side of the patient, and the assistant comfortably

C. Esposito et al. (eds.), *Pediatric Robotic Assisted Surgery*,
https://doi.org/10.1007/978-3-031-99532-3_8

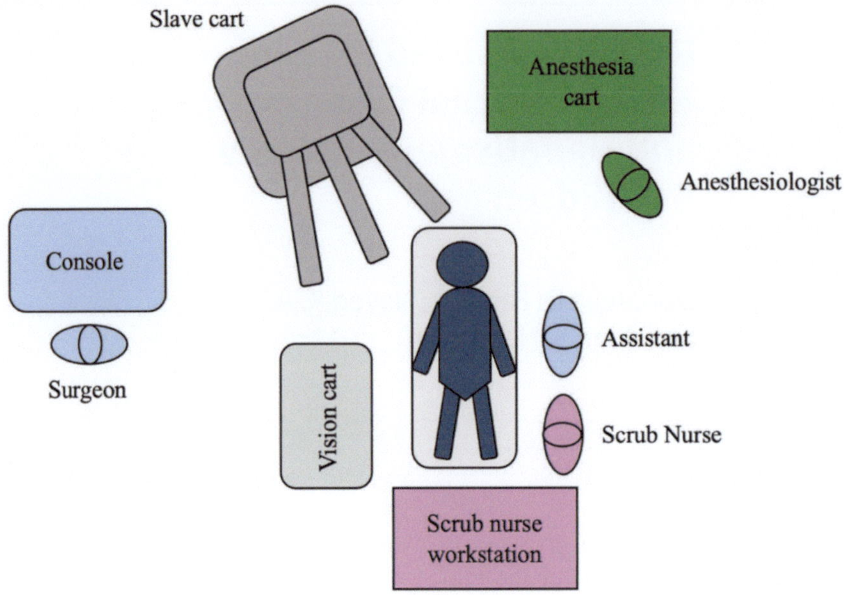

Fig. 1 Theatre set-up for a da Vinci system (previous generations)

occupies a position at the patient's left. The scrub nurse and instrument trolley are positioned on the left, close to the foot of the table (Fig. 1).

3 Port Placement

Given the limited working surface and space in infants and small children, versatility of larger telescope and instruments and the advantages of having an accessory conventional laparoscopic port (traction/retraction instrument, suction/irrigation, sutures in/out and cut, flexible mini-scope if required), we prefer the use of three arms of the da Vinci system: telescope (12-mm 30 degree), two robotic working ports (8 mm) and one accessory laparoscopic (3–5 mm).

In children older than 1 year of age, the procedure starts by making a suitable sized sub-umbilical curved incision and placement of a medium-sized Alexis® laparoscopic system wound protector/retractor (Applied Medical in Rancho Santa Margarita, California, USA). The telescope port is placed through the lid of the protector/retractor while maintaining a pneumoperitoneum (CO_2 pressure 8–10 mmHg). Smaller devices are without a lid, therefore unsuitable to use in infants and smaller children. Here, the sub-umbilical incision is made small (1.5 cm and a purse string suture) initially to accommodate a 12-mm optic port, which needs to be extended (to 3–4 cm) at the latter stage of the procedure for the formation of the Roux loop extracorporeally. Once the loop is reduced back into the peritoneal cavity, the wound is partially closed to reaccommodate the optic port, a pneumoperitoneum is reestablished, and the final robotic manipulation and the anastomosis are completed intracorporeally.

The position of working ports is dependent on the size of the patient and cyst. Typically, the right port is positioned at or slightly below the level of the umbilicus, while the left port is placed slightly higher, at or lateral to the midclavicular lines. The accessory laparoscopic port is placed in a far left lateral position, just below the costal margin. A Nathanson's retractor is inserted through a small right subcostal incision stab incision to retract the liver gently exposing the porta hepatis (Fig. 2). As always, all ports, instruments, retractors and sutures are placed in and out under vision.

Fig. 2 Port placement

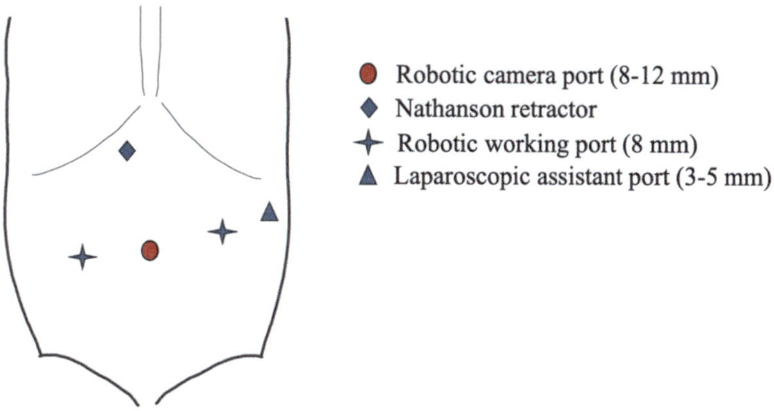

4 Procedure Steps

To maximize working space and safety, large cysts are aspirated with an under-vision percutaneously inserted wide bore long needle. Sometimes cyst aspiration may become necessary after the insertion of camera port, in order to be able to insert the working ports safely.

The dissection is performed using an atraumatic grasper in one hand and either the plasmakinetic (PK) or bipolar forceps (grasp, seal/burn, tease/divide and spread technique - GSTST) or an insulated monopolar curved thin-bladed scissors on the other side. Sometimes, a combination of the mentioned modalities proves helpful. The dissection is commenced by opening the hepatico-duodenal ligament over the anteromedial surface of the cyst, which is then continued strictly on the surface and around the cyst well away from the portal vein and hepatic artery. The dissection is continued caudal behind the first part of duodenum to the distal aspect of the cyst as it tapers into the pancreas (Fig. 3), while the assistant retracts the duodenum downward using an atraumatic forceps through the accessory port. Typically, this is the easiest point to get around the back of cyst, and ultra-care is taken not to damage the vessels, pancreas and the pancreatic duct. A patent distal end is then divided in between ligatures, transfixation sutures or clips, while a clearly visible atretic distal common bile duct is divided without the need to ligate.

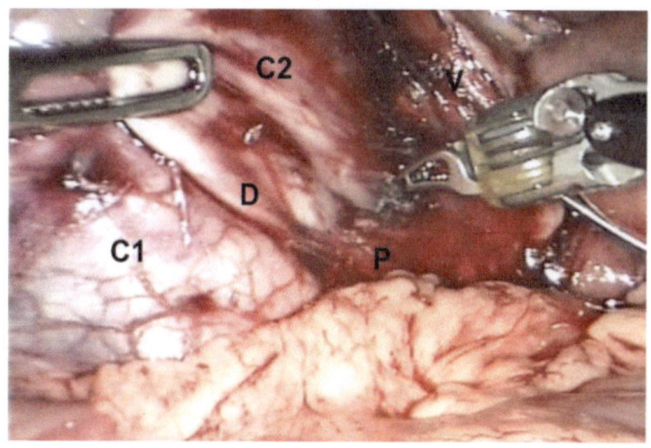

Fig. 3 Blunt dissection strictly on the cyst wall using a bipolar grasp, seal, teas and spread technique. C1, anterior wall of a partially aspirated giant cyst; C2, postero-medial aspect of the cyst; D, distal common duct tapering into pancreas; P, pancreas thinned out by the large cyst; V, major vessels

The choledochal cyst is completely mobilized off the portal vein cephalad to and beyond the common hepatic duct with the dissection being strictly on the cyst well away from the vessels. The gall bladder is then mobilized off its bed leaving the fundus attached to the liver to prevent it from falling into the operative field. The common hepatic duct is then divided well below the confluence of the left and right ducts (Fig. 4). The hepatic ducts are inspected within, flushed if required, and the common duct is trimmed sufficiently high leaving a sleeve to allow for a safe anastomosis. Before and after preparing the proximal end of the common hepatic duct, it is important that the porta hepatis is carefully inspected for signs of low inserting segmental (accessory)

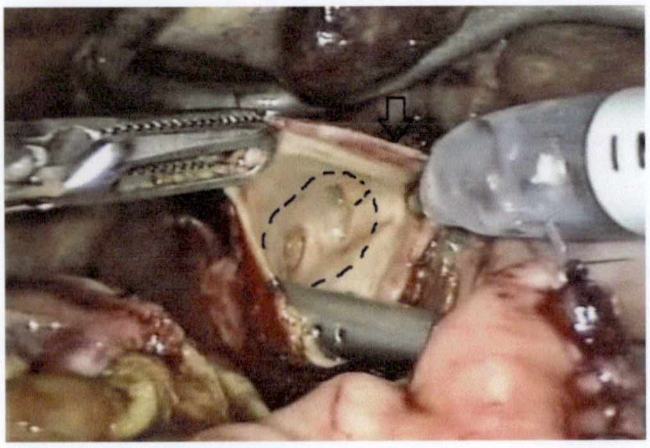

Fig. 4 Transected lower common hepatic duct. Instruments holding the edge with a suction probe inside and a clearly visible left and right hepatic duct openings. Broken line denotes the line of final trimming which is extended to near but not the edge of left duct

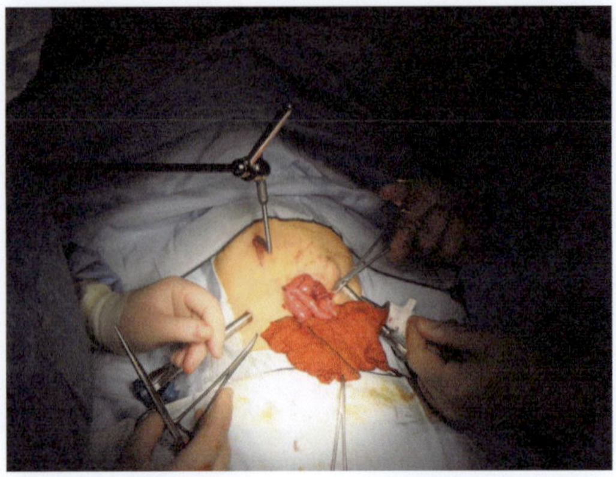

Fig. 5 Extracorporeal Roux-en-Y loop formation

duct branches. Care is taken not to divide the duct too high and ending up separating the left and right hepatic ducts. Once the correct anatomy is ensured, the proximal cut end is bevelled slightly toward but not into the left duct (Fig. 4). This manoeuvre allows for a wide oblique anastomosis which in turn minimizes the risk of stricture occurring postoperatively. If the left and right hepatic ducts are separated, they can either be anastomosed separately or joined together (pantaloon shape), before performing a single hepaticojejunostomy.

The next step is to create the Roux loop (Fig. 5). The assistant gently lifts the transverse colon using an atraumatic grasper with a ratchet (Johan) through the accessory port, while the operator identifies the duodenojejunal (DJ) flexure. Proximal jejunum is then carefully oriented, followed for about 30 cm and guided into the assistant's grasper. The assistant must make every effort not to disengage, twist, or disorientate the gently grasped jejunal loop, while the robot is undocked, the lid of Alexis retractor removed, and the grasped loop of jejunum is exteriorized through the retractor by the assistant. In infants and very small children without an Alexis retractor, the subumbilical port incision is extended sufficiently to allow for the grasped loop to be delivered externally. A 30-cm Roux loop is then fashioned externally, using staplers and hand sutures; the mesenteric defect is closed and returned into the abdominal cavity. Alexis lid is replaced (or subumbilical incision is partially closed to reintroduce the telescope port in small children), pneumoperitoneum is reestablished, robot is redocked, and the final stage of the procedure is commenced.

A small window in the transverse mesocolon facilitates a retrocolic route for the Roux loop. Here, transverse colon is held against the anterior abdominal wall with mesocolon facing the camera by the assistant's atraumatic grasper, while the operator is pointing toward the camera gently from behind at the chosen site with a robotic instrument, and a window is made with a second robotic instrument (PK or bipolar forceps). Care is taken not to damage colic vessels or other structures behind. The Roux loop is then identified; its correct orientation is ensured and pulled cephalad through the window and placed in the proximity of the previously transected hepatic duct. The loop must sit comfortably at the porta hepatis without any signs of tension in particular that of the mesentery, constriction at the window, torsion, or ischaemia.

An antimesenteric enterotomy is now made, using the tip of a thin-bladed monopolar diathermy scissors, several millimetres away from the end of the Roux loop, to match the size of the prepared hepatic duct. A tension-free anastomosis is created using interrupted 5/0 absorbable sutures, starting at the 6 o'clock position on the posterior wall preferably with the suture knots being outside. Few carefully positioned fine interrupted sutures between the Roux loop and free edge of the mesocolic window minimizes the risk of a postoperative internal hernia occurring.

Finally, the peritoneal cavity is thoroughly aspirated and irrigated with warm saline if thought necessary. A suction drain is then placed near the anastomosis using the Nathanson retractor site. The fundus of gall bladder is detached from the liver, and the free specimen is now removed in one or multiple pieces. Appropriate local anaesthetic agent is instilled and all wounds are closed in layers.

5 Postoperative Care

The urinary catheter is usually removed at the end of the procedure. Intravenous prophylactic antibiotics are continued for 48 h postoperatively. Intravenous morphine infusion is continued at the anaesthetist's discretion. The nasogastric tune may be retained for 1–2 days as thought necessary, while oral feeding is typically initiated on day 3. The drainage tube is commonly removed on day 4, and patients are discharged home between day 4 and 6, depending on patient's circumstances and comorbidity. A long-term follow-up is essential in all.

6 Tips and Tricks

Management of a choledochal cyst is a challenging process. Although great advantages are conferred to the operating surgeon through the robot, attention to details during pre-, per and postoperative periods as well as long follow-up minimizes the risks of complications and improves outcome. Many tips and tricks highlighted below are similar to those learnt during open, conventional laparoscopic and general robotic techniques, while some have already been described within the "procedure steps".

6.1 Limitation of Workspace

Working space can be limited due to patient's size, cyst size, the presence of pre-existing comorbidities such as inflammatory oedema and a large liver and intermittent loss of pneumoperitoneum. Complete muscle relaxation throughout the procedure, strategic positioning of the ports/retractor and aspiration of the cyst are essential to maximize workspace. The use of a fixed subhepatic retractor such as Nathanson is essential during biliary surgery. However, care must be taken to avoid prolonged forceful retraction that interferes with ventilation and liver circulation.

6.2 Arms and Instrument Collisions

These risks can be minimized by increasing the arc of movements of arms and instruments. This is achievable by appropriately positioned patients and ports. The former is accomplished with either an operating table tailored to the patient's size or raising the patient off standard tables with a suitably sized several centimetres or more thick, soft mattress thus avoiding collisions between the robot and table's edges. This has been our practice for all minimal invasive and robotic procedures for three decades.

6.3 Dissection

The use of PK or bipolar forceps during dissection (grasp, seal, teas and spread technique strictly on the surface of cyst) increases safety by minimizing the risks of bleeding and unintended monopolar diathermy injury. This is particularly so while separating the cyst from major vessels and pancreas and in small children, complex anatomy, or the presence of inflammation and scarring. In rare circumstances, the cyst may be opened through the lower part of its anterior wall to facilitate dissection within (inner layer plane) during the early and difficult stages of mobilization. Once the difficult part is safely mobilized, dissection is then continued on the outer surface of the cyst toward the hepatic duct.

6.4 Stones and Sludge

Common channel stones and sludge, a rare occurrence, may be cleared through the lower anterior wall using a flexible choledochoscope via the accessory port.

6.5 Handling Bile Ducts and Major Vessels

Anatomical anomalies are not uncommon occurrences and can easily be missed on preoperative imaging. The almost complete lack of tactile sensation in robotic surgery complicates the matter further. Once the upper limit of the cyst is reached, minimal dissection at and beyond the common hepatic duct is required. It is always better to transect common hepatic duct just above the cyst, well below the confluent of left and right ducts (Fig. 4). Once the lumen is inspected, and position of left and right ducts, and accessory duct, if any, are checked, further common duct excision is safely performed as thought necessary. Such an approach minimizes the risk of duct wall ischaemia, and collateral injuries which may also involve aberrant vessels and accessory hepatic duct. The final duct transection should be straight, made by a single stroke if possible, using thin-bladed sharp scissors. This and atraumatic duct handling facilitate easy and safe anastomosis.

Above left and right hepatic ducts confluent transection, mandate either individual or pantaloon type duct anastomosis to the loop. An accessory duct may be anastomosed separately to the loop if at all possible, or ligated.

6.6 Eye on the Anastomosis

The anastomosis must be very close to the end of the customized loop to minimize risks of elongation and redundancy of the closed end which may predispose to postoperative bile stagnation and stone formation within the loop and bile ducts.

To minimize the risks of stricture, the ratio between the diameters of the common hepatic duct and the proximal Roux-en-Y jejunal lumen should be equal to or less than 1 (common hepatic duct) to 2.5 (jejunum), the anastomosis is completed with interrupted absorbable sutures, and the suture knots are kept outside.

7 Discussion and Conclusions

Robotic surgery has revolutionized the landscape of paediatric surgery, offering better visualization of the operative field, precision, dexterity and minimally invasive approach for surgery in general, challenging procedures such as choledochal cyst in particular [6–8].

Hepaticoduodenostomy and hepaticojejunostomy restore bile flow in patients undergoing choledochal cyst excision. The former is considerably easier to perform due to the shorter distance required to reconnect the bile duct to the digestive tract; therefore, a loop formation and multiple intestinal anastomosis are avoided. This results in shorter operating time and hospital stay; reducing risks of potential complications such as leak, redundant loop syndrome and stricture; and allowing postoperative endoscopic access to the anastomosis in cases of stricture or stone occurrence. However, the technique increases the risks of two-way flow (bile into the duodenum and duodenal contents into bile ducts) and long-term complications of recurrent cholangitis and bile gastritis [9].

On the other hand, Roux-en-Y hepaticojejunostomy is technically much more challenging but facilitates bile flow directly into the small intestine, thereby reducing the risks of long-term complications [9]. Like most paediatric surgeons, we believe hepaticoduodenostomy should be reserved for patients in whom hepaticojejunostomy is not achievable.

The choice of Roux-loop formation, intra- or extra-corporally, is largely dependent on the patients' size and surgeons' preference [10]. Like most surgeons, we favour extra-corporal loop formation which is reproducible at all ages, technically easier to perform and saves the operating time significantly.

High-volume paediatric laparoscopic choledochal cyst surgery centres advocate a learning curve span of 37 cases [11]. Given the positive impact of robotic-assisted technique in laparoscopy, particularly the complex procedures, it is hardly surprising that a lesser number of 14 patients have been suggested in robotic-assisted approach [12]. In our experience of robotic-assisted choledochal cyst excision and hepaticojejunostomy, the learning phase did not impact the conversion or complication rates [13, 14].

A recent metanalysis of robotic-assisted choledochal cyst surgery in children reported a conversion rate of 0.2–10.5% and postoperative complication 1.9–12%, including intestinal obstruction 0.7–10.5%, bleeding 0.1–4.5%, anastomotic leak 0.6–4.1% and anastomotic stricture 0.3–3.5% [15]. In our prospective study of the first 60 robotic choledochal cysts (age 0.3–15, 43% less than 2 years) over a 9-year period, the mean console time was 302 minutes (range 220–394), conversion rate 13.3% with ½ being due to anaesthetic related factors and the other ½ complex anatomy or pre-existing comorbidities (none from an intraoperative complication). In the same study, significant postoperative complications included redo surgery for anastomotic stricture in 6%, adhesive intestinal obstruction 2%, but no significant leak or bleeding [13, 14].

In conclusion, robotic technology is safe, effective and advantageous in the treatment of choledochal cyst. The conversion and complication rates are comparable favourably to conventional surgery. The importance of surgical conditions and technique cannot be overemphasized.

References

1. Stringer MD, Dhawan A, Davenport M, Mieli-Vergani G, Mowat AP, Howard ER. Choledochal cysts: lessons from a 20 year experience. Arch Dis Child. 1995;73:528–31. https://doi.org/10.1136/adc.73.6.528.
2. Farello GA, Cerofolini A, Rebonato M, Bergamaschi G, Ferrari C, Chiappetta A. Congenital choledochal cyst: video-guided laparoscopic treatment. Surg Laparosc Endosc. 1995;5:354–8.
3. Liem NT, Pham HD, Dung le A, et al. Early and intermediate outcomes of laparoscopic surgery for choledochal cysts with 400 patients. J Laparoendosc Adv Surg Tech A. 2012;22:599–603.
4. Qiao G, Li L, Li S, et al. Laparoscopic cyst excision and roux-Y hepaticojejunostomy for children with choledochal cysts in China: a multicenter study. Surg Endosc. 2015;29:140–4.
5. Woo R, Le D, Albanese CT, Kim SS. Robot-assisted laparoscopic resection of a type I choledochal cyst in a child. J Laparoendosc Adv Surg Tech A. 2006;16(2):179–83. https://doi.org/10.1089/lap.2006.16.179. PMID: 16646713
6. Alizai NK, Dawrant MJ, Najmaldin AS. Robot-assisted resection of choledochal cysts and hepaticojejunostomy in children. Pediatr Surg Int. 2014;30(3):291–4. https://doi.org/10.1007/s00383-013-3459-5. Epub 2014 Jan 24. PMID: 24458067
7. Chen S, Lin Y, Xu D, Lin J, Zeng Y, Li L. Da vinci robotic-assisted treatment of pediatric choledochal cyst. Front Pediatr. 2022;10:1044309. https://doi.org/10.3389/fped.2022.1044309.
8. Koga H, Murakami H, Ochi T, Miyano G, Lane GJ, Yamataka A. Comparison of robotic versus laparoscopic hepaticojejunostomy for choledochal cyst in children: a first report. Pediatr Surg Int. 2019;35(12):1421–5. https://doi.org/10.1007/s00383-019-04565-3.
9. Hinojosa-Gonzalez DE, Roblesgil-Medrano A, Leon SUV, Espadas-Conde MA, Flores-Villalba E. Biliary reconstruction after choledochal cyst resection: a systematic review and meta-analysis on hepaticojejunostomy vs hepaticoduodenostomy. Pediatr Surg Int. 2021;37(10):1313–22. https://doi.org/10.1007/s00383-021-04940-z. Epub 2021 Jun 11. PMID: 34115175
10. Xie X, Li K, Xiang B. Total versus conventional robotic-assisted cyst excisions and hepaticojejunos-

tomies in children with choledochal cysts: a case-control study. J Robot Surg. 2023;17(3):869–76. https://doi.org/10.1007/s11701-022-01484-9. Epub 2022 Nov 2. PMID: 36324048
11. Wen Z, Liang H, Liang J, Liang Q, Xia H. Evaluation of the learning curve of laparoscopic choledochal cyst excision and Roux-en-Y hepaticojejunostomy in children: CUSUM analysis of a single surgeon's experience. Surg Endosc. 2017;31(2):778–87. https://doi.org/10.1007/s00464-016-5032-5. Epub 2016 Jun 23. PMID: 27338584; PMCID: PMC5266761
12. Xie X, Feng L, Li K, Wang C, Xiang B. Learning curve of robot-assisted choledochal cyst excision in pediatrics: report of 60 cases. Surg Endosc. 2021;35(6):2690–7. https://doi.org/10.1007/s00464-020-07695-1. Epub 2020 Jun 15. PMID: 32556766
13. Cundy TP, Fabrizio DD, Alizai NK, Najmaldin AS. Conversions in pediatric robot-assisted laparoscopic surgery. J Pediatr Surg. 2022;57(8):1637–41. https://doi.org/10.1016/j.jpedsurg.2021.10.056. Epub 2021 Nov 16. PMID: 34924187
14. Di Fabrizio D, Alizai NK, Najmaldin AS. Early and long-term complications of robotic assisted laparoscopy in infants and children. J Pediatr Surg. 2023;58(9):1832–7. https://doi.org/10.1016/j.jpedsurg.2023.02.061. Epub 2023 Mar 4. PMID: 36997389
15. Zhang MX, Chi SQ, Cao GQ, Tang JF, Tang ST. Comparison of efficacy and safety of robotic surgery and laparoscopic surgery for choledochal cyst in children: a systematic review and proportional meta-analysis. Surg Endosc. 2023;37(1):31–47. https://doi.org/10.1007/s00464-022-09442-0. Epub 2022 Aug 1. PMID: 35913517

Liver Cyst

Naved Alizai, Melania Matcovici,
and Sarah Vecchione

1 Introduction

Liver cysts are relatively rare in pediatric population and should be regarded as a separate entity from choledochal and parasitic liver cysts, when considering surgical management. Liver cysts present with a diverse histopathological spectrum, ranging from simple cysts to more complex forms such as ciliated hepatic foregut cysts, cysts of biliary origin, and mesenchymal hamartomas [1]. Most of the simple cysts are asymptomatic and a conservative, and clinical and radiological monitoring approach is the recommended standard management [2]. Intervention is typically indicated for cyst enlargement, the presence of symptoms, description of septae on imaging, or suspicion of malignancy [3].

Various treatment modalities are described including aspiration, sclerotherapy, deroofing, partial or complete enucleation/excision, and partial hepatectomy [3, 4]. While laparoscopic approach has been documented in a small number of case reports and series, robotic excision remains relatively rare. In our center, we approach these cases robotically and always aim for complete excision. We published our experience with robotic resection of pediatric liver cysts, representing the largest reported series of minimally invasive surgery (MIS) resection in the literature [5], and we present our technique in this chapter.

1.1 Patient Selection and Preoperative Assessment

A large number of liver cysts are found incidentally on ultrasound scan (USS), when patients are being investigated for other pathologies, while others are suspected on antenatal scans. US allows for initial characterization of the cyst, but to further delineate the anatomy and to ensure an adequate preoperative preparation and avoid surprises during the surgical procedure, magnetic resonance cholangiopancreatogram (MRCP) is the investigation of choice. A hepatobiliary iminodiacetic acid (HIDA) might be indicated in some cases to exclude or confirm connection with the biliary tract.

Age and weight at operation varies greatly, with the youngest patient operated in our series being 5 months old and 5.1 kg in weight at the time of surgery.

N. Alizai (✉) · M. Matcovici · S. Vecchione
Paediatric Liver Unit and Department of Paediatric Surgery, Leeds Children's Hospital, Leeds, UK
e-mail: naved.alizai@nhs.net; sarah.vecchione@nhs.ne

C. Esposito et al. (eds.), *Pediatric Robotic Assisted Surgery*,
https://doi.org/10.1007/978-3-031-99532-3_9

2 Patient Positioning

Patients are positioned supine on the operating table. Nasogastric tube and urinary bladder catheter are inserted after the induction of anesthesia.

Da Vinci® Robot System (Intuitive Surgical, Sunnyvale, CA, USA), component positioning is illustrated in Fig. 1. Careful attention is given to the anesthetic machine's position, which needs to be well away on the right side of the patient. It is also important to put the drip stand beside the anesthetic machine to avoid obstruction of the arms of the robot.

One of the problems, especially in small-sized children, is the clash of the external part of robotic arms to the table. In most operating rooms, the theater table is wide, and the arms of the robot hit the table when operating on a ***small size child lying in the middle of the table. The authors overcome this problem by either raising the child on a thick piece of gel pad or by using a narrow or a neonatal table. If using a neonatal table, the scrub staff has to use an additional trolley to rest the camera and diathermy cables, which normally lie on the operating table.

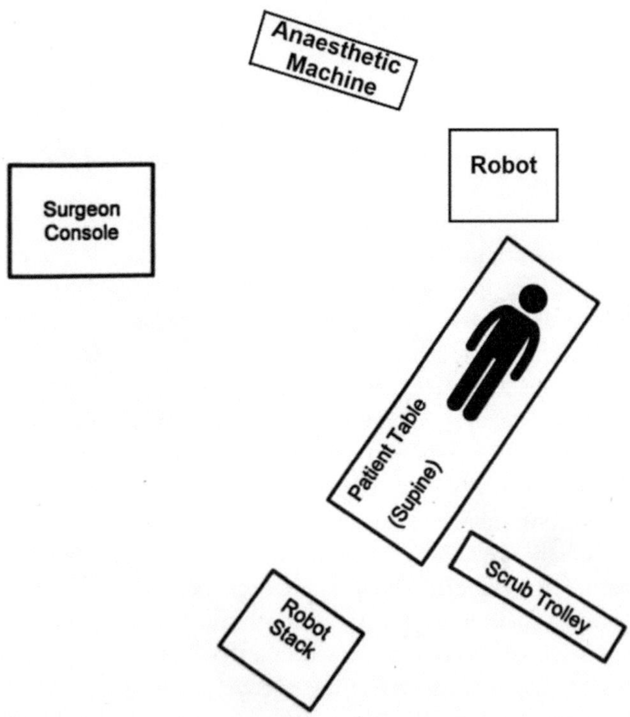

Fig. 1 Operating room setup

3 Robot Settings

We utilize the four-arm da Vinci® Robot System (Intuitive Surgical, Sunnyvale, CA, USA), specifically the da Vinci® X system. However, we only use three arms for the excision of liver cysts. Optimal settings include low pressures between 8 and 12 mmHg and a flow rate between 0.5 and 4 liters per minute, depending on the size of the patient, with higher flow rate for larger children. The robotic instruments used include a Cadiere grasping forceps in surgeon's left hand and monopolar scissors or bipolar dissector for effective dissection.

4 Port Placements

We use three 8-mm ports. The primary/camera port is inserted using Hasson/open technique, through an "intra-umbilical" curved incision, in the inferior skin fold of the umbilicus. This site provides a good cosmetic result, as it gets incorporated into the umbilicus and is hardly visible, when seen in the postoperative follow-up clinic.

Pneumoperitoneum is established, and two additional 8-mm robotic working ports are inserted under direct vision. The site of the working ports varies according to the location of the cyst and also according to the size of the patient. The aim is to try and triangulate the working ports and provide enough room for the length of the working part of the instrument. In small patients, the working port sites may need to be further down on the abdomen, while in bigger children, it may be at a higher site on the abdomen. The placements of the ports are not aimed at any specific distance between the ports, as suggested by the company, to be 8 cm, but is eyeballed, both internally and externally, to provide enough mobility, without an external clash of robotic arms. In smaller children, this may restrict the range of movement of the working arms.

On occasions, an additional instrument may be required for assistance. This can be achieved by inserting a laparoscopic port (3–5 mm) usually on the left lateral side of the abdomen, as posteriorly as possible, just below the margin of the ribs, to provide maximum range of movements for the assistant, without clashing with surgeon's right arm, externally. The accessory port helps facilitate tissue retraction, suction, irrigation, removal of the cyst, and application of hemostatic sealants. If required, depending on the cyst location and size, a Nathanson retractor is inserted through a stab incision in the right subcostal region to retract the liver.

5 Procedure Steps

To facilitate improved visualization and dissection, aspiration of the cyst is recommended, where the cyst is large. This is performed transabdominally, under direct vision, with a long, large bore needle (Fig. 2).

For exophytic cysts, the external portion of the cyst is resected first using monopolar scissors (Fig. 3). For the remaining part of the cyst attached to the liver bed, dissection is continued by identifying the plane between the cyst and the liver (Fig. 4). In cases where the cyst is in proximity of major vascular and biliary structures, the dissection is performed with bipolar forceps, while in other cases monopolar scissors are used for the resection (Fig. 5). A wet small swab is

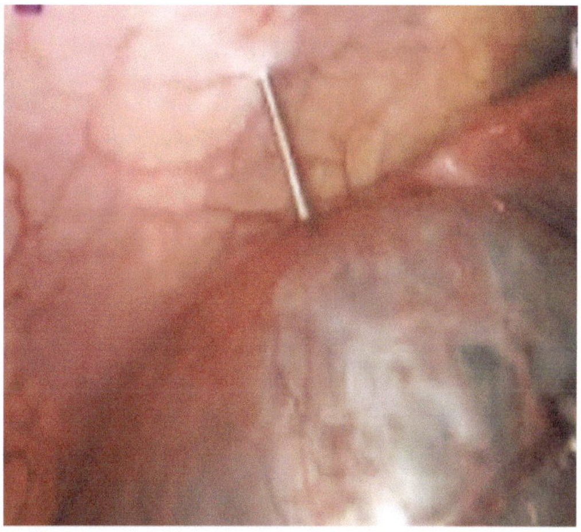

Fig. 2 Percutaneous cyst aspiration

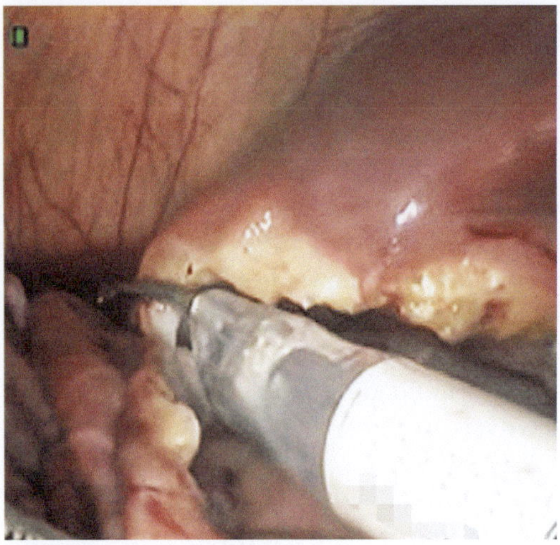

Fig. 3 Excision of the cyst exophytic component using monopolar scissors

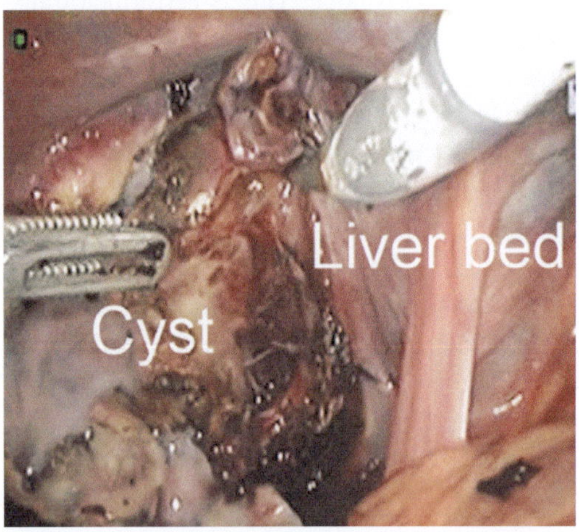

Fig. 4 Dissecting the remaining cyst off the liver bed

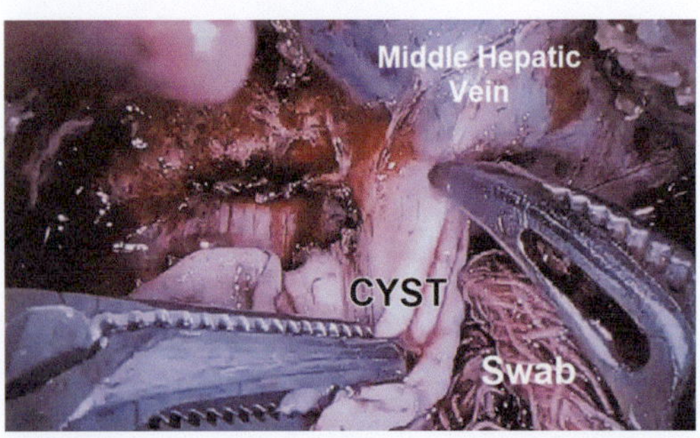

Fig. 5 Cyst dissection off the middle hepatic vein (MHV)

always kept inside to assist dissection or to be used for applying pressure in case of bleeding (Picture 4). In all cases, we ensure complete resection is achieved. Specimen is removed through the umbilical port; an Endo Bag may be used in some cases.

Preoperative evaluation of the association of the cyst with major vascular structures is crucial to plan a safe excision. It is also crucial to find out, preoperatively, if any part of the cyst is visible on the surface of the liver. If the cyst is not visible on the surface of the liver, there can be an option of using a laparoscopic intraoperative USS; however, the width and length of the instrument are fairly large requiring additional port and are quite cumbersome. It is not practical for the laparoscopic ultrasound to be used in small patients. Hence, all efforts should be made to find the exact location of the cyst. It is also feasible for the cyst site to be marked preoperatively under ultrasound guidance, by an interventional radiologist, using a dye. If used, only a very small volume of the dye should be used to avoid the mark spreading.

In author's experience, if the cyst has recently enlarged in size, the parenchyma is very "wet," and diathermy dissection produces large amount of moisture. In such situations, a low-pressure suction, through the accessory port, and increasing the CO_2 insufflation flow rate helps the dissection.

Authors prefer to use a prophylactic hemostatic sealant, predominantly TISSEEL or FLOSEAL® (Baxter International Inc., Deerfield, IL, USA), to cover the liver bed following cyst excision, even if there is no obvious bleeding as this further ensures hemostasis and would reduce postoperative bleeding complications.

Authors do not use a drain. However, it can be used if necessary. Authors would recommend using one of the robotic or retraction port sites. The defect will need to be narrowed around the drainage catheter; otherwise, fluid will leak around the drain.

6 Postoperative Management

Postoperative management involves close monitoring of vital signs, pain control, and assessment for potential complications such as bleeding or infection.

The postoperative pain is generally managed by a morphine loading dose at the end of the procedure and PRN postoperatively, supported by nonsteroidals and paracetamol. It is preferable not to use infusion of patient- or nurse-controlled (PCA or NCA) narcotic analgesia. This involves a frank discussion with the anesthetist.

Depending on the extent of bowel handling, if done at all, the nasogastric tube is typically removed the following morning, along with the urinary catheter unless the patient is on PCA or NCA, which slows the recovery. For smaller cysts and shorter operation duration, the nasogastric tube is removed at the end of the procedure.

A rapid return to a normal diet is encouraged as tolerated. Usually, day 1 or 2 postoperatively patients are ready for discharge.

The typical follow-up includes a visit after 1 year, with USS on arrival. If the USS is clear, the patient is discharged, with no further follow-ups. If there is a suggestion of recurrence, which can happen if the cyst was not removed completely or if there was another unrecognized cyst, which may have been missed on the preoperative scan, the patient should be assessed with MR scan and redo resection arranged, which can be robotic again.

The authors do not believe in reviewing the patients on regular intervals or keep an eye for many years, if there is no recurrence after 1 year.

7 Tips and Tricks

- Preoperative imaging is extremely important to delineate anatomy of the cyst's location and planning port placement.
- Carefully planned patient and port positioning and meticulous dissection along a precise plane between the cyst wall and the liver parenchyma, and/or blood vessels are very important steps to ensure good ergonomics, access to the cyst, and efficient operating.
- Aspiration of the cyst prior to dissection can aid in reducing its size, facilitating better visualization, and reducing operative time.
- For completely intraparenchymal cysts, preoperative ultrasound-guided marking by the radiologist or intraoperative ultrasound scan can be used to determine cyst location.
- In cases where cysts are in the vicinity of biliary or vascular structures, the use of bipolar forceps rather than scissor is recommended to allow finer dissection and to avoid injuring these structures. Special considerations in dissection should be taken when the cyst is near the gallbladder wall.
- The use of hemostatic agents like TISSEEL and FLOSEAL® can mitigate bleeding risks and promote a smoother postoperative recovery.

8 Conclusion

The advantages offered by the robotic approach are multiple [5, 6]. Although studies have demonstrated equivalent outcomes to both laparoscopic and open approaches, there is no doubt that the robotic approach provides improved surgical exposure and dexterity [5, 6].

The robotic approach to resect liver cysts in children offers a minimally invasive alternative with potential benefits in terms of precision, reduced postoperative pain, and faster recovery.

References

1. Rogers TN, Woodley H, Ramsden W, Wyatt JI, Stringer MD. Solitary liver cysts in children: not always so simple. J Pediatr Surg. 2007;42:333–9. https://doi.org/10.1016/j.jpedsurg.2006.10.024.
2. Charlesworth P, Ade-Ajayi N, Davenport M. Natural history and long-term follow-up of antenatally detected liver cysts. J Pediatr Surg. 2007;42:494–9. https://doi.org/10.1016/j.jpedsurg.2006.10.041.
3. Celebi S, Kutluk G, Bestas CB, Kuzdan Ö, Sander S. Current diagnosis and management of simple

hepatic cysts detected prenatally and postnatally. Pediatr Surg Int. 2014;30:599–604. https://doi.org/10.1007/s00383-014-3509-7.
4. Ramanujam TM, Ramesh JC, Goh DW, Wong KT, Ariffin WA, Kumar G, Taib NA. Malignant transformation of mesenchymal hamartoma of the liver: case report and review of the literature. J Pediatr Surg. 1999;34:1684–6. https://doi.org/10.1016/s0022-3468(99)90644-9.
5. Vecchione S, Matcovici M, Bhishma P, Dawrant MJ, Alizai NK. Robotic liver cyst excision: 13 year experience of a paediatric hepatobiliary surgical centre in the UK. J Pediatric Endoscopic Surgery. 2024;6:123–31. https://doi.org/10.1007/s42804-024-00230-2.
6. Yamada S, Koga H, Seo S, Ochi T, Shibuya S, Yazaki Y, Takeda M, Fujiwara N, Lane GJ, Yamataka A. Comparison of robotic assistance and laparoscopy for pediatric choledochal cyst: advantages of robotic assistance. Pediatr Surg Int. 2023;40:1. https://doi.org/10.1007/s00383-023-05588-7.

Robotic Splenectomy

Arnaud Bonnard and Louise Montalva

1 Introduction

In children with sickle cell disease (SCD), the spleen is altered early in life and may also be the site of serious complications such as acute splenic sequestration (ASS) or hypersplenism. When such complications occur, surgical removal of the spleen, or splenectomy, may be necessary but may expose to subsequent infectious or thromboembolic risk. Moreover, the age at which splenectomy may be safely performed remains unclear. The use of laparoscopy for pediatric splenectomy in 1993 by Tulman and Holcomb was one of the major changes in splenic surgery. Despite the challenges in adopting robotic approaches in the pediatric population, it was successfully applied in many pediatric specialties [1, 2]. A recent meta-analysis comparing laparoscopic and robotic splenectomy in pediatrics has reported that complication and conversion rates were similar with both approaches [3].

Laparoscopic splenectomy can be sometimes challenging, especially if the spleen is large, and if the patient has received many red blood cell transfusions, resulting in an increased number of lymph nodes hiding the pedicle. Laparoscopic splenectomy can be performed using two approaches: the anterior approach starting with the dissection of the splenic pedicle and the posterior approach starting with the dissection of the splenic ligament, followed by a posterior dissection of the pedicle once the spleen has fallen in the right hypochondrium. For these two approaches, the patient position is very different, requiring you to prepare and plan your procedure.

2 Patient Positioning and Planning

The position is highly dependent on the way you want to approach the spleen.

- Anterior approach: The patient is in supine position. A pad is placed at the base of the chest to elevate the left hypochondrium. To use hidden incisions as we will describe, the legs are placed in boots, slightly lower than the table to help with the docking and the movements of the robotic arms (Fig. 1).
- Posterior approach: The patient is placed in almost complete right decubitus allowing the spleen to fall down once the posterior ligament has been divided. A tilt during the procedure can be useful to expose the splenic area.

A. Bonnard (✉) · L. Montalva
Department of Pediatric Surgery, Robert Debré Children's University Hospital and UMR1141 Inserm, Paris Cité university, Paris, France
e-mail: arnaud.bonnard@aphp.fr; louise.montalva@aphp.fr

C. Esposito et al. (eds.), *Pediatric Robotic Assisted Surgery*,
https://doi.org/10.1007/978-3-031-99532-3_10

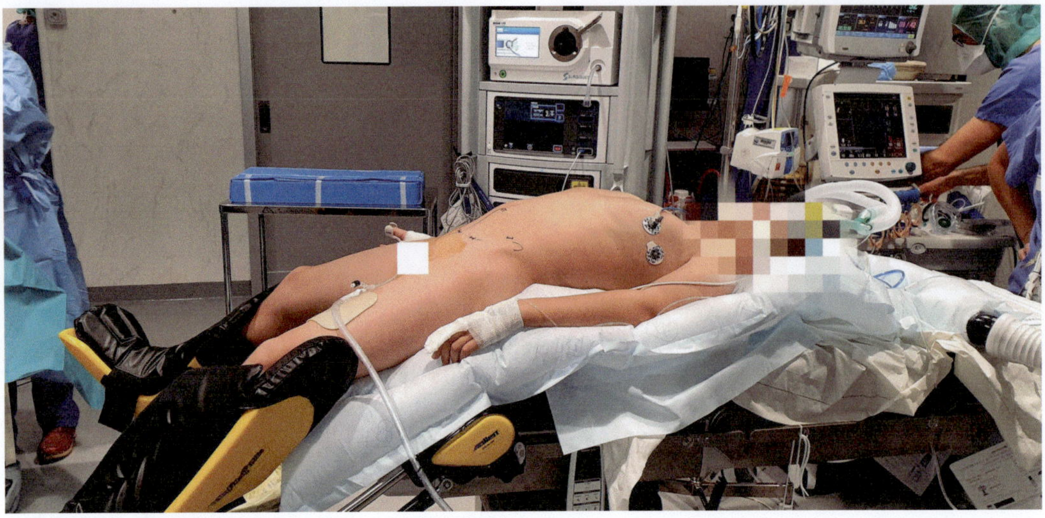

Fig. 1 Patient positioning modified

3 Incision and Port Placement (Fig. 2)

We will describe here the anterior approach, which we believe is safer. There are two possible port placements using a Xi Da Vinci Robot:

1. On an oblique line, separated from 4 to 6 cm, with the following:
   - The camera port in the umbilicus
   - One port in the left iliac fossa
   - Two ports in the right hypochondrium
2. Hidden incision: Ports are placed in the Pfannenstiel line (SLIP placement) [4]
   - Three 8-mm ports in the Pfannenstiel line
   - One 3-mm extra port in the xyphoid area

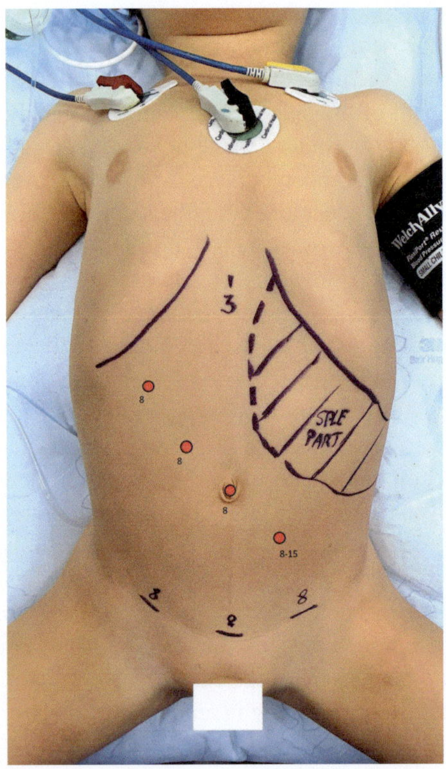

Fig. 2 Port placement

4 Robot Positioning

Using the Xi system, the placement of the robot and the boomer does not matter. It can be placed on the right or on the left side of the patient; robotic settings must be set on superior quadrant. It could be convenient to place an extra monitor for the assistant. Before starting the procedure, conflicts between the robotic arms should be solved and/or anticipated.

5 Procedure Steps

A few landmarks need to be known to gain time during the procedure. First, the spleno-gastric ligament will be the first to be divided to enter the lesser sac. The tail of the pancreas is incarcerated in the splenic hilum with the splenic vein immediately behind or just above. The left colonic angle is sometimes attached to the lower splenic pole, and a careful division of the spleno-colic ligament needs to be performed to avoid a colonic perforation. At last, the spleen can be also tightly attached to the diaphragm, and the risk is to perforate the diaphragm while dividing the posterior ligament.

A first port is inserted through the umbilicus, and insufflation is started at 1.5 l/min for a pressure of 10–12 mmHg. The three 8-mm operative ports are then inserted in the Pfannenstiel line under direct vision respecting a distance between the ports of 4–6 cm. Once these are inserted, the optical is placed in the port situated in the middle of the Pfannenstiel line, the umbilical port is removed, and the umbilicus closed. You can then proceed with the docking and the insertion of the instruments. The assistant on the operative field can insert a bowel grasper through the 3-mm extra port placed under the xiphoid to expose the surgical field by grabbing the stomach.

Different steps need to be followed to decrease the operative time and avoid any intraoperative complications:

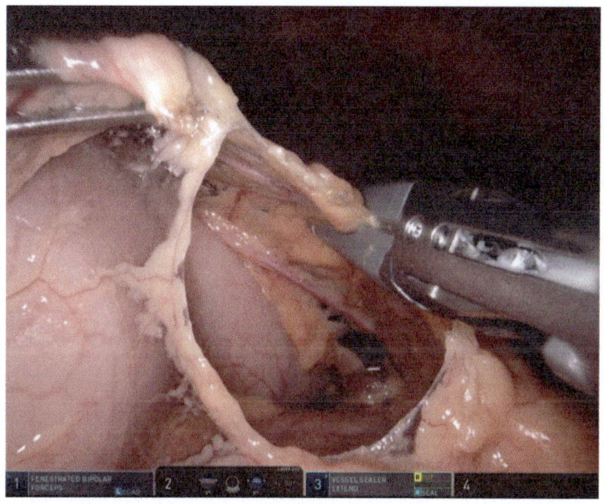

Fig. 3 Opening the lesser sac

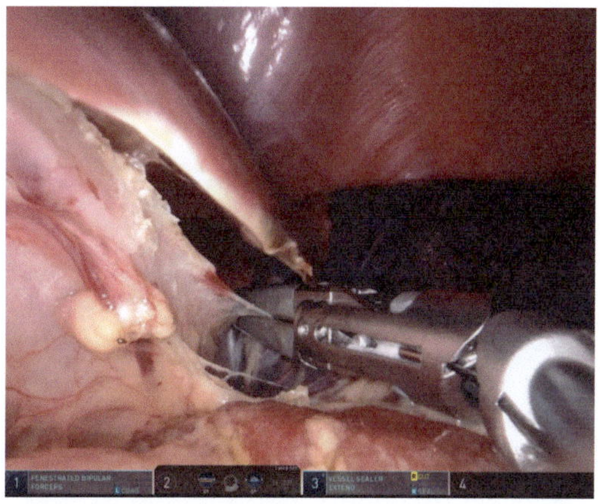

Fig. 4 Dissection of the main artery

1. Division of the gastro-splenic ligament to open the lesser sac (Fig. 3). This is performed using the vessel sealer in the right hand and the fenestrated bipolar forceps in the left hand. The extra 3-mm port holds the stomach to expose the ligament. During this step, the dissection is carried out by dividing the short gastric vessel until the upper pole is separated from the stomach.
2. Dissection of the splenic pedicle (Fig. 4). The main splenic artery is found immediately on the superior edge of the pancreas. Sometimes, many lymph nodes are present, and grasping them will facilitate finding the artery right behind. The dissection is better carried out using the monopolar hook or spatula cautery. To ensure that the main trunk is dissected, and not one of the branches, the dissection should

be carried out close to the hilum. The artery is better controlled using knotting with absorbable stitches.

3. After the artery has been controlled, the vein should not be controlled immediately in order to allow the spleen to wash out through the splenic vein, which will facilitate the specimen fragmentation. During this washout, the division of the spleno-colic ligament should be performed in order to detach the spleen from the colonic angle, followed by the dissection of the pancreatic tail. Special care should be taken in separating the pancreatic tail from the spleen without causing injury to the pancreas. Throughout this dissection, the assistant holds up the lower pole of the spleen using the 3-mm bowel grasper. The vein will then be visualized once the pancreatic tail has been dissected (Fig. 5) and may be controlled using absorbable stitches and knotting or the vessel sealer.
4. Division of the posterior splenic ligament: Using the vessel sealer, division of the ligament will be started from the lower pole and going up following the spleen until the upper pole is reached. It can be tricky, especially if the volume of the spleen is important. Take your time to avoid diaphragmatic injury.
5. The spleen is then placed in an Endocatch (Fig. 6). To do this, you will need to switch the 8-mm port on the left side of the Pfannenstiel line to a 15-mm port to insert the Endocatch. You will lose one robotic arm which can make this step a bit difficult using only one robotic arm and the 3-mm bowel grasper. Once the spleen is in the Endocatch, fragmentation is used to extract the spleen from the abdomen.

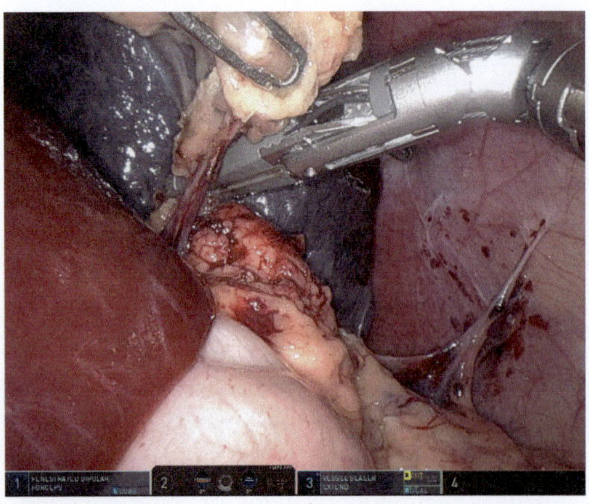

Fig. 5 Splenic vein control

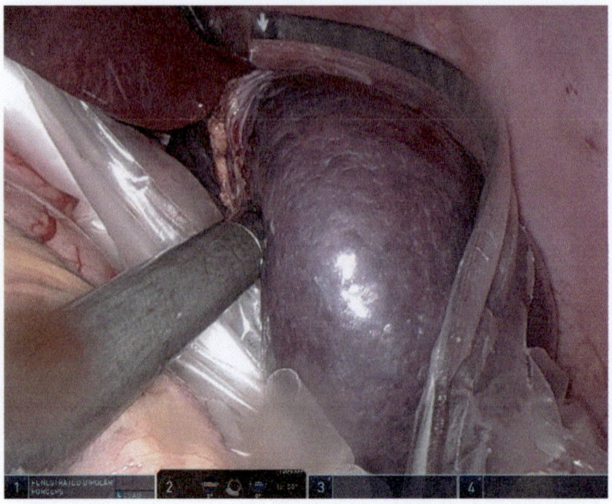

Fig. 6 Endocatch

The alternative is to place the port following the oblique line. Another alternative would be to use a posterior approach with the patient placed in right decubitus. It could be easier to have a connecting operating table to use a tilt without the need to redock the robot.

6 Postoperative Period

The postoperative course depends highly on the indication for splenectomy. In case of sickle cell disease, the risk of complications is more related to the disease itself than the surgery: acute chest syndrome and vaso-occlusive crisis. The main complication related to surgery is bleeding. A pleural effusion may also occur and can require a chest X-ray for assessment. The patient is monitored in intensive care for 24 hours and then discharged in conventional hospitalization for another 24 hours. Feeds can be started 6 hours after surgery. On postoperative day 2, the patient can be discharged from the hospital.

7 Tips and Tricks

It is essential to respect the different steps in order to avoid wasting time or taking any risks. The main pitfall here is to make the dissection too close to the hilum, which will result in the need to control several branches instead of only one artery and one vein. The other pitfall is to injure the pancreatic tail which can be responsible for subphrenic and pleural effusion with a risk of acute chest syndrome in patients with sickle cell disease [5]. This time of dissection needs to be slow and cautious, ensuring the absence of lesion on the pancreatic tail.

8 Discussion and Conclusion

Splenectomy is a procedure that can be performed in children using a robotic approach with a suprapubic placement of the trocars. This approach offers a precise dissection of the pedicle, good ergonomic conditions, and postoperative course similar to the laparoscopic approach. Starting by controlling the main artery first is a safe strategy in order to avoid any intraoperative bleeding. Knotting is the safest way to control the artery and allow the resident and fellows to acquire minimally invasive knotting as a surgical skill.

References

1. O'Brien LP, Hannan E, Antao B, Peirce C. Paediatric robotic surgery: a narrative review. J Robot Surg. 2023;17(4):1171–9.
2. Krebs TF, Schnorr I, Heye P, Häcker FM. Robotically assisted surgery in children-a perspective. Children (Basel). 2022;9(6):839.
3. Ghidini F, Bisoffi S, Gamba P, Fascetti Leon F. Robot-assisted versus laparoscopic approach for splenectomy in children: systematic review and meta-analysis. J Laparoendosc Adv Surg Tech A. 2022;32(11):1203–10.
4. Del Conte F, Montalva L, Ali L, Langeron M, Colas AE, Bonnard A. Scarless laparoscopic incisions in Pfannenstiel (slip): the first 50 cases using an innovative approach in pediatric robotic surgery. J Robot Surg. 2023;17(1):215–21.
5. Bonnard A, Masmoudi M, Boimond B, Capito C, Holvoet L, Skhiri A, El Ghoneimi A. Acute chest syndrome after laparoscopic splenectomy in children with sickle cell disease: operative time dependent? Pediatr Surg Int. 2014;30(11):1117–20.

Robotic-Assisted Proctectomy and Ileal Pouch

Michela Cing Yu Wong, Maria Grazia Faticato, and Girolamo Mattioli

1 Introduction

Restorative proctocolectomy (RPC) with ileal pouch-anal anastomosis (IPAA) is the gold standard surgical treatment for patients with ulcerative colitis (UC) unresponsive to medical therapy and those with familial adenomatous polyposis (FAP) [1–3]. The procedure has three surgical stages, which can be performed over one, two, or three separate operations based on patient conditions: subtotal colectomy, proctectomy and IPAA with ileostomy, and lastly the reversal of the ileostomy. Minimally invasive surgery is usually performed. Robotic-assisted laparoscopic surgery (RALS) has been shown to have great merits in colorectal procedures involving the pelvis. In 2011, Pedraza et al. reported the first initial experience of five consecutive patients who underwent RALS RPC with IPAA, assessing the safety and feasibility of robotic technology for reconstruction surgery in UC [4]. Recently, Romeo et al. revealed that robotic IPAA is a safe and feasible option for the surgical treatment of UC in children [5]. This chapter aims to illustrate the aspects of technique, step by step, surgical indications, success rate, tips and tricks, and complications.

2 Patient Positioning and Planning

The operating theater and robotic Xi Da Vinci technology are set as shown in Fig. 1. The patient is placed in supine position, in slight Trendelenburg to allow the small bowel to fall cephalad, with spread legs, having a contemporary abdomen and perineum exposure. Arms are positioned along the body, and limbs are blocked in order to avoid slipping during the surgery. Then the operative field is prepared from nipples to thighs, including the perineum, and drapes applied. Bladder catheter is positioned in a sterile way after setting the operating field. The surgical plan consists first of unmooring the stoma and constructing the ileal J-pouch, then the robotic phase begins, and the proctectomy is performed; finally, the ileo-anal J-pouch anastomosis is created.

M. C. Y. Wong (✉) · M. G. Faticato · G. Mattioli
IRCCS Gaslini, Genoa, Italy
e-mail: michelawong@gaslini.org; mariagraziafaticato@gaslini.org; girolamomattioli@gaslini.org

C. Esposito et al. (eds.), *Pediatric Robotic Assisted Surgery*,
https://doi.org/10.1007/978-3-031-99532-3_11

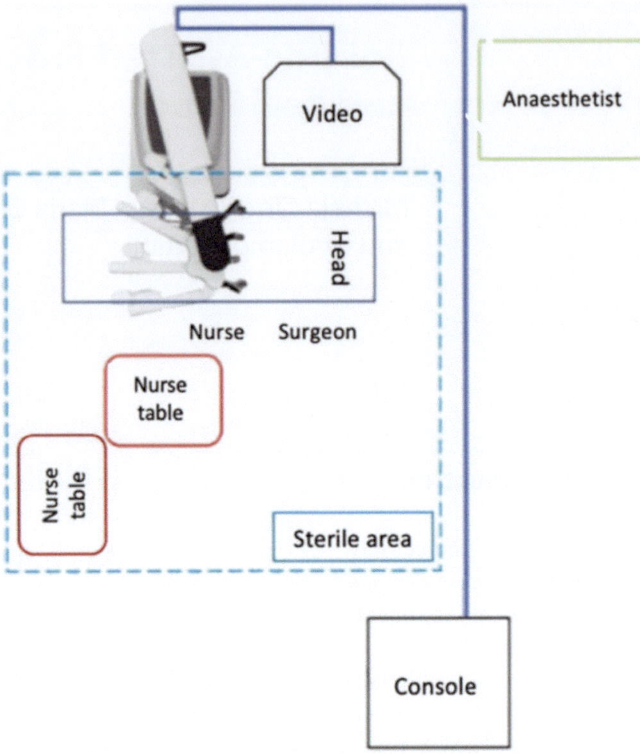

Fig. 1 Operating theatre and robotic Xi Da Vinci disposition

3 Incision and Port Placement

After freeing the ileostomy, the ileal pouch is created and pushed into the abdomen. The camera port should be placed through an incision in the umbilicus. Under direct visualization, other three robotic ports are placed on the umbilical transverse line, and each trocar is placed 4–6 cm apart to prevent robotic arms conflicts. A 12-mm Airseal trocar is usually positioned as extra working port in the ileostomy site (Fig. 2).

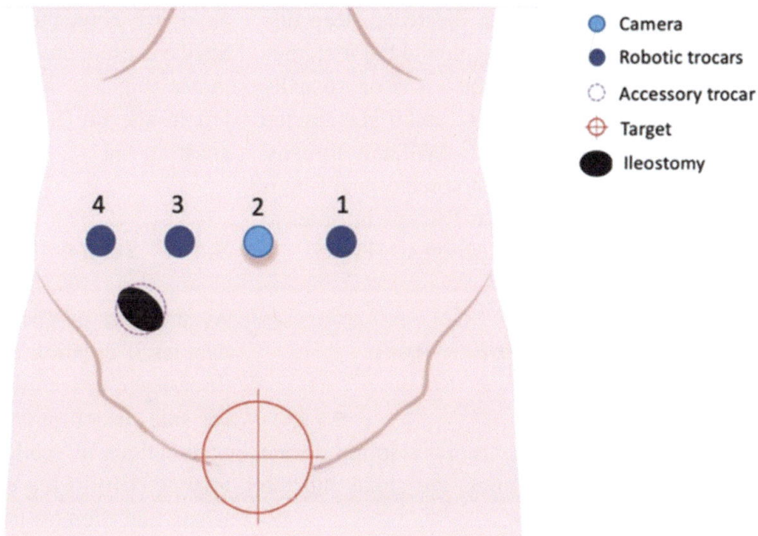

Fig. 2 Port placement

4 Robot Positioning

The robotic DaVinci Xi system is set, and docking is performed. For this procedure, the robot is side-docked, and the cart advances at an almost perpendicular angle to the operative table (Fig. 1). In our experience, we prefer always to use all the four robotics arms, adding a fifth 12-mm trocar for the Airseal system. In the learning curve period, it is always preferable to have a robot specialist inside the operating room to help in case of issues with the docking process.

5 Procedure Steps

5.1 Step 1: Liberation of the Ileostomy and Ileal-Pouch Creation

Ileostomy is freed from the abdominal wall using sharp dissection and electrocautery, and a linear stapler device is used to close the terminal ileum. The ileum is bent on itself, and a small incision is created in the apex of the folded ileum, a linear stapling device is inserted with one arm in each limb, and the J-pouch is created (4–6 cm). The J-pouch is pulled down to the pubis to assess whether it easily reaches the anal plane. The pouch apex should reach the pubis bone, and, if necessary, the surgeon can incise the mesenteric peritoneum in order to earn some centimeters and to reduce the vascular compression. The anvil of the circular stapling device (when mechanical anastomosis will be created) is inserted in the ileal enterotomy, a purse-string suture is fashioned around it, and the pouch is pushed into the abdomen.

5.2 Step 2: Robotic Proctectomy

The rectum is dissected down to the pelvic floor level taking care not to damage adjacent structures such as nerves, vessels, vagina (in females), and bladder neck (in males). The proctectomy usually starts dissecting the presacral space from the posterior side to preserve the hypogastric nerves. It is important to pull the rectal stump with the left hand to provide an appropriate tension to facilitate the dissection, which continues laterally with the mesentery detachment. After adequate dissection bilaterally, the dissection is performed on the anterior plane (Fig. 3). As for the instruments, we usually use a Cadiere forceps in the left hand (arm 1), a monopolar scissor (arm 3), and a Maryland bipolar forceps (arm 4) in the right hand. We prefer to perform the rectal dissection using the monopolar scissor and/or Maryland bipolar forceps. The surgeon assistant measures the distance from the rectal deep dissection to the skin anal margin, and the rectum is transected with monopolar scissor usually 3–4 cm from the skin (Fig. 4), and it is extracted directly from the anus with a Williams forceps. After the rectal transection, the recto-anal side is freed with Maryland bipolar forceps in order to ensure the space for the anastomosis (Fig. 5).

5.3 Step 3: Ileal-Pouch-Anal Anastomosis

The blunt portion of the circular stapling device is inserted through the anus, the spike and the anvil are connected, and the circular stapling device is fired, creating the ileo-anorectal anastomosis (Fig. 6). Sometimes an ileoanal probe is left in site for 2–3 days in order to protect the anastomosis.

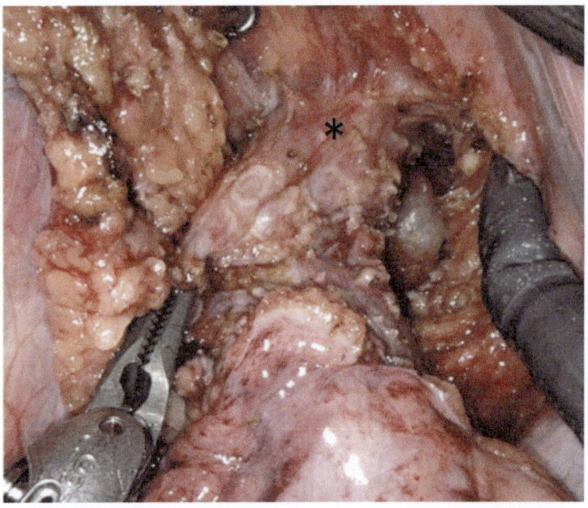

Fig. 3 Rectal dissection. The asterisk indicates the anterior wall of the rectum during dissection

5.4 Step 4: Ileostomy Creation

At the end of the anastomosis, the surgeon decides if creating an ileostomy. Up to date, a three-stage procedure is recommended to allow for safe discontinuation of immunosuppressive medications as well as reduction of inflammatory activity in the rectum and adjacent pelvic tissue and thereby lower perioperative morbidity [6]. The feasibility of IPAA without ileostomy has been demonstrated in selected patients, in the so-called modified two-stage approach [7, 8]. Ileostomy for IPAA seems not to be related to reduction of morbidity, leakage rate and reoperation [9]. The modified two-stage approach has been described also in pediatric population, with comparable complication rates, similar functional outcome, and fewer total hospital days [10, 11].

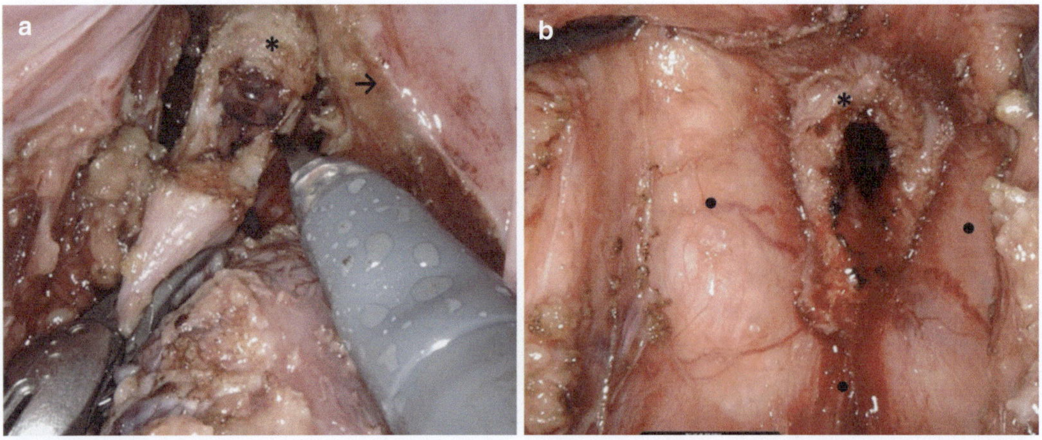

Fig. 4 Rectal transection with monopolar scissors. In (**a** and **b**), the asterisk indicates the rectal stump; in (**a**) the arrow indicates the peritoneal reflection; in (**b**) the rounds indicate the levator ani muscle

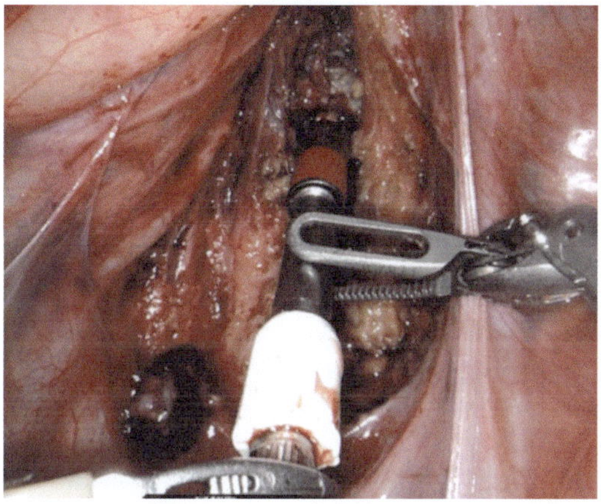

Fig. 5 Positioning of circular stapler

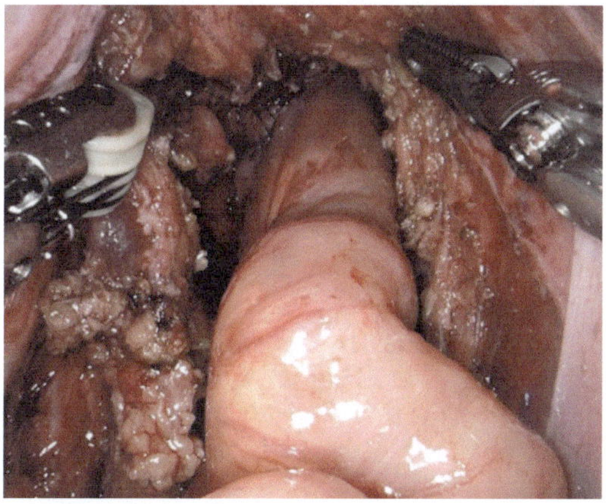

Fig. 6 Ileal J-pouch-rectal anastomosis

6 Postoperative Period

The patient can resume full oral diet when the ileostomy starts to work. If the ileostomy is not created, the full oral diet starts usually in second to third postoperative day. The ileoanal probe is usually left in site for 2–3 days, favoring the exit of liquid ileal stool. Prophylactic antibiotics should be routinely used in the first 24 h and then stopped. Morphine or epidural catheter is usually maintained for 2–3 days. The patient is normally discharged 4–5 days after surgery.

The most feared short-term complication after IPAA is the anastomosis dehiscence which, if not recognized, can lead to a pelvic abscess with high risk for the survival of the pouch. It usually appears with fever, pelvic and/or anal pain, and elevated infection indices. When a dehiscence is suspected, drainage of the collection and ileostomy (if not present) have to be immediately performed. Other short-term complications include stoma site complications (when ileostomy is performed), wound infection, bowel obstruction, and twist of the pouch. Long-term complications include stoma site complications (when ileostomy is performed), bowel obstruction, anastomotic stenosis, pouchitis, cuffitis, pouch-vaginal fistula, and pouch failure. Derderian et al. and Bismar et al. did not observe differences in early and late complication rate between patients who performed three- vs. two-stage approach [10, 11].

A physiatrist expert in pelvic floor rehabilitation usually evaluates the patient before and after surgery, and a pelvic physiotherapy program is usually organized. The gastroenterologist usually recommends some fecal thickener to improve the consistency of the stool, so that it is less liquid.

7 Tips and Tricks

On the basis of our experience, we always place four robotic trocars with a 30° optic and one 12-mm trocar to put the Airseal to facilitate the smoke escape and reduce the risk of fogging the camera by working in a very deep area. It is important to underline that a skilled bedside surgeon is needed in the robotic team.

For the rectal dissection, we suggest to stay very close to the visceral wall in order to reduce the risk of perirectal nerve damage. For the type of cautery, we usually prefer monopolar scissors in the first phase, in the plane of peritoneal reflection, and then we prefer to use Maryland bipolar forceps to reduce the risk of thermal dispersion.

In the posterior rectal wall, the dissection is easier, while in the anterior rectal wall, the surgeon must be cautious especially in girls where the risk of vaginal lesion is present, with subsequent risk of pouch-vaginal fistula.

A circular stapler is usually used to perform the J-pouch-rectal anastomosis. A minimal residual of rectal stump is left (1–2 cm from the dentate line) in order to avoid to damage nerve and subsequent risk of incontinence.

We usually record all robotic procedures. This is helpful to analyze the steps of the operative procedures. It can be used as a didactic tool to show to the trainees the details of the operative technique and eventually the mistakes that may happen.

8 Discussion and Conclusion

Based on our experience, we believe that in patients with UC and FAP, the robotic RPC with IPAA should be the technique of choice if the robotic technology is available. In centers without robotic system, laparoscopy can be adopted. Robotic assistance in small and deep working areas as the pelvis provides the surgeon an excellent ergonomics, a 3-D magnified view, and the ability to perform a fine and deep dissection in a similar or less time compared to laparoscopy. The view of the muscles is clear, and the ability to descend to the plane of the levator ani allows leaving a minimal residual rectal cuff.

A recent systematic review of the literature identified nine studies comparing the robotic with the laparoscopic approach for IPAA in adults. Mean blood loss, return of the bowel movement, mean hospital stay, and conversion to open were found to be significantly lower in the robotic approach as compared to both laparoscopic and conventional open techniques [12]. In our pediatric experience, the three-stage procedure has been the preferred choice for years, with a single senior surgeon with high laparoscopic skills managing this kind of surgery. The possibility to switch from a three- to a two-stage option was a big challenge for the senior surgeon, and the introduction of the robotic system represented the keystone on the decision to switch from the three-stage to the modified-two stage procedure in our center, in selected patients. Regarding the hospital stay, laparoscopy and robotics provide shorter hospital stay compared to open surgery.

References

1. Ng KS, Gonsalves SJ, Sagar PM. Ileal-anal pouches: a review of its history, indications, and complications. World J Gastroenterol. 2019;25(31):4320–42.
2. Mattioli G, Barabino A, Aloi M, Arrigo S, Caldaro T, Carlucci M, Cucchiara S, De Angelis P, Di Leo G, Illiceto MT, Impellizzeri P, Leonelli L, Lisi G, Lombardi G, Martelossi S, Martinelli M, Miele E, Randazzo A, Romano C, Romeo C, Romeo E, Selvaggi F, Valenti S, Dall'Oglio L. Paediatric ulcerative colitis surgery: Italian survey. J Crohns Colitis. 2015;9(7):558–64.
3. Mattioli G, Guida E, Pini-Prato A, Avanzini S, Rossi V, Barabino A, Coran AG, Jasonni V. Technical considerations in children undergoing laparoscopic ileal-J-pouch anorectal anastomosis for ulcerative colitis. Pediatr Surg Int. 2012;28(4):351–6.
4. Pedraza R, Patel CB, Ramos-Valadez DI, Haas EM. Robotic-assisted laparoscopic surgery for restorative proctocolectomy with ileal J pouch-anal anastomosis. Minim Invasive Ther Allied Technol. 2011;20(4):234–9.
5. Romeo C, Di Fabrizio D, Impellizzeri P, Arena S, Dipasquale V, Palo F, Costa S, Pellegrino S, Antonuccio P, Romano C, Mattioli G. Laparoscopic robotic-assisted restorative proctocolectomy and ileal J-pouch-anorectal anastomosis in children. Pediatr Surg Int. 2022;38(1):59–68.
6. Grobler SP, Hosie KB, Keighley MR. Randomized trial of loop ileostomy in restorative proctocolectomy. Br J Surg. 1992;79(9):903–6.
7. Luo WY, Singh S, Cuomo R, Eisenstein S. Modified two-stage restorative proctocolectomy with ileal pouch-anal anastomosis for ulcerative colitis: a systematic review and meta-analysis of observational research. Int J Color Dis. 2020;35(10):1817–30.
8. Marulanda K, Purcell LN, Egberg MD, Mangat SA, McCauley CJ, Chaumont N, Sadiq TS, Hayes-Jordan AA, Phillips MR. Analysis of a modified two-stage approach to Ileal pouch-anal anastomosis without fecal diversion in pediatric patients. Am Surg. 2022;88(1):103–8.
9. Ahmed O, Lefevre JH, Collard MK, Creavin B, Hor T, Debove C, Chafai N, Parc Y. Is ileostomy mandatory for ileal pouch-anal anastomosis? A propen-

sity matched analysis of 388 procedures. Surgery. 2020;168(1):113–8.
10. Bismar N, Knod JL, Patel AS, Schindel DT. Outcomes following two-stage surgical approaches in the treatment of pediatric ulcerative colitis. J Pediatr Surg. 2019;54(8):1601–3.
11. Derderian SC, Phillips R, Acker SN, Bruny J, Partrick DA. Pediatric ulcerative colitis: three- versus two-stage colectomy with ileal pouch-anal anastomosis. Pediatr Surg Int. 2020;36(2):171–7.
12. Khawaja Z, Jamal Z, Zafar N, Adnan N, Haider MI, Zafar A, Siddiqi NN. Role of robotic approach in ileal pouch-anal anastomosis (IPAA): a systematic review of the literature. J Robot Surg. 2022;17:941.

Urology

Robotic-Assisted Surgery in Pediatric Urology: Current Status and Future Directions

Deepansh Dalela and Craig A. Peters

1 Background

Ever since the Food and Drug Administration (FDA) approval of the surgical robot for performing cardiac surgery in 2000, robotic surgery has been one of the most path-breaking developments in the field of surgical sciences. As of April 2023, Intuitive Surgical, the company that makes the da Vinci Surgical System, had installed nearly 7800 da Vinci robots in 69 countries around the world. Urology was one of the first disciplines to adopt robotic surgery, with Menon and colleagues developing the first robotic prostatectomy program in the world in 2001 [1]. With its three-dimensional vision, smooth and tremor-free movements, superior articulation and seven degrees of freedom, and the ability to operate in small spaces, usage and indications for the robot have rapidly expanded in pediatric urology as well. The initial reports for robotic pyeloplasty emerged two decades ago [2]. While upper tract surgeries (such as pyeloplasty and nephrectomy) remain the most common procedures to be done robotically, multiple centers have successfully performed lower urinary tract (ureteral reimplants and ureteroureterostomy) surgeries and are increasingly pushing the envelope with more complex reconstructive procedures (such as robotic augmentation cystoplasties, continent catheterizable channels, and bladder neck reconstruction). While this review does not go into nuances of individual robotic procedures, we focus on the potential advantages of the robotic platform, some of the potential concerns and limitations, and advent of some new tools to augment robotic surgery.

2 Lessons Learned

From the early reports of pediatric robotic pyeloplasty in the mid-2000s, several key elements have been integral to the progression and refinement of robotic pediatric urological surgery, likely shared by all early adopters as the field developed.

2.1 Progressive Capability

As Robert Gross, considered to be the "father" of pediatric surgery in the USA, would say: "If an operation is difficult, you are not doing it prop-

D. Dalela
Department of Urology, Children's Medical Center Dallas, University of Texas Southwestern, Dallas, TX, USA

Division of Pediatric Urology, University of Iowa, Iowa City, IA, USA

C. A. Peters (✉)
Department of Urology, Children's Medical Center Dallas, University of Texas Southwestern, Dallas, TX, USA
e-mail: craig.peters@utsouthwestern.edu

C. Esposito et al. (eds.), *Pediatric Robotic Assisted Surgery*,
https://doi.org/10.1007/978-3-031-99532-3_12

erly," the ideal goal of using the robot in any given surgery would be to make it easier: for the patient, for trainees, and for the performing surgeon. In order to achieve that, it is critical to have *progressive capability*: attaining proficiency in one surgery and applying those skills to a similar surgery. Pyeloplasty was the first pediatric surgery performed in children, based largely on its frequency and prior experience with laparoscopic pyeloplasty. In turn, robotic pyeloplasty facilitated confidence with hemi- and partial nephrectomy, ureteroureterostomy [3], and reoperative pyeloplasty [4]. Similarly, skills learned from ureteral reimplant translate into more complex procedures, such as megaureter repair and continent catheterizable channels [5].

While each procedure can have its own learning curve considerations (Planchamp and colleagues, for instance, noted an inflection point in outcomes after performing 30 robotic pyeloplasties [6]), acquisition of robotic surgery skills is not a linear process. Skill acquisition can transcend subspecialties: Surgeons from Europe reported safely resecting intra-abdominal tumors in 100 pediatric patients robotically (including 24 with unilateral Wilms tumor), within a multi-institutional, guideline-driven framework [7]. This "transition of skills" is obviously predicated on ability to perform the same surgery open and strict adherence to surgical principles.

2.2 Flexibility

Pediatric disease, both congenital and acquired, can be very diverse, necessitating adapting to the child. Beyond the anatomical and pathological variations within the body, performing robotic surgery additionally mandates navigating a tool that was initially designed for adult patients. For instance, Finkelstein et al. [8] noted increasing robotic arm collisions (using the da Vinci Si platform) in infants with distance between both anterior superior iliac spines less than 13 cm or pubo-xiphoid distance less than 15 cm, but no significant association between age, weight, or site of surgery (upper vs. lower tract) and frequency of collisions. Our experience, however, has been quite different, and we were able to avoid collisions with careful attention paid to port placement and patterns of movement. With the introduction of the Xi DaVinci system, and now single-port and da Vinci 5 platforms, improved robotic ergonomics and less stringent port placement requirements have afforded the flexibility to safely perform robotic surgery in the smallest of patients [9].

The pediatric urologist must be comfortable performing multiple different types of procedures to fully realize the advantages of this technology. There is great variation in the anatomy of similar conditions, clinical contexts and presentation, as well as simply patient size. We must be flexible enough to manage a 5 kg infant as well as a 100 kg adolescent.

2.3 Imagination and Innovation

Given the variability of pediatric conditions, anatomy, and size, the pediatric robotic surgeon had to have robust imagination and a spirit of innovation. Building on the elements of progressive capability and flexibility, multiple centers have reported techniques to improve cosmesis (such as hidden incision endoscopic surgery "HIDeS" approach [10] or using the single-port robotic platform through an infraumbilical or retroperitoneal approach [11]), intraoperative ultrasound imaging for more precise identification and excision of masses [12], the use of fluorescent dyes such as indocyanine green (ICG) for delineation of vascular supply [13], or perioperative modifications to allow robotic pyeloplasty and extravesical ureteral reimplants in the outpatient setting [14].

Techniques to place ureteral stents in small infants have been devised [15] as well as novel exposure techniques such as a bladder hitch stitch.

2.4 Teaching the Next Generation

One of the key features of robotic surgery is the relative ease of skill dissemination: The prime example for this has been radical prostatectomy. Once a challenging operation with a rather steep learning curve, whether performed open or laparoscopically, radical prostatectomy has now become the commonest approach for treatment of localized prostate cancer, and >80% of all radical prostatectomies are performed robotically in the USA. Graduating urology residents are increasingly comfortable and facile with the robotic platform, and this affords a ripe opportunity for pediatric urology trainees (fellows and residents) to acquire and improve robotic surgery skills. Indeed, in a Society of Pediatric Urology (SPU) survey, 58% of the respondents reported performing robotic surgery, of which over half received robotic training either during residency or fellowship, and another one-third attended formal robotic learning and simulation courses [16]. Once again taking the example of robotic pyeloplasty as an index procedure for robotic proficiency, it can take fellows up to 37 cases to achieve proficiency at the level of experienced pediatric urologist performing robotic pyeloplasties [17].

3 Challenges with Pediatric Robotic Surgery

Despite the potential benefits of the robotic platform, there are certain limitations hindering its widespread acceptance, especially in the pediatric surgery and urology community. For one, there are certain procedural inefficiencies with the robot: the longer operative time (and room/surgical personnel setup), need for an additional port for dynamic retraction, inefficient suturing (especially in operations involving significant suturing such as bladder augmentation or megaureter tailoring [18]), and lack of miniaturized instruments adapted for use in pediatric population and second, the high costs needed to purchase and maintain a robot and its supplies [19], necessitating a critical volume of robotic cases to offset the financial investment made by the hospital. While "modular" robots may provide a cheaper alternative and allow more flexibility by adapting to the target anatomy, the da Vinci system has essentially monopolized the robot market for the last two decades. Lastly, while the current robotic platform allows overlaying intraoperative ultrasound and fluorescence imaging for better anatomical delineation, "real-time" integration of information (such as CT and MRI scans) to aid in challenging/scarred fields and provide surgical navigation is still limited. On a global scale, most of the intra-abdominal pediatric urology procedures continue to be performed open or laparoscopically. However, we have been able to progressively develop robust pediatric urological robotic surgery programs. At our center, all surgeons have robotic privileges, and one of the faculty is a second-generation trainee of the senior author.

4 What's on the Horizon

4.1 New Robotic Platforms

While the da Vinci ® system remains the most utilized and most studied platform for robotic surgery over the last two decades, there has been a flurry of novel robotic platforms in recent years, most of which have been developed and used outside of the USA. While the Da Vinci system obtained FDA approval for pediatric surgery in 2005 and is the global market leader, no other robotic platform in the USA was commercially available and FDA approved until March 2023, when Senhance Surgical System (Asensus Surgical, Morrisville, NC) was approved for pediatric surgery. There are some important differences between the two: (a) while the Xi Da Vinci system has all arms connected to one patient cart, instruments that are all specific to the Da Vinci system and has no haptic feedback, the Senhance system is a modular platform with surgeon console and three robotic arms each on their own cart (with 3-mm, 5-mm, and 10-mm instruments). The camera system is cross-compatible (5-mm Stryker [Stryker Corp, Kalamazoo, MI] and a 10-mm Conmed [Conmed Corporation, Largo, FL] have been used), and there is the ability to use commercially available trocars. Haptic feedback and eye-tracking camera control are also included. These design features combined may reduce the financial and physical footprint of the robot and potentially allow safer surgery for novice surgeons [20]. However, availability of the Senhance system is likely to be limited in the foreseeable future, given the widespread permeation of the Da Vinci system in US hospitals. Furthermore, as of Nov 2023, the FDA has issued a class I recall of the Senhance system due to malfunctions causing unintended movement of one of the robotic arms (https://www.fda.gov/medical-devices/medical-device-recalls/asensus-surgical-inc-recalls-senhance-surgical-system-due-malfunctions-unintended-movement)

4.2 The Use of Quality Improvement Tools and Objective Metrics

Current models of robotic surgery training largely hinge on dry lab training and/or da Vinci Skills Simulator in preparation for live surgery. Realizing the absence of focused training on tissue handling, manipulation, and force interaction, the Global Evaluative Assessment of Robotic Skills (GEARS) score, a five-domain score incorporating depth perception, bimanual dexterity, efficiency of motion, force sensitivity, and robotic control (each graded from 1 through 5, higher being better), has been extensively studied and correlated with surgical outcomes [21].

Inherent drawbacks of the GEARS scoring system are its time-consuming nature, lack of domain−/procedure-specific metrics, and subjectivity of the grading scale. In order to address these concerns, novel, more objective approaches have been studied. The most common of these are automated performance metrics (APM): for a given surgical step (e.g., performance of urethrovesical anastomosis in a robotic radical prostatectomy), these refer to instrument kinematic data (such as instrument travel time, path length, velocity) and events data (clutch usage, camera movements, third-arm swap, and energy use), captured via the dV Logger ®. Gill and colleagues at the University of Southern California [22] showed that 5 APMs (completion time, ratio of dominant to nondominant arm instrument path length, frequency of camera use, frequency of energy use, and dominant instrument EndoWrist angular frequency) were significantly different between experts (prior experience of median 150 robotic cases) and super-experts (prior experience of median 3000 robotic cases) and correlated with surgical outcomes (higher lymph node yield, less blood loss, fewer 30-day readmissions and nonsignificantly better biochemical recurrence and continence outcomes for super experts vs. experts). Other groups have similarly used kinematics data to create an "operative robotic index" to identify proficiency (based on a predetermined benchmark value) and ability to distinguish between novice and more advanced surgeons [23]. The fundamentals of robotic surgery (FRS) curriculum were developed to evaluate five basic robotic skills (knot tying, continuous suturing, cutting, dissection, and vessel coagulation: skills that are universal to any robotic procedure) and showed its effectiveness in training inexperienced surgical trainees within a randomized controlled trial [24].

While none of these metrics have been explored specifically for pediatric urological surgery, they will arguably be even more important in this arena, as the robotic surgical volume for most pediatric urologists is significantly less (median 0–4 cases/month) than their adult counterparts [16].

4.3 Incorporation of Artificial and Augmented Intelligence

With ever-increasing amounts and complexity of medical data, "augmented" intelligence and artificial intelligence (AI) have the potential to revolutionize the field, and robotic surgery is no exception. Using the APM described earlier, machine learning algorithms can be trained to identify "outliers": Patients likely to have prolonged length of stay [25] or postoperative complications and readmissions. Similarly, multitask convolutional neural networks can rapidly, and perhaps more objectively, assign GEARS scores to individual parts of robotic surgery, with an 86% accuracy in corresponding with manual assignment of scores by experts [26]. Knudsen and colleagues [27] have proposed a theoretical model of how AI can have widespread ramifications in robotic surgery training and skills dissemination. AI algorithms can be iteratively fed data from patient characteristics, intraoperative video footage, instrument movements and the built-in robotic sensors, and clinical outcomes, which could then be used to allow varying degrees of "autonomous" surgery, intraoperative assistance for difficult dissections, real-time intraoperative feedback, and error prediction and allow surgical skills assessment for training and quality improvement purposes (Fig. 1).

While currently available robotic features such as FireFly® mode for visualizing ICG-avid areas [13] or using the TilePro ® for intraoperative ultrasound to better delineate masses prior to resection [12] (Fig. 2) allow the surgeon to make "intelligent" decisions, it is fascinating to envision going a step further: using augmented reality to project anatomical structures from preoperative imaging or warn the surgeon of critical structures hidden imperceptibly beneath native or distorted tissue planes. Indeed, teams at various medical centers (such as Maryland, Stanford, Duke and Johns Hopkins) are working on bringing "augmented reality" into real-time surgery and decision-making [28]. It remains to be seen if, and how, currently available robotic platforms will adapt to this possibility.

Autonomous or semiautonomous robotic surgical systems have been explored to offer the potential for more efficient and reproducible procedures [29–31]. There are numerous challenges

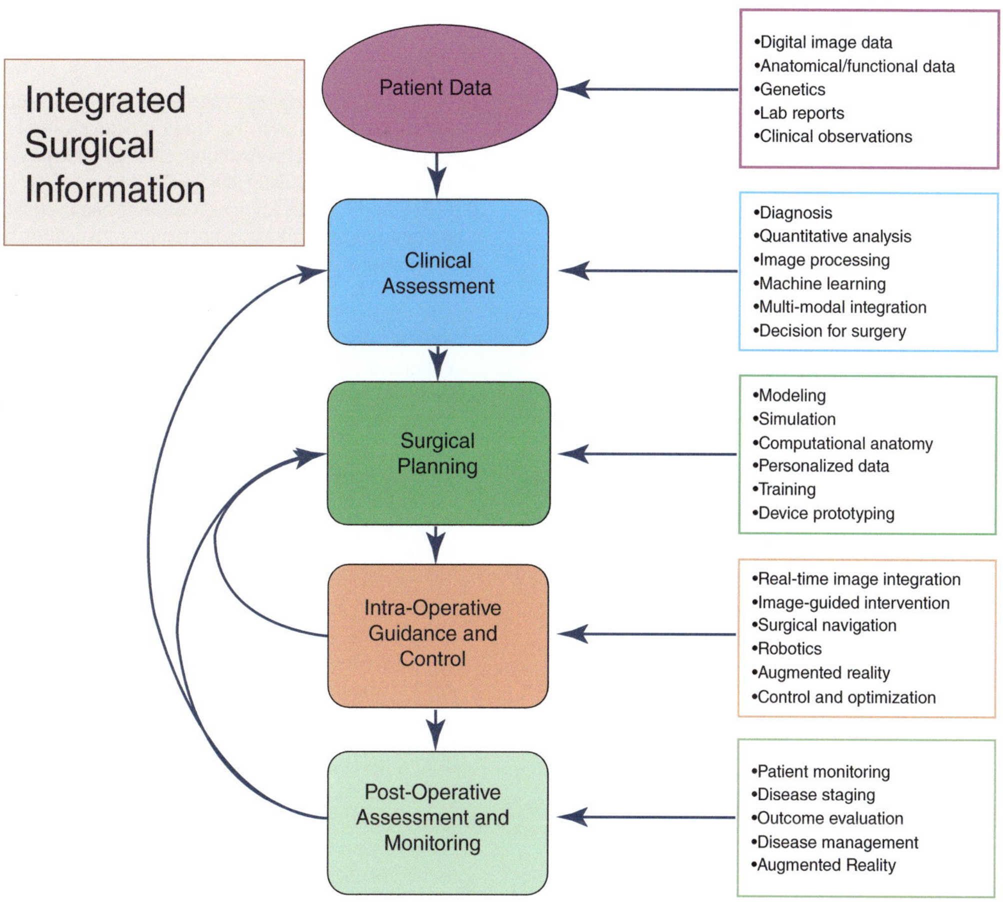

Fig. 1 Figure showing integration of different data points into an artificial intelligence model and its potential uses to refine surgical outcomes based on patient, surgical, and outcomes parameters of relevance. Patient characteristics, surgical performance, and clinical outcomes data are continuously integrated back into the learning system to enhance its potential utility

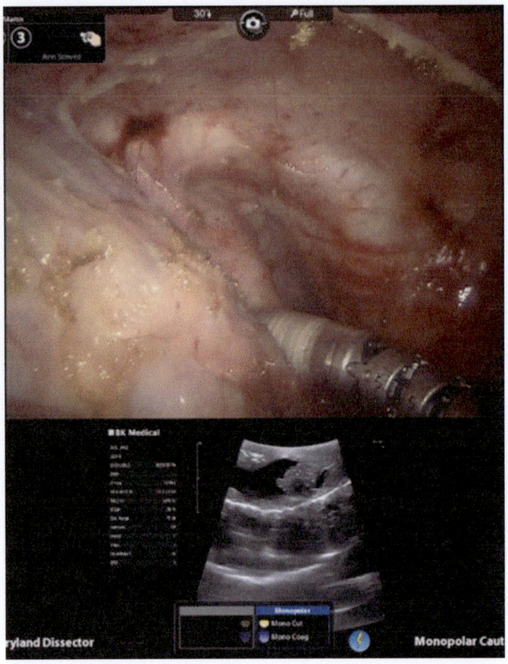

Fig. 2 Partial cystectomy for residual rhabdomyosarcoma post-chemotherapy with intraoperative transvaginal US guidance

to effectively applying this concept to human surgery, but pilot studies and technologies are promising. Currently, the model of supervised autonomy is the most realistic, and it remains to be proven how well this can advance robotic surgical capabilities. The STAR system currently being tested at Johns Hopkins has been used in human surgery, based on the surgeon defining the targets for suturing and monitoring progress [29]. Significant effort has been applied to dealing with issues of real-time computer recognition of deformable tissues and responding appropriately.

References

1. Menon M, Shrivastava A, Tewari A, Sarle R, Hemal A, Peabody JO, et al. Laparoscopic and robot assisted radical prostatectomy: establishment of a structured program and preliminary analysis of outcomes. J Urol. 2002;168(3):945–9.
2. Peters CA. Robotically assisted paediatric pyeloplasty: cutting edge or expensive toy? BJU Int. 2004;94(9):1214–5.
3. Sahadev R, Rodriguez MV, Kawal T, Barashi N, Srinivasan AK, Gundeti M, et al. Upper or lower tract approach for duplex anomalies? A bi-institutional comparative analysis of robot-assisted approaches. J Robot Surg. 2022;16(6):1321–8.
4. Jacobson DL, Shannon R, Johnson EK, Gong EM, Liu DB, Flink CC, et al. Robot-assisted laparoscopic Reoperative repair for failed pyeloplasty in children: an updated series. J Urol. 2019;201(5):1005–11.
5. Nguyen HT, Passerotti CC, Penna FJ, Retik AB, Peters CA. Robotic assisted laparoscopic Mitrofanoff appendicovesicostomy: preliminary experience in a pediatric population. J Urol. 2009;182(4):1528–34.
6. Planchamp T, Bento L, Mouttalib S, Belbahri I, Coustets B, Aissa DA, et al. Robotic pyeloplasty learning curve for a pediatric surgeon without previous laparoscopic pyeloplasty experience. J Robot Surg. 2023;17(6):2955–62.
7. Blanc T, Meignan P, Vinit N, Ballouhey Q, Pio L, Capito C, et al. Robotic surgery in pediatric oncology: lessons learned from the first 100 tumors-a Nationwide experience. Ann Surg Oncol. 2022;29(2):1315–26.
8. Finkelstein JB, Levy AC, Silva MV, Murray L, Delaney C, Casale P. How to decide which infant can have robotic surgery? Just do the math. J Pediatr Urol. 2015;11(4):170.e1–4.
9. Andolfi C, Rodríguez VM, Galansky L, Gundeti MS. Infant robot-assisted laparoscopic pyeloplasty: outcomes at a single institution, and tips for safety and success. Eur Urol. 2021;80(5):621–31.
10. Gargollo PC. Hidden incision endoscopic surgery: description of technique, parental satisfaction and applications. J Urol. 2011;185(4):1425–31.
11. Smith JM, Hernandez AD, DeMarco RT, Bayne CE. Early experience with pediatric single-port robotic pyeloplasty compared to multiport robotic cohorts. J Urol. 2023;210(2):236–8.
12. Antar A, Bachtel HA, Bates JN, Kim SJ, Saleem A, Bhatia V, et al. Robotic partial nephrectomy in the pediatric population: cumulative experience at a large pediatric hospital. J Pediatr Urol. 2022;18(4):538–40.
13. Esposito C, Coppola V, Del Conte F, Cerulo M, Esposito G, Farina A, et al. Near-infrared fluorescence imaging using indocyanine green (ICG): emerging applications in pediatric urology. J Pediatr Urol. 2020;16(5):700–7.
14. Neheman A, Kord E, VanderBrink BA, Minevich EA, Noh PH. Outpatient robotic surgery in pediatric urology: assessment of feasibility and short-term safety. J Urol. 2022;207(4):894–900.
15. Caldwell KM, Coco CT, Ammah CN, Batie SF, Peters CA. A novel technique for ureteral orifice dilatation in the infant. Videourology. 2022;36(1):36.
16. Berrondo C, Makari JH. Current practice in robotic surgery among pediatric urologists: a survey study. J Endourol. 2022;36(6):740–4.
17. Tasian GE, Wiebe DJ, Casale P. Learning curve of robotic assisted pyeloplasty for pediatric urology fellows. J Urol. 2013;190(4 Suppl):1622–6.

18. Herz D, Smith J, McLeod D, Schober M, Preece J, Merguerian P. Robot-assisted laparoscopic management of duplex renal anomaly: comparison of surgical outcomes to traditional pure laparoscopic and open surgery. J Pediatr Urol. 2016;12(1):44.e1–7.
19. Mahida JB, Cooper JN, Herz D, Diefenbach KA, Deans KJ, Minneci PC, et al. Utilization and costs associated with robotic surgery in children. J Surg Res. 2015;199(1):169–76.
20. Puentes MC, Rojnica M, Sims T, Jones R, Bianco FM, Lobe TE. Senhance robotic platform in pediatrics: early US experience. Children (Basel). 2023;10(2)
21. De Groote R, Puliatti S, Amato M, Mazzone E, Larcher A, Farinha R, et al. Discrimination, reliability, sensitivity, and specificity of robotic surgical proficiency assessment with global evaluative assessment of robotic skills and binary scoring metrics: results from a randomized controlled trial. Ann Surg Open. 2023;4(3):e307.
22. Hung AJ, Oh PJ, Chen J, Ghodoussipour S, Lane C, Jarc A, et al. Experts vs super-experts: differences in automated performance metrics and clinical outcomes for robot-assisted radical prostatectomy. BJU Int. 2019;123(5):861–8.
23. Lyman WB, Passeri MJ, Murphy K, Siddiqui IA, Khan AS, Iannitti DA, et al. An objective approach to evaluate novice robotic surgeons using a combination of kinematics and stepwise cumulative sum (CUSUM) analyses. Surg Endosc. 2021;35(6):2765–72.
24. Satava RM, Stefanidis D, Levy JS, Smith R, Martin JR, Monfared S, et al. Proving the effectiveness of the fundamentals of robotic surgery (FRS) skills curriculum: a single-blinded, multispecialty, multi-institutional randomized control trial. Ann Surg. 2020;272(2):384–92.
25. Hung AJ, Chen J, Gill IS. Automated performance metrics and machine learning algorithms to measure surgeon performance and anticipate clinical outcomes in robotic surgery. JAMA Surg. 2018;153(8):770–1.
26. Wang Y, Dai J, Morgan TN, Elsaied M, Garbens A, Qu X, et al. Evaluating robotic-assisted surgery training videos with multi-task convolutional neural networks. J Robot Surg. 2022;16(4):917–25.
27. Knudsen JE, Ghaffar U, Ma R, Hung AJ. Clinical applications of artificial intelligence in robotic surgery. J Robot Surg. 2024;18(1):102.
28. Murthi S, Varshney A. How augmented reality will make surgery safer. Harv Bus Rev. 2018;20
29. Saeidi H, Opfermann JD, Kam M, Wei S, Leonard S, Hsieh MH, et al. Autonomous robotic laparo scopic surgery for intestinal anastomosis. Sci Robot. 2022;7(62):eabj2908.
30. Ge J, Saeidi H, Opfermann JD, Joshi AS, Krieger A. Landmark-guided deformable image registration for supervised autonomous robotic tumor resection. Med Image Comput Comput Assist Interv. 2019;11764:320–8.
31. Shademan A, Decker RS, Opfermann JD, Leonard S, Krieger A, Kim PC. Supervised autonomous robotic soft tissue surgery. Sci Transl Med. 2016;8(337):337ra64.

Robotic-Assisted Laparoscopic Pyeloplasty (RALP)

Ciro Esposito, Mariapina Cerulo, Fulvia Del Conte, Giorgia Esposito, Louise Montalva, Vincenzo Coppola, Francesco Tedesco, Roberta Guglielmini, Francesca Carraturo, Benedetta Cesaro, Marialuisa Pirone, and Maria Escolino

1 Introduction

Ureteropelvic junction obstruction (UPJO), caused, respectively, by fibrosis/stenosis of the proximal ureter or aberrant lower pole vessels, is a common issue in pediatric urology.

UPJO is usually detected by ultrasonography (US) at antenatal screening, whereas sometimes this pathology is discovered later in life, in older children with flank abdominal pain and Dietl's crisis. As for diagnostic point of view, US is the first-line diagnostic exam adopted to measure the anteroposterior diameter (APD) of renal pelvis and grade UPJO according to international guidelines. Then to determine the suitability for surgery, other diagnostic exams as dynamic scintigraphy (e.g., MAG-3) or MRI to identify a crossing vessel are performed [1]. The gold standard procedure for the treatment of UPJO remains the Anderson–Hynes dismembered pyeloplasty, traditionally performed with an open flank approach, which has an overall success rate ranging from 90 to 100% [2]. In 1995, the first reported pediatric laparoscopic pyeloplasty (LP) was performed. Some years later, the technique was confirmed as a safe and effective minimally invasive treatment alternative for UPJO, but LP is a challenging procedure in terms of intracorporeal suturing and knotting, ergonomics, and learning curve [3, 4].

In the last 20 years in pediatric surgery, there was the robotic revolution, and the robotic-assisted laparoscopic pyeloplasty (RALP) has become a natural evolution from the development of open and then laparoscopic procedures to treat UPJO [5–8].

In the recent years, in pediatric patients with more than 3 years of age (or with a body weight of more than 10–15 kgs), RALP has become the most performed robotic procedure in pediatric urology, with reported success rates of 95–100% [9, 10].

This chapter aims to illustrate the aspects of technique, step by step, surgical indications, success rate, tips and tricks, and complications.

C. Esposito (✉) · M. Cerulo · F. Del Conte · V. Coppola · F. Tedesco · R. Guglielmini · F. Carraturo · B. Cesaro · M. Pirone · M. Escolino
Pediatric Surgery and Urology Unit, University of Naples, Federico II Naples, Naples, Italy
e-mail: ciroespo@unina.it; mariapina.cerulo@unina.it; maria.escolino@unina.it

G. Esposito
Internal Medicine Unit, University of Naples, Federico II Naples, Naples, Italy

L. Montalva
Pediatric Surgery Unit, University Hospital of Paris Robert Debré, Paris, France
e-mail: louise.montalva@aphp.fr

C. Esposito et al. (eds.), *Pediatric Robotic Assisted Surgery*,
https://doi.org/10.1007/978-3-031-99532-3_13

2 Patient Positioning and Planning

We always adopt a transperitoneal approach. The patient is placed on the operating table in a supine semilateral position with a rolled up cloth positioned under the patient. A padded buttress, attached to the operating table, is placed, with appropriate padding, on the upper arm and upper thigh of the contralateral side. Straps are also placed over the chest and knees to stop patient roll. A soft head ring can be used to keep the head steady. At this point, a test tilt is completed, where the operating table is tilted, so that the patient is in the mid-lateral position with the affected kidney uppermost. Then the operative field is prepared from nipples to thighs, including the perineum, and drapes applied. Once the area is sterile, a Foley catheter is placed into the bladder to avoid any upper tract dilatation and to ease pelvic mobilization. A sterile drape covers the genitals. Intraoperative analgesia can be achieved with epidural, TAP, or local anesthetic using TOF means, dependent upon local protocol.

3 Incision and Port Placement

The camera port should be placed through an incision in the umbilicus (Fig. 1). The port is placed under direct vision, and insufflation achieved with appropriate flow rate and pressure. We prefer to record all the robotic procedures for didactic purposes. The optic can then be inserted to assess the anatomy. One working port should be placed in the midline of the epigastrium as shown and the other in the iliac fossa of the affected kidney. This should be at a distance (7–8 cm) equal to that of the umbilicus-epigastric ports and offset from the midline by approximately 5–10 degrees, avoiding the inferior epigastric vessels. For this reason, it is important always to perform the abdominal wall transillumination (as in laparoscopy) to avoid damaging the parietal vessels. In addition, we always place a fourth 5-mm trocar for the bedside surgeon. The role of bedside surgeon is essential during robotic procedures to insert and remove needles and sutures, cut sutures, and expose the anatomic structures. Once the ports have been placed, the mid-lateral position can again be adopted in preparation for robot docking.

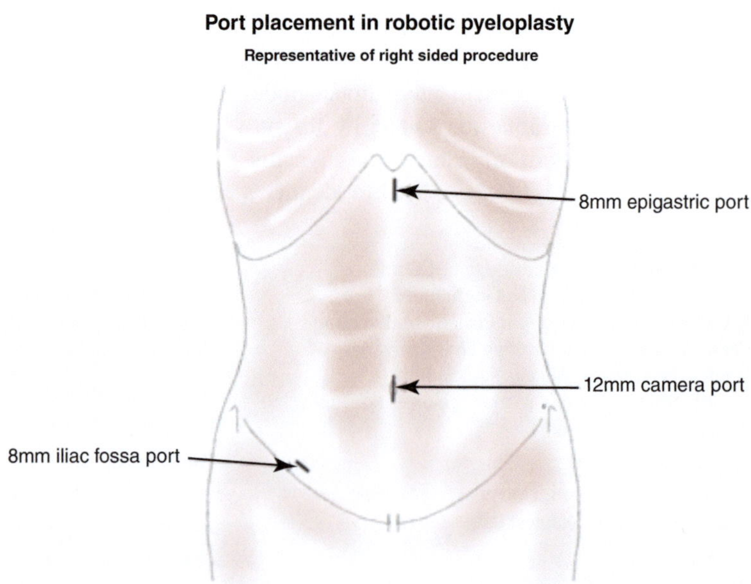

Fig. 1 Port placement for robotic pyeloplasty (RALP)

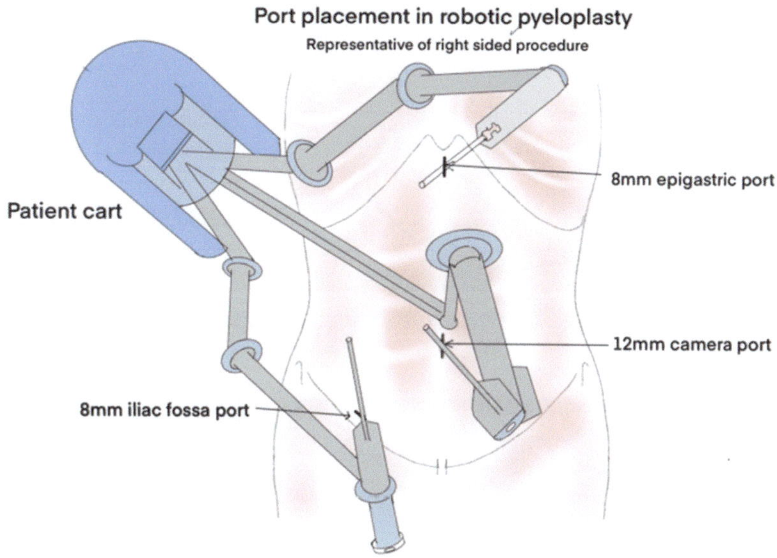

Fig. 2 Robotic positioning for robotic pyeloplasty (RALP)

4 Robot Positioning

For this procedure, the robot is side-docked. The cart advances at an almost perpendicular angle to the operative table, although allowance of a few degrees of angulation toward the head allows for the slightly superior position of the renal pelvis above the transumbilical plane. The arms pass over the semi-laterally lying patient and reflect back to be docked with the ports (Fig. 2). In our experience, we prefer always to use three robotics arms, excluding the fourth robotic arm and to add always a fourth trocar for the bedside surgeon. In the learning curve period, it is always preferable to have a robot specialist inside the operating room to help in case of issues with the docking process [11, 12].

5 Procedure Steps

5.1 Step 1: Decide How to Approach the Pelvis

Also if some teams prefer to approach the kidney to perform RALP through the mesocolon, creating a mesocolic window [13], we always prefer to dissect and mobilize the colon from the lateral abdominal wall. In this way, the colon slides down, and the ureter and the kidney can be easily approached.

As for the instruments, we prefer to perform the dissection using the robotic vessel sealer. In general, we use a fenestrated grasping forceps or Maryland bipolar forceps in the left hand and scissors or needle holder in the right hand. Sometimes you can use ICG fluorescence technology with Firefly system to assess the presence of crossing vessels.

However, more extensive mobilization of the colon either up to hepatic or splenic flexures may be necessary to improve field of view or access to a difficult kidney such as malrotated kidney or in fatty children (Fig. 3) [14].

5.2 Step 2: Establish the Anatomic Situation and the Clinical Problem

Once the UPJO has been identified, by seeing the bulging of the pelvis, the cause of the obstruction should be identified and confirmed. It is important to evaluate the caliber of the ureter and

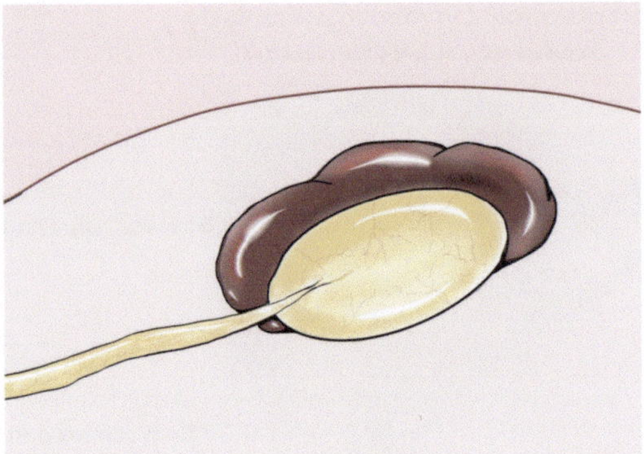

Fig. 3 The first step is to identify the anatomy and how to approach the pelvis

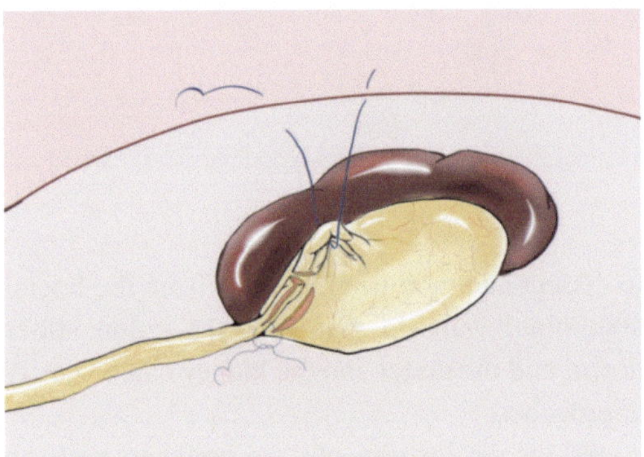

Fig. 4 A stay suture can be positioned in case of malrotade kidney to easy dissection phase. The ureter is spatulated. We prefer to use four or five interrupted sutures to stabilize the ureter to the pelvis

peristaltic effort. Additionally, the presence of an extrinsic obstruction due to aberrant lower pole vessels should be identified. In case of malrotated kidney or intrarenal small pelvis, to help surgeon with mobilization, a transabdominal stay suture (e.g., 4/0 or 5/0 dyed monofilament) using a straight or a long 3/8 circle needle may be placed [14]. The suture is passed superficially through the UPJ, and back outside, to be clipped under tension by the assistant. This trick permits a good visualization of the pelvis, UPJ, and ureter (Fig. 4).

5.3 Step 3: Incise Ureter and Pelvis

Using a scissor, a transverse cut is made in the posteromedial aspect of normal ureter, distally to the obstruction. Lack of urine flow confirms the obstruction. During this step, the role of bedside surgeon with a suction aspiration device is essential. The ureter spatulation should be made in this same plane, for a length of approximately 1–1.5 cm (the length of the scissor head). The length of the spatulation can be longer, if the caliber of the ureter is too small. The most dependent portion of the pelvis should be identified and a longitudinal incision made, reducing the volume of the pelvis as necessary, but taking care not to enter the calyces laterally.

5.4 Step 4: Anastomosis

We prefer to use a standard robotic needle holder, and the bedside surgeon has the role to cut the suture. However, some surgeons prefer to adopt a suture-cut robotic device for the anastomosis. The bedside surgeon passes a 5/0 Monosyn suture via the bedside port using a manual needle holder. The length of the suture should be stipulated beforehand and is determined by personal preference and how many throws are envisaged. The apex of the ureteric spatulation is sutured to the most dependent portion of the open pelvis using the "outside-in, inside-out" method, so the knot lies on the serosal surface. Correct lie of the knots is essential. We first place four or fivde interrupted sutures to stabilize the ureter to the pelvis. Thereafter, a running suture is performed to anastomose the posterior wall of the ureter to the pelvis. The double-J stent is placed, and a second running suture closes the anterior wall of the anastomosis. Finally, the pelvis is closed with some interrupted stitches.

5.5 Step 5: Positioning the JJ Stent in the Ureter

Using an extracorporeal approach, the assistant inserts a device capable of admitting a Ch 3.7 or 4.7 stent. We usually adopt a Ch5 suprapubic catheter cannula. This should be inserted at an angle so the cannula, once the needle is removed, is able to be brought close, and parallel to the ureter, which is still hitched up. Obviously, it is important to measure the approximate distance from pelvis to bladder, so that one knows when the guidewire should have been expected to have passed through the vesicoureteral junction (VUJ) and also not to enable it to pass into the bladder neck. Once the guidewire is deemed to be in the bladder, the stent is passed through and, with the help of a colored pusher, traverses into the bladder. It is mandatory to use a colored pusher to avoid having confusion if the pusher has the same color of the JJ stent. Lift the sterile drape regularly to expose the genitals to see whether the guidewire or stent has emerged from the urethra. Pressure over the bladder should result in a spurt of urine from the proximal stent fenestrations.

5.6 Step 6: End of the Procedure

As already reported in the step 4, after inserting the JJ stent, the anterior wall of anastomosis is closed in a continuous fashion (Fig. 5). Once the first knot of the pelvic closure has been placed, the UPJO can be excised completely and removed through one of the working ports (Fig. 6). The rest of the pelvis is closed with separated sutures. Using a suction aspiration device, any residual urine can be aspirated before undocking the robot. We usually leave a drain tube through the bedside surgeon port for 24 hours postoperatively. Conversely, some authors do not leave any drainage at the end of the procedure.

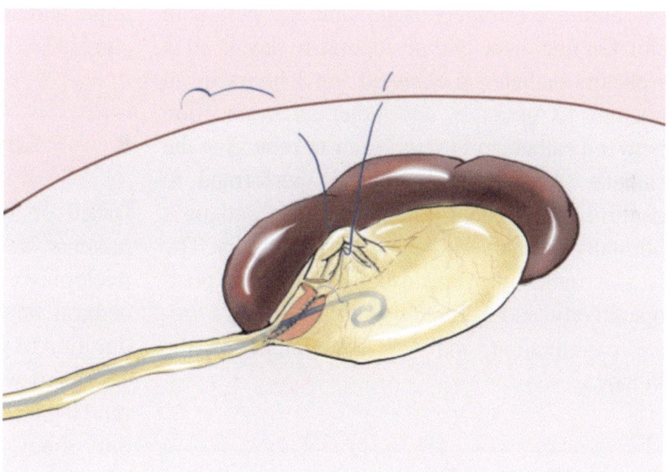

Fig. 5 After completing the running suture on the posterior wall, the JJ stent is positioned

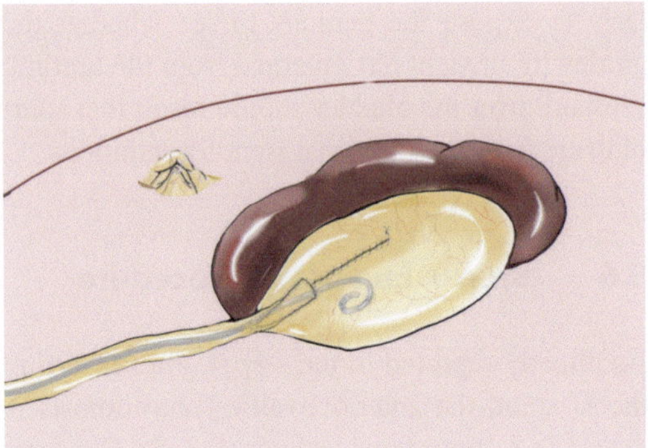

Fig. 6 Final aspect of the pyeloplasty after closing the anteriol wall with another running suture and after closing the upper part of the pelvis

6 Postoperative Period

The patient can resume full oral diet the same day when they feel well enough to do so. The urethral catheter is placed on free drainage overnight, and it is important to inform parents that the urine should be seen red colored. Prophylactic antibiotics should be routinely used, while the stent is in situ. On first or second postoperative day, if all is well, the catheter is clamped for 3 hours in an attempt to untangle any potential connection between catheter and stent, prior to removing the catheter. An ultrasonography is performed to confirm correct stent positioning. The patient is normally discharged 2–3 days after surgery. The stent is removed by cystoscopy 4–8 weeks postoperatively, and follow-up is continued by clinical examination and US assessment of the kidney.

7 Tips and Tricks

On the basis of our experience, we always place use three robotic trocars with a 30° optic and one 5-mm trocar for the bedside surgeon. It is important to underline that a skilled bedside surgeon is needed in the robotic team, with a key role in introducing, removing, cutting the sutures, and in the exposure of the anatomic structures. In RALP, it is preferable to always use a colored suture, easy to identify in contrast with the background. Another important device that you need during RALP is the suction device, because aspiration of urines allows to keep a clear field all the time. If available, Airseal device should be preferentially adopted to remove the fog and keep constant the intra-abdominal pressure while using the suction device. In our mind, JJ stent is mandatory to avoid anastomotic stricture. There are several JJ stents on the market. It is also worth to have available different types of guidewires. In our experience, hydrophilic guidewires work better.

Regarding the learning curve period, it is fundamental to work with a double console system. In this way, the surgeon seated on the second console can perform parts of the procedure. A dedicated nurse staff is crucial to decrease the docking time.

As our surgical unit is a training center for Robotics and Center of Reference for Robotics, we always record all robotic procedures. This is helpful to analyze the steps of the operative procedures. It can be used as a didactic tool to show to the trainees the details of the operative technique and eventually the mistakes that may happen [15].

8 Conclusion

Based on our experience, we believe that in patients weighing less than 15 kgs, the open pyeloplasty is still preferable, as the main procedural benefit in such patients is the shorter duration of general anesthesia. In patients above 15 kgs of weight, we believe that RALP is currently the technique of choice. In centers without robot availability, laparoscopy can be adopted in patients above 10–15 kgs of weight. If the center has the robotic system, laparoscopy has no role [8].

Robotic assistance during pyeloplasty provides the surgeon an excellent ergonomics, a 3-D magnified view, the ability to perform fine and precise sutures in a significantly less time compared to laparoscopy. RALP is also particularly indicated in case of redo pyeloplasty. Analyzing the international literature, there are several papers about comparison of open, laparoscopic, and robotic pyeloplasty, reporting that the three procedures give equal success rates and complications rates [3–6]. Regarding the hospital stay, laparoscopy and robotics provide shorter hospital stay compared to open surgery. By 2009, RALP became the most used modality to treat UPJO in pediatrics and will continue to grow in popularity [7].

References

1. Vemulakonda VM. Ureteropelvic junction obstruction: diagnosis and management. Curr Opin Pediatr. 2021;33(2):227–34.
2. Szavay P, Zundel S. Surgery of uretero-pelvic junction obstruction (UPJO). Semin Pediatr Surg. 2021;30(4):151083.
3. Masieri L, Sforza S, Cini C, Escolino M, Grosso A, Esposito C, Minervini A, Carini M. Minilaparoscopic versus open pyeloplasty in children less than 1 year. J Laparoendosc Adv Surg Tech A. 2019;29(7):970–5.
4. Esposito C, Masieri L, Castagnetti M, Sforza S, Farina A, Cerulo M, Cini C, Del Conte F, Escolino M. Robot-assisted vs laparoscopic pyeloplasty in children with uretero-pelvic junction obstruction (UPJO): technical considerations and results. J Pediatr Urol. 2019;15(6):667.e1–8.
5. Autorino R, Eden C, El-Ghoneimi A, Guazzoni G, Buffi N, Peters CA, et al. Robot-assisted and laparoscopic repair of ureteropelvic junction obstruction: a systematic review and meta-analysis. Eur Urol. 2014;65:430–52.
6. Turner MA, Salahuddin S, Subramaniam R. In: Esposito, Subramaniam, Varlet, Masieri, editors. Robotic pyeloplasty, minimally invasive technique in pediatric urology. Springer Publisher; 2022. p. 83–9.
7. Esposito C, Autorino G, Castagnetti M, Cerulo M, Coppola V, Cardone R, Esposito G, Borgogni R, Escolino M. Robotics and future technical developments in pediatric urology. Semin Pediatr Surg. 2021;30(4):151082.
8. Esposito C, Masieri L, Castagnetti M, Pelizzo G, De Gennaro M, Lisi G, Cobellis G, Gamba P, Di Benedetto V, Escolino M. Current status of pediatric robot-assisted surgery in Italy: epidemiologic National Survey and future directions. J Laparoendosc Adv Surg Tech A. 2023;33(6):610–4.
9. Castagnetti M, Iafrate M, Esposito C, Subramaniam R. Searching for the least invasive management of pelvi-ureteric junction obstruction in children: a critical literature review of comparative outcomes. Front Pediatr. 2020;8:1–6.
10. Esposito C, Cerulo M, Lepore B, Coppola V, D'Auria D, Esposito G, Carulli R, Del Conte F, Escolino M. Robotic-assisted pyeloplasty in children: a systematic review of the literature. J Robot Surg. 2023;17(4):1239–46.
11. Tasian GE, Wiebe DJ, Casale P. Learning curve of robotic assisted pyeloplasty for pediatric urology fellows. J Urol. 2013;190(4 Suppl):1622–6.
12. Ashraf J, Krishnan J, Turner A, Subramaniam R. Robot docking time: cumulative summation analysis of a procedure-independent learning curve in pediatric urology. J Laparoendosc Adv Surg Tech. 2018;28:1139–41.
13. Gupta NP, Mukherjee S, Nayyar R, Hemal AK, Kumar R. Transmesocolic robot-assisted pyeloplasty: single center experience. J Endourol. 2009;23(6):945–8.
14. Esposito C, Masieri L, Blanc T, Musleh L, Ballouhey Q, Fourcade L, Escolino M. Robot-assisted laparoscopic pyeloplasty (RALP) in children with complex pelvi-ureteric junction obstruction (PUJO): results of a multicenter European report. World J Urol. 2021;39(5):1641–7.
15. Coppola V, Autorino G, Cerulo M, Conte FD, Ricci E, Borgogni R, Cardone R, Escolino M, Esposito C. Video-based coaching: an efficient learning and teaching modality for pediatric surgery and pediatric urology training program. J Laparoendosc Adv Surg Tech. 2021;31(5):594–7.

Nephrectomy: Robotic Approach

Lorenzo Masieri

Learning Objectives
- To describe surgical steps of robot-assisted radical nephrectomy (RARN).
- To report the updates about the indications for RARN in pediatric urology.
- To describe tips and tricks of RARN in pediatric urology.
- To show a video of RARN technique.

1 Introduction

Radical nephrectomy (RN) is the surgical recommended approach in several diseases, in both adults and children.

In pediatric age, the indications for RN include benign diseases as follows:

- Multicystic or dysplastic kidneys with or without renal hypertension
- Nonfunctioning kidneys associated with reflux nephropathy
- Nonfunctioning hydronephrotic kidney/infected kidney
- Kidney-mediated hypertension not responding to pharmacological therapy
- Xanthogranulomatous pyelonephritis
- Protein-losing nephropathy (pretransplantation nephrectomy)

And malignant diseases as follows:

- Wilms tumor
- Other renal tumors (renal cells carcinoma, RCC, etc.) [1]

Currently, nephrectomy can be performed by different surgical approaches such as open surgery or mini-invasive surgery.

Open RN can be performed via retroperitoneal access (posterior or lateral) or with an anterolateral transperitoneal approach.

Regards on mini-invasive surgery, laparoscopic transperitoneal nephrectomy is a well-standardized procedure; more recently, robotic approach gained popularity also in pediatric field [2].

This chapter is focused on the operative technique of robot-assisted laparoscopic radical nephrectomy (RALN).

2 Preoperative Assessment

Preoperative examination should focus on clinical evaluation and patient's history. Anatomic characteristics of kidney and urinary tract, renal vessels, and locoregional nodes are defined with

L. Masieri (✉)
Department of Urology, University of Florence, Florence, Italy
e-mail: lorenzo.masieri@unifi.it

C. Esposito et al. (eds.), *Pediatric Robotic Assisted Surgery*,
https://doi.org/10.1007/978-3-031-99532-3_14

radiological investigations: renal ultrasonography (US), abdominal MRI scan, or CT scan. Renal scintigraphy is used to evaluate residual renal function and the contralateral kidney.

It is important to emphasize that every patient is evaluated in a multidisciplinary team with pediatric nephrologists, radiologists, and oncologists in addition to urologists in order to define the appropriate pathway.

Surgical procedure is discussed and described to parents and patients during the outpatient evaluation. A specifically formulated informed consent is administered during the last visit and has to be signed before the procedure. We endorse and apply, before during and after any surgery, the WHO Surgical Safety Checklist. We check using a validated Italian translation of the original version [3].

Children are hospitalized the day before surgery. Regarding on the prompt preoperative management, we usually do not prescribe intestinal preparation, but fasting from food or artificial milk is needed for at least 6 h, from breastfeeding for at least 4 h, from clear liquids for 1 h [4].

Patients receive a general anesthesia with orotracheal intubation, myorelaxation, and transversus abdominis plane (TAP) block.

A Foley catheter is positioned into the bladder using sterile precautions just before surgery and is usually removed in first to second postop day, after complete mobilization of the patient. A nasogastric tube is placed in order to keep empty the stomach during the procedure and removed at the end of the surgery.

All patients receive antibiotic prophylaxis at the induction of anesthesia with broad-spectrum antibiotic (usually third-generation cephalosporin).

3 Patient Positioning

The patient is placed in a semi-lateral decubitus close to the edge of the table, rotating the operative side up by 45° axially with the help of silicone pads underneath (Figs. 1 and 2). This position, allowing the retraction of the colon, provides a clear dissection of the ureter and a safe access to the renal pedicle.

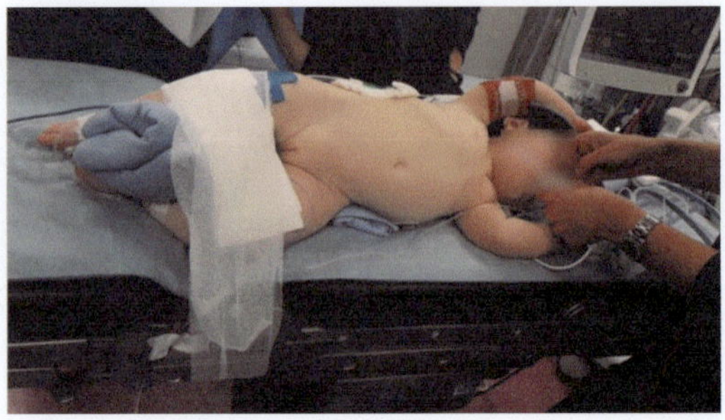

Fig. 1 Left flank position

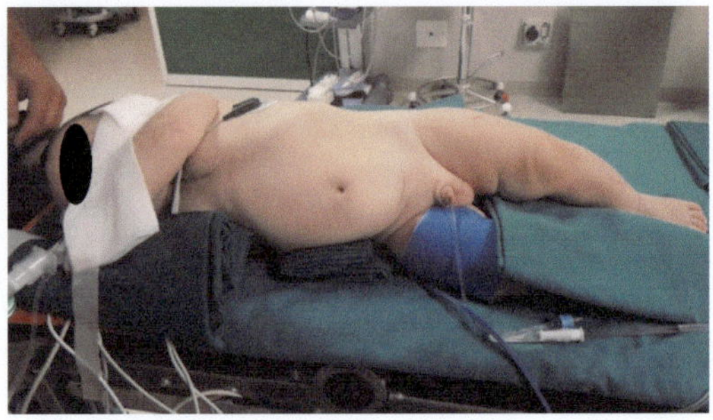

Fig. 2 Right flank position

Both the robotic console DaVinci® Xi and Si (Intuitive Surgery, Sunnyvale, CA) are available in our center. The surgeon sits at the console, and the assistant stands at the operative table facing the monitor for the laparoscopic assistance.

Three-arm configuration is usually set for a simple nephrectomy with a 5-mm port for the assistant. An additional trocar, if needed, can be placed more often on the right side to retract the liver or on the left side to retract the spleen.

4 Trocars and Instruments

We adopt an 8-/10-mm trocar for 30-degree camera and 8 mm-robotic ports, while assistant usually has a 5-mm trocar. We use monopolar curved scissors for the right robotic arm and Maryland fenestrated bipolar forceps for the left robotic arm. A robotic needle driver is rarely adopted for this procedure. The assistant may use laparoscopic Johann atraumatic fenestrated grasping forceps, suction device, clip applier, curved Metzenbaum scissors, endo-clinch or needle holder, Hem-o-lok applier.

The hilar vessel control is usually performed using 5-mm titanium clips, or alternatively, using hemostatic devices such as Hem-o-lok, depending on vessels' size. An endo-bag is needed to remove the kidney, which is usually exteriorized through a mini-Pfannenstiel incision or through the umbilical port depending on the dimension of the kidney.

5 Technique

RARN can be carried out through either a retroperitoneal or transperitoneal approach.

5.1 Transperitoneal Approach

We first place the 8-/10-mm camera trocar infraumbilically: after the induction of pneumoperitoneum (8–10 mmHg), we insert the two 8-mm robotic trocars under vision. Robotic ports are placed on the emiclavear line, one 2 cm under the subcostal arch, and the other 3 cm above the inguinal ligament. The 5-mm assistant port is positioned on the pararectal line and mean 6 cm caudal to the robotic camera port.

The ports are positioned in a sort of "kite-like" appearance and as far apart as possible to reduce collisions (Fig. 3). Moreover, a slight traction of trocars, tenting the abdominal wall, appears to us useful to create some extra room and have adequate working space [5].

The da Vinci Xi or Si robot is then docked.

The colon is detached in correspondence of the Toldt's line and lowered. We then open the Gerota's fascia in order to have access to the kidney. The ureter is identified, isolated, and clipped. The next step is to identify and isolate hilar vessels and possible accessory vessels. In dysplastic kidneys, aberrant arterial supply is common.

After the kidney is completely isolated, hilar vessels are clipped with titanium clip or Hem-o-lock and divided. Another option to manage the vessels is to seal them using sealing device, but we usually prefer the first technique.

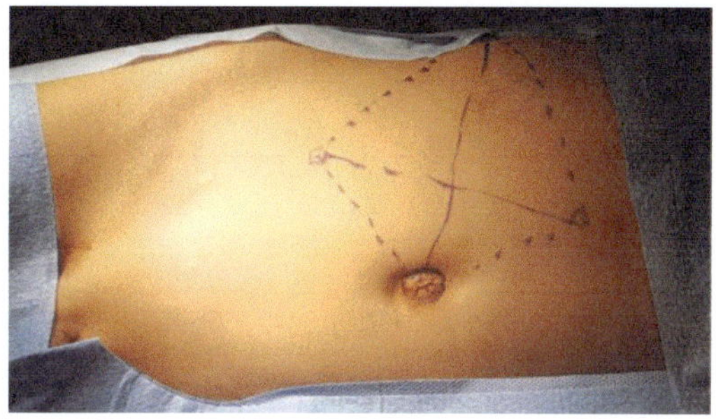

Fig. 3 Kite-like positioning of trocars

Once resected, the kidney is placed into an endo-bag and then removed through a mini-Pfannenstiel incision or through the umbilical port depending on the size. An abdominal drainage can be left to check postoperative leakage, even if usually it is not necessary. Urethral catheter is usually removed in first to second postop day, after complete mobilization of the patient.

5.2 Retroperitoneal Approach

The 11th and 12th ribs, the iliac crest, and the lumbar muscles are identified (Fig. 4).

An incision (1–1.5 cm) at the tip of the 12th rib following the anterior margin of the rib itself is performed, and the posterior fascia is opened to access the retroperitoneum. The retroperitoneal space is created performing a blunt dissection with gauzes, a dissection balloon, or finger-guided maneuvers. These maneuvers have to be extremely delicate to avoid accidental lesions to the peritoneum that would allow the passage of gas in the abdomen, consequently losing the retroperitoneal space. An 8-mm trocar is positioned.

An 8–10 mm trocar for the camera is positioned on the iliac crest along the midaxillary line. An 8-mm robotic trocar is then positioned along the psoas muscle below the 12th rib-vertebra angle.

Once all the trocars are positioned, pneumoperitoneum is induced, and the da Vinci Si® or

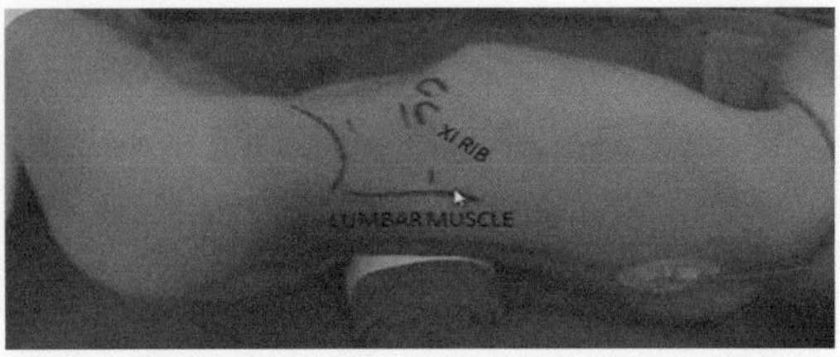

Fig. 4 Landmarks for retroperitoneal approach

Xi® robotic surgical system (Intuitive Surgical, Sunnyvale, CA) is positioned and docked [6].

The kidney is retracted anteriorly, and the dissection proceeds along the psoas muscle until the underlying renal vessels are identified. The renal hilum is then dissected and ligated using suture ligation, clips, and/or robotic Hem-o-lok clips. The resected kidney is placed in an endo-bag and then removed through a mini incision, or through the camera port depending on the size. An abdominal drainage can be left to check postoperative leakage. Urethral catheter is usually removed in first to second postop day, after complete mobilization of the patient.

We use to perform both techniques, despite the transperitoneal approach is the preferred for simple nephrectomy, especially with lymphadenectomy, as it offers a wider working space compared to the retroperitoneal one.

6 Postoperative Care

Patients start liquid intake few hours postoperatively and following oral feeding. Analgesic therapy is prescribed by the anesthesiologist according to our internal pain management protocol: Paracetamol (dosage 15 mg/kg at 6–8-hour interval) and Tramadol (dosage 1 mg/kg at 8 hours interval) are administered in the first 24–48 hours postoperatively.

A short-term antibiotic therapy is performed for 48–72 hours postoperatively.

Patients are usually discharged on second or third postoperative day (POD). An early postoperative outpatient control is scheduled on seventh to tenth POD to evaluate the surgical wound.

The subsequent follow-up depends on the underlying pathology that lead to surgery, being preferred a multidisciplinary follow-up of all patients (urologists, nephrologists, oncologists, radiologists).

7 Results

Even if the robotics learning curve is flatter than the laparoscopic one, it is important to underline that the surgeon needs a significative robotic experience before performing a robot-assisted nephrectomy, especially for vessels management. Due to this, literature is still poor regarding robotic radical nephrectomy in pediatric patients.

In literature, robotic RN are performed especially and almost exclusively for Wilms tumors (small ones) and nonfunctioning atrophic kidneys [7–12].

Regarding on the age of patients, in our center, we perform RARN and robot-assisted urological surgery preferably in children over 1 year of age, due to logistic (DaVinci® Robot is located in another pavilion), anesthesiologist's, and surgeon's comfort.

However, in literature are emerging many articles describing robot-assisted urological procedures even in children younger than 1 year of age [13, 14].

8 Complications and Management

Main complications in a mini-invasive RN are represented by bleeding (immediate for intraoperative vessel damage or in the postoperative period for clips dislodgment) or damage to abdominal structure such as bowel, liver, spleen, or wound infection [1].

Complications could be managed, depending on which occurs, by redo surgery or explorative laparotomic surgery.

In our experience, to date, we have not experienced any intraoperative and postoperative complications, nor particular difficulties in performing the surgical technique described above.

9 Tips and Tricks

Semilateral decubitus, with the operative side up by 45° with pads underneath, is crucial to optimize the surgery: the intestinal loops slide down and allow to have an excellent exposure of the renal lodge. Detaching the colon is important to easily expose the kidney and to isolate the ureter. At the end of the procedure, it is not necessary to reattach the colon to the abdominal wall.

Ports positioned in a sort of "kite-like" appearance, as far apart as possible help to reduce robotic arms collisions. Moreover, a slight traction of trocars, tenting the abdominal wall, appears to us useful to create some extra room and have adequate working space.

An additional trocar may be useful especially when working on the right side to retract the liver, but sometimes it can be needed also on the left side, depending on the spleen's size and on the surgeon's preference.

The use of sealing devices for tissue dissection makes the procedure bloodless, faster, and safer.

Regarding on the management of hilar vessels, despite sealing devices have the FDA approval to seal vessels of 5–7 mm in diameter, we believe that it is safer to ligate separately hilar vessels with endoscopic clips (titanium or Hem-o-lok). If titanium clips are applied on vessels, it is forbidden to use monopolar energy or sealing devices to seal the vessels in order to avoid the risk of clips dislodgement.

10 Discussion

Advanced robotic procedures in pediatric urology field are now promoted by the use of new technologies available such as HD optics, miniaturized instruments, sealing devices, etc., and thanks to the robot-assisted surgical experience of adult urologists.

However, to date, robot-assisted radical nephrectomy is not the gold standard in pediatric patients.

Indications for robotic approach in pediatric renal surgery are limited to clinical cases requiring nephrectomy with associated lymphadenectomy, partial nephrectomy, or heminephrectomy/nephroureterectomy in duplication of the renal system, also, anatomical situations for which the robotic approach is more comfortable for the surgeon.

This procedure has not gained wider acceptance compared to the laparoscopic or the open approach, due to the high costs related to robotic surgery and because it is mostly indicated for reconstructive procedures. Da Vinci robotic system, moreover, is not available in all centers, and only few pediatric surgeons and urologists have experience with robotic surgery.

The advantages of the robotic approach are the 3D vision with a complete and clear view of all the urinary tract and the robotic arms seven degrees of freedom allowing to more fine movements especially in more challenging passages as the exposure of renal hilar vessels.

Robotic nephrectomy is, anyway, a challenging procedure that can be performed only in pediatric centers with a very strong experience in minimally invasive surgery.

Take-Home Points

- Literature is still poor regarding robotic radical nephrectomy in pediatric patients.
- The learning curve for robotic nephrectomy is flatter than for the laparoscopic technique.
- The surgeon needs a significative robotic experience before performing a robot-assisted nephrectomy, especially for vessels management.
- The advantages of the robotic approach are the 3D vision with a complete and clear view of all the urinary tract and the robotic arms seven degrees of freedom allowing to more fine movements especially in more challenging passages as the exposure of renal hilar vessels.
- The correct positioning of the patient and the robotic ports is already half the work.

References

1. Chiarenza SF, Bleve C, Esposito C, Escolino M, Beretta F, Cheli M, Di Benedetto V, Scuderi MG, Casadio G, Marzaro M, Fascetti LF, Bagolan P, Vella C, Conighi ML, Codric D, Nappo S, Caione P. Guidelines of the Italian Society of Videosurgery in infancy for the minimally invasive treatment of pediatric nephrectomy and partial nephrectomy. Pediatr Med Chir. 2019;41 https://doi.org/10.4081/pmc.2019.231.
2. Cerulo M, Escolino M, Turrà F, et al. Benefits of retroperitoneoscopic surgery in pediatric urology. In: Weiss D, editor. . Pediatric Urology; 2018.
3. WHO. www.who.int/patientsafety/topics/safe-surgery/checklist/en/. [Online].
4. Anderssona H, Schmitzb A, Frykholm P, et al. Preoperative fasting guidelines in pediatric anesthesia: are we ready for a change? Curr Opin Anaesthesiol. 2018;3:342–8.
5. Masieri L, Sforza S, Grosso AA, et al. Does the body weight influence the outcome in children treated with robotic pyeloplasty? J Pediatr Urol. 2020;16:109.e1.
6. Rogers C, Laungani R, Krane LS, et al. Robotic nephrectomy for the treatment of benign and malignant disease. BJU Int. 2008;
7. Briony K. Vardaa, Patricia Choa, Andrew A. Wagnerb, and Richa. B. K. Vardaa, P.Choa, A. A. Wagnerb et al. 2018. Collaborating with our adult colleagues: a case series of robotic surgery for suspicious and cancerous lesions in children and young adults performed in a free-standing children's hospital. J Pediatr Urol.
8. Andolfi C, Kumar R, Boysen WR, et al. Current status of robotic surgery in pediatric urology. J Laparoendoscopic Adv Surgical Techniques. 2019;
9. Kibar Y, Yalçın S, Kaya E, et al. Our experiences with robot-assisted laparoscopic surgery in pediatric patients: the first case series from Turkey. Turk J Urol. 2017;
10. Cost NG, Liss ZJ, Bean CM, et al. Prechemotherapy robotic-assisted laparoscopic radical nephrectomy for an adolescent with Wilms tumor, vol. 37. J Pediatr Hematol Oncol; 2015.
11. Waterloos M, Ploumidis A, Pappas A, et al. Robot-assisted resection of ectopic kidney in children: anatomical illustration. J Pediatr Urol. 2019;
12. Blanc T, Pio L, Clermidi P, et al. Robotic-assisted laparoscopic management of renal tumors in children: preliminary results. Pediatric Blood Cancer. 2019;
13. Avery DI, Herbst KW, Lendvay TS, et al. Robot-assisted laparoscopic pyeloplasty: multi-institutional experience in infants. J Pediatr Urol. 2015;11:139.e1.
14. Finkelstein JB, Levy AC, Silva MV, et al. How to decide which infant can have robotic surgery? Just do the math. J Pediatr Urol. 2015;11:170.e1.

Robotic-Assisted Partial Nephrectomy

Marco Castagnetti and Alfredo Berrettini

1 Introduction

Partial nephrectomy is generally performed in the scenario of a nonfunctioning moiety in a complex duplex system [1]. The partial nephrectomy can concern either the upper or the lower pole. An upper pole partial nephrectomy is generally performed for either a duplex system ureterocele or an ectopic upper pole ureter [1]. The major indication for a lower pole partial nephrectomy is a symptomatic primary vesicoureteral reflux (VUR) in a dysplastic, poorly functioning moiety [1]. Partial nephrectomy can also be performed for oncological indications in order to perform a nephron-sparing surgery [2], but this topic is beyond the scope of present chapter.

As far as preoperative work-up is concerned [1], it generally starts with an ultrasound scan to define the anatomy of the dilated reno-ureteral units and grade the severity of the dilatation. A voiding cystourethrography is performed to assess the VUR status. Moiety function is, finally, assessed by a renal nuclear scan. In our practice, a dynamic scan is the scan of choice for this purpose. Occasionally, when the standard workup mentioned above is not conclusive, additional imaging can be required such as a Uro-MRI or a preoperative retrograde pyelography.

Partial nephrectomy is a variable option in the scenario of a complicated renal duplication. Under these circumstances, moiety function is often negligible, and an upper tract approach avoids any bladder manipulation and the associated risks. Partial nephrectomy can be performed open, by conventional laparoscopy, also via a retroperitoneal approach, or by robotic-assisted surgery. As for many other minimally invasive procedures, the robot assistance makes the procedure easier. However, it must be appreciated that many strategies alternative to partial nephrectomy do exist to treat complicated renal duplication anomalies including endoscopic procedures, primary lower urinary tract reconstruction, ureteroureterostomy, and ureteral clipping [3–6].

Present chapter aims to illustrate the aspects of technique, step by step, surgical indications, success rate, tips and tricks, and complications.

2 Patient Positioning and Planning

The surgery is performed under general anesthesia. Analgesia can be achieved with epidural, TAP, or local anesthetic using TOF means.

M. Castagnetti (✉)
University of Roma Tor Vergata, Rome, Italy

Pediatric Urology Unit, Bambino Gesù Children Hospital, Rome, Italy
e-mail: marco.castagnetti@opbg.net

A. Berrettini
Department of Pediatric Urology, Fondazione IRCCS Ca' Granda Ospedale Maggiore Policlinico, Milan, Italy

C. Esposito et al. (eds.), *Pediatric Robotic Assisted Surgery*,
https://doi.org/10.1007/978-3-031-99532-3_15

2.1 Preoperative Endoscopy

The procedure generally starts with an endoscopy. With the patient in frog leg position, an endoscope of suitable size (a size between 8 and 9.5 Fr is adequate in most of the cases) is introduced into the urethra and the anatomy identified. In case of an ectopic ureter, the ectopic orifice is not always visible, and the dilated ureter imprinting the posterior wall of the bladder can be seen during cystoscopy and is called pseudo-ureterocele. In every case, we prefer to leave a stent indwelling into the ureter of the moiety that is going to be preserved, namely, the lower pole ureter in case of upper pole partial nephrectomy, and the upper pole ureter in case of a lower pole partial nephrectomy. This is normally within the bladder. The favorite tube is a 3–5 Fr ureteral catheter. Usually, the largest fitting into the ureter is selected. This tube is anchored to a transurethral Foley catheter, and the two are kept sterile during subsequent patient repositioning and preparation for the robotic surgery in order to make them accessible for the assistant during the procedure.

2.2 Positioning

We always prefer a transperitoneal approach. As for almost any robotic renal surgery in our practice, the patient is placed on the operating table in a supine semilateral decubitus with the flank corresponding to the kidney to be operated upward. A padded buttress, attached to the operating table, is placed. Straps are also placed over the chest and knees to prevent patient displacement during the procedure and after any table tilt. A soft head ring can be used to keep the head steady (Fig. 1).

The operative field is finally prepared from nipples to thighs.

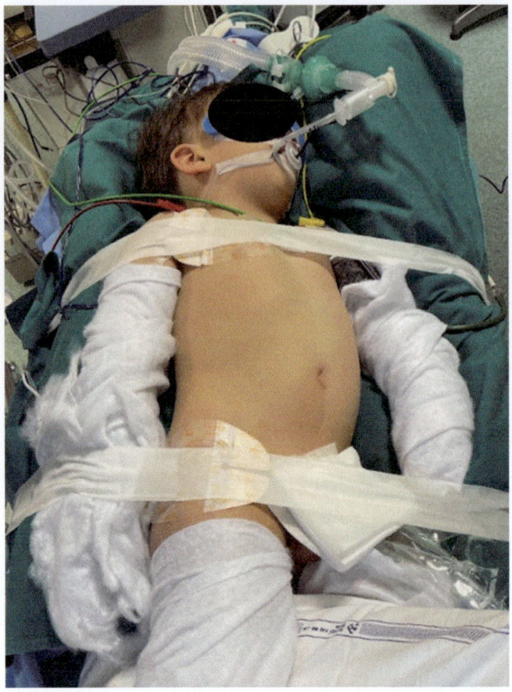

Fig. 1 Patient positioning

3 Incision and Port Placement

A partial nephrectomy requires four ports. The camera port is placed using an open approach through a periumbilical incision on the side of the kidney to be operated (Fig. 2). Insufflation is started at appropriate flow rate and pressure, usually 8–10 cm of water and a flow of 6–10 liters per minute. The optic is inserted to assess the anatomy and rule out any injuries to intra-abdominal organs. Two operating ports are placed on the midline, one in the epigastrium and the other in the hypogastrium, each at around 8 cm from the camera port. This generally corresponds to a fist. As in laparoscopy, transillumination can help avoiding injuring parietal vessels during port placement. The fourth port is to be used

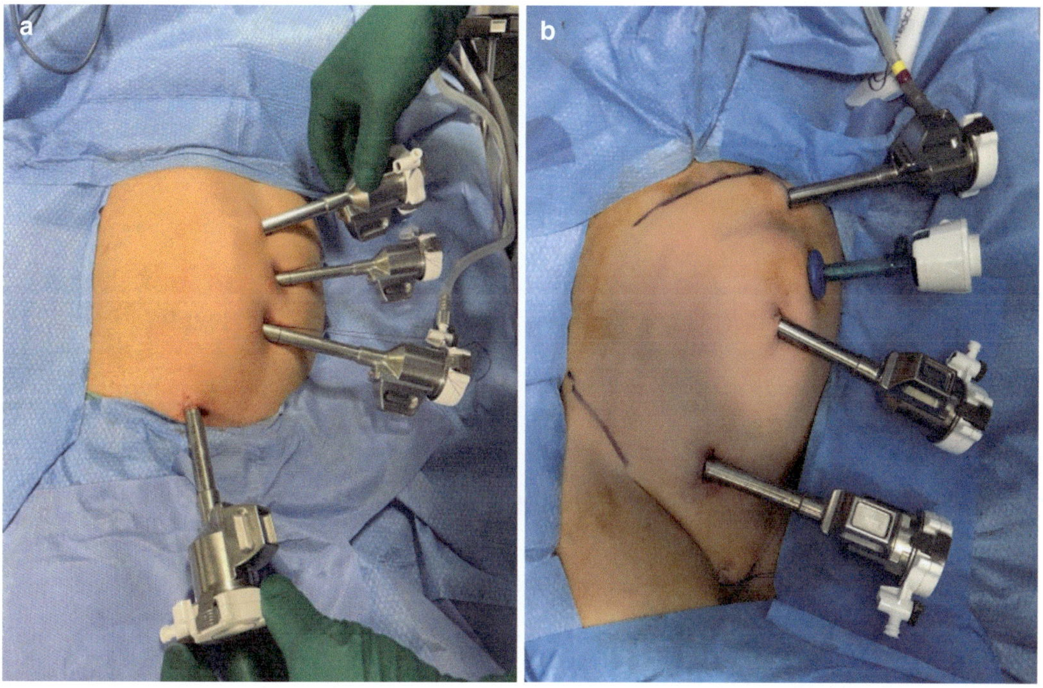

Fig. 2 Port placement. (**a**) Using all four robotic trocars. (**b**) Using one 5-mm laparoscopic trocar as fourth port

either for the fourth robotic arm or by the bedside surgeon. It is placed in the epigastrium as far as possible from the operating port as space permits. If the airSeal system is available, this could be a viable alternative to the fourth robotic port as it allows introducing any device into the abdomen without losing intra-abdominal pressure. This fourth port is essential to expose the anatomic structures, such as lifting the liver up during right upper pole partial nephrectomy, or for flashing and suctioning in the operating field in case of bleeding. It is also used to introduce clips and hemolocks inside the abdomen.

Once the four ports have been placed, robot docking is performed.

4 Robot Positioning

The robot is side-docked. The cart advances at a perpendicular angle to the operative table from the back of the patient. If the fourth robotic arm is excluded, one of the two central arms are docked with the camera port and the two next to is to operating ports. Whether to exclude the first or fourth arm depends mainly on practical reasons.

5 Procedure Steps

5.1 Access to the Kidney and Ureters

The colon is mobilized from the lateral abdominal wall to expose the kidney and the ureter. For this dissection, we generally use a fenestrated grasping forceps in the left hand, and a Maryland bipolar forceps or scissors electrified with monopolar energy in the right hand. We recommend to extend the colic mobilization from the hepatic or splenic flexures down to the pelvis in order to have a good control of the anatomy.

The following step is to identify the ureters, the lower and the upper pole one. The one of the diseased moieties is generally dilated, and the one of the healthy moiety is generally nondilated. A notable exception to this principle is a duplex system ureterocele with a lower pole-associated obstruction or reflux. Under these circumstances, both ureters can be dilated. The presence of the ureteral catheter can help in identifying preserving the ureter corresponding to the healthy moiety. ICG fluorescence technology with Firefly system performed injecting the dye via the ureteral catheter can help in the process [7, 8].

Once the ureter of the moiety to be removed is identified and dissected off the other ureter, it can be ligated and sectioned and be used as a traction during the rest of the procedure.

5.2 The Partial Nephrectomy

The kidney is then mobilized. In case of an upper pole partial nephrectomy, it is important to fully mobilize the upper pole in order to get access to the pedicle, and the upper pole ureter is passed behind the vessels upward. The urinary tract is used to identify the potential line of demarcation of the two moieties. The ileum is dissected, and selective ligature of the vessels, possibly the artery first, is performed. Several instruments can be used for closure of the vessels. Our preferred options are clips or hemlocks. Either instrument is introduced by the assistant via the fourth port. This should be followed by a discoloration of the ischemic moiety. Intravenous injection of ICG can further enhance the difference between the ischemic and the healthy moiety [7, 8]. This confirms meantime a good vascular supply to the preserved moiety.

The parenchyma is cut along the line of demarcation using carefully a sealing device such as a Maryland bipolar forceps. The margins of the healthy moiety are carefully inspected to detect any leakage of urine from any calyx that could have been opened inadvertently. A new injection of ICG via the ureteral catheter inserted preoperatively can further confirm the absence of injury to the urinary tract of the preserved moiety [7, 8].

A sealant glue and sponge are applied on the section margin, and two or three stiches can be applied to approximate the renal capsule.

A drainage is then passed through the lowest trocar into the abdominal cavity and placed in the paracolic gutter next to the kidney close to the branch of section. The colon is relocated into its initial location to cover the kidney. It is generally not necessary to re-suture the colic gutter in our experience.

5.3 Specimen Retrieval

Extraction of the removed pole form the abdomen is generally easier using a standard laparoscopic technique. Therefore, the robot is undocked, the camera is moved to the epigastric port, and an endo-bag is introduced via the umbilical port. The removed pole is caught into the endo-bag, and an additional trocar introduced can help in this maneuver. Depending on the size, it may be necessary to slightly enlarge the umbilical incision. Personally, we do not like and perform morcellation of the specimen.

6 Postoperative Period

The patient can resume full oral diet the same day when they feel well enough to do so.

The ureteral and urethral catheters placed on free drainage for 48–72 h to garantee urinary drainage. The surgical drainage can be removed after 48 h, and the transurethral catheter and the ureteral catheter anchored to it be removed at the same time. The patient is normally discharged 2–3 days after surgery.

Follow-up is continued by clinical examination and US assessment of the kidney 3–4 months after surgery. This confirms the absence of perirenal collections. By the way, asymptomatic cysts have been describer after partial nephrectomy and do not need drainage as long as they do not tend to increase in size and remain asymptomatic. The US should also include a Doppler to document viability of the moiety left in place. In case of doubt, a renal nuclear scan can be performed postoperatively to assess the function of the residual moiety. Reportedly, a damage to the vasculature of the preserved pole results in function loss in about 6% of cases, and infants are at increased risk.

7 Tips and Tricks

Irrespective of the approach, the robotic partial nephrectomy follows the same steps of the open procedure. A major innovation is the use of ICG fluorescence technology with Firefly system [7, 8]. The latter can be used in three different steps of the procedure: first, during the identification of the upper and lower pole ureter to avoid any injury to the ureter of the moiety to be preserved. In this case, the ICG has to be injected via the transurethral catheter inserted before starting the robotic procedure. Second, after division of the vessels of the moiety to be removed, in order to enhance the line of demarcations between the healthy moiety and the one to remove ICG has to be injected intravenously. Finally, the ICG can be injected again via the transurethral catheter of the preserved moiety to detect any leakage from the brunch of section of the preserved moiety due to an inadvertent injury to the calyx.

8 Discussion and Conclusion

As for any laparoscopic procedures, the robot has made partial nephrectomy much easier compared to the procedure performed with standard laparoscopy. Results are overall comparable [9–11]. The 3D vision, the seven degrees of freedom of the instruments, and the availability of powerful sealing devices can account for this. On the other side, the use of the robot, and the related costs, require special considerations for partial nephrectomy [12].

First of all, the robot shows its greatest value when suturing is required during the surgical procedure, and this is usually not the cases in partial nephrectomies, unless a calyx is inadvertently opened. Different is the setting of an atypical resection of a renal mass, where the robot can play an important role [2]. In case of partial resection of a nonfunctioning moiety in a duplex system, instead, the standard laparoscopic approach is cost saving and can be performed using smaller incisions or even as single-site procedure.

Second, also the indication for partial nephrectomy per se can be questioned [3–8]. Indeed, accumulating evidence suggests that nonfunctioning renal moieties can safely be left in situ, if asymptomatic and well decompressed. Therefore, refluxing lower poles can be managed conservatively, if asymptomatic. If the VUR is symptomatic, instead, endoscopic treatment can be attempted and often fixes the problem, further limiting the need for a lower pole partial nephrectomy in this scenario. The situation is not much different for urological conditions affecting the upper pole. Endoscopic puncture has become a popular minimally invasive option for upper pole ureteroceles. If the ureterocele is associated with a lower pole reflux, the upper pole nonfunctioning moiety can be reimplanted at the same time of the lower pole refluxing one, if primary lower urinary tract reconstruction is deemed necessary. Ureteroureterostomy and ureteral clipping are other options for upper pole ureteroceles and ectopic ureters too. For the latter, also dismembered extra-vesical reimplantation is possible.

In contrast to these alternative options, partial nephrectomy carries two important risks. The first one is the risk of persistent urinary leakage from the branch of section. Even when no leakage occurs, formation of cysts at the renal pole is common [13]. The latter is more probably of serosal origin and can generally be managed conservatively; US follow-up is however recommended [13]. The second, and most concerning complication, is a vascular damage and subsequent loss of the preserved moiety [14]. The latter complication seems more common when the procedure is performed in infants. Therefore, if this is the surgical strategy elected, waiting until the child get older is advisable.

Single-site robotic partial nephrectomy could represent the future evolution of the robotic partial nephrectomy [15].

In conclusion, robotic-assisted laparoscopic partial nephrectomy is feasible and safe for the treatment of renal duplication anomalies. Indications remain scant, and a number of alternative procedures exist. Major complications of partial nephrectomy include persistent urinary leakage due to a damage to a calyx of the preserved kidney and a vascular injury resulting in functional loss of the preserved kidney. The use of ICG fluorescence technology with Firefly system can help in several steps of the procedure.

References

1. Castagnetti M, Rigamonti W. Ureteral duplications and ureteroceles. In: Lima M, Manzoni G, editors. Pediatric urology: contemporary strategies from fetal life to adolescence. © Springer-Verlag Italia; 2014. https://doi.org/10.1007/978-88-470-5693-0_11.
2. Antar A, Bachtel HA, Bates JN, Kim SJ, Saleem A, Bhatia V, Link RE, Koh CJ. Robotic partial nephrectomy in the pediatric population: cumulative experience at a large pediatric hospital. J Pediatr Urol. 2022;18(4):538–40. https://doi.org/10.1016/j.jpurol.2022.06.029.
3. Castagnetti M, Canali R, Mastrocinque G, Esposito C, Rigamonti W. Dismembered extravesical reimplantation of dilated upper pole ectopic ureters in duplex systems. J Pediatr Surg. 2013;48(2):459–63. https://doi.org/10.1016/j.jpedsurg.2012.11.050.
4. Castagnetti M, Vidal E, Burei M, Zucchetta P, Murer L, Rigamonti W. Duplex system ureterocele in infants: should we reconsider the indications for secondary surgery after endoscopic puncture or partial nephrectomy? J Pediatr Urol. 2013;9(1):11–6. https://doi.org/10.1016/j.jpurol.2012.06.016.
5. Castagnetti M, El-Ghoneimi A. Management of duplex system ureteroceles in neonates and infants. Nat Rev Urol. 2009;6(6):307–15. https://doi.org/10.1038/nrurol.2009.82.
6. Lopes RI, Fernandez N, Koyle MA, Dos Santos J, Perez J, Romao R, Lorenzo AJ. Clinical outcomes of the upper urinary tract after ureteral clipping for treatment of low functioning or nonfunctioning renal moieties. J Urol. 2018;199(2):558–64. https://doi.org/10.1016/j.juro.2017.09.080.
7. Esposito C, Autorino G, Coppola V, Esposito G, Paternoster M, Castagnetti M, Cardone R, Cerulo M, Borgogni R, Cortese G, Escolino M. Technical standardization of ICG near-infrared fluorescence (NIRF) laparoscopic partial nephrectomy for duplex kidney in pediatric patients. World J Urol. 2021;39(11):4167–73. https://doi.org/10.1007/s00345-021-03759-6.
8. Esposito C, Masieri L, Cerulo M, Castagnetti M, Del Conte F, Di Mento C, Esposito G, Tedesco F, Carulli R, Continisio L, Chiodi A, Escolino M. Indocyanine green (ICG) fluorescence technology in pediatric robotic surgery. J Robot Surg. 2024;18(1):209. https://doi.org/10.1007/s11701-024-01968-w.
9. Neheman A, Kord E, Strine AC, Vander Brink BA, Minevich EA, DeFoor WR, Reddy PP, Noh PH. Pediatric partial nephrectomy for upper urinary tract duplication anomalies: a comparison between different surgical approaches and techniques. Urology. 2019;125:196–201. https://doi.org/10.1016/j.urology.2018.11.026.
10. Varda BK, Rajender A, Yu RN, Lee RS. A contemporary single-institution retrospective cohort study comparing perioperative outcomes between robotic and open partial nephrectomy for poorly functioning renal moieties in children with duplex collecting systems. J Pediatr Urol. 2018;14(6):549.e1–8. https://doi.org/10.1016/j.jpurol.2018.06.011.
11. Batra NV, Dangle P. A review of robotic-assisted laparoscopic partial nephrectomy in the management of renal duplication anomalies. Front Surg. 2024;11:1364246. https://doi.org/10.3389/fsurg.2024.1364246.
12. Roshan A, Mac Neily AE. Dorsal lumbotomy for pediatric upper pole hemi-nephrectomy: Back (door) to the future? J Pediatr Urol. 2020;16(4):480.e1–7. https://doi.org/10.1016/j.jpurol.2020.04.031.
13. Esposito C, Escolino M, Troncoso Solar B, Iacona R, Esposito R, Settimi A, Mushtaq I. Diagnosis and long-term outcome of renal cysts after laparoscopic partial nephrectomy in children. BJU Int. 2017;119(5):761–6. https://doi.org/10.1111/bju.13698.
14. Wallis MC, Khoury AE, Lorenzo AJ, Pippi-Salle JL, Bägli DJ, Farhat WA. Outcome analysis of retroperitoneal laparoscopic heminephrectomy in children. J Urol. 2006;175(6):2277–80.; discussion 2280–2. https://doi.org/10.1016/S0022-5347(06)00338-7.
15. Ditonno F, Licari LC, Franco A, Bologna E, Manfredi C, Soputro NA, Ramos R, Antonelli A, Nelson RJ, Ahmed M, Stifelman M, Badani K, Kaouk J, Crivellaro S, Autorino R. Current expectations and opinions on single-port robotic surgery: a survey among European experts by the SPARC collaborative group. Eur Urol Open Sci. 2024;60:54–7. https://doi.org/10.1016/j.euros.2024.01.007.

Robotic-Assisted Laparoscopic Extravesical Ureteral Reimplantation (REVUR)

Kristina Gam and Mohan Gundeti

1 Introduction

Vesicoureteral reflux (VUR) is defined as the retrograde flow of urine from the bladder to the ureter and possibly to the kidney during voiding [1]. It is caused by a dysfunctional ureterovesical junction (UVJ) and is one of the most common congenital abnormalities of the urinary tract [1]. The estimated incidence of VUR in healthy children is approximately 1%, while the estimated incidence of VUR in children with urinary tract infection (UTI) is between 25% and 40% [2, 3].

VUR is usually diagnosed in the following scenarios: UTI workup, hydronephrosis workup, or screening a sibling of a child with VUR [2]. The gold standard imaging to diagnosis VUR is a voiding cystourethrogram (VCUG). Radionuclide cystogram (RNC) can also be utilized but is not as commonly used.

The natural history of VUR is highly variable as it may spontaneously resolve (especially low grade VUR), lead to severe infection including pyelonephritis, and/or cause permanent renal damage from scarring [4–6]. The management options for VUR include surveillance for low-grade VUR, expectant management with antibiotic prophylaxis, and surgical correction [2].

K. Gam (✉) · M. Gundeti
Comer Children's Hospital Chicago,
Chicago, IL, USA
e-mail: kgam@uchicagomedicine.org; mgundeti1@uchigaco.edu

Open surgical techniques for ureteral reimplant were first developed in the 1950s and 1960s through intravesical and extravesical methods [5, 7, 8]. The initial success rates for open ureteral reimplant were favorable, ranging from 93% to 96% [9, 10]. The high success rate for open reimplant has persisted, leading to its remaining as the gold standard treatment for the surgical treatment of VUR.

However, with the development of laparoscopic and robotic surgical procedures, minimally invasive techniques have emerged. The first description of extravesical ureteral reimplant was published in 2004. Since then, robotic extravesical ureteral reimplant (REVUR) has been adopted as a minimally invasive surgical option for patients with VUR. The success rates have been variable, ranging from 72% to 98.5%, leading to a slower adoption of REVUR [11, 12]. Nevertheless, REVUR remains a minimally invasive surgical option for the treatment of VUR. In this chapter, we describe our "LUAA" technique for robotic extravesical ureteral reimplantation.

The LUAA technique is named after the steps to create an ideal detrusor tunnel and detrusorrhaphy (Table 1) [13].

Table 1 LUAA technique

L	Length of the submucosal detrusor tunnel (4 cm)
U	U-stitch
A	Apical alignment stitch
A	Adventitia of the ureter incorporated into detrusorrhaphy

C. Esposito et al. (eds.), *Pediatric Robotic Assisted Surgery*,
https://doi.org/10.1007/978-3-031-99532-3_16

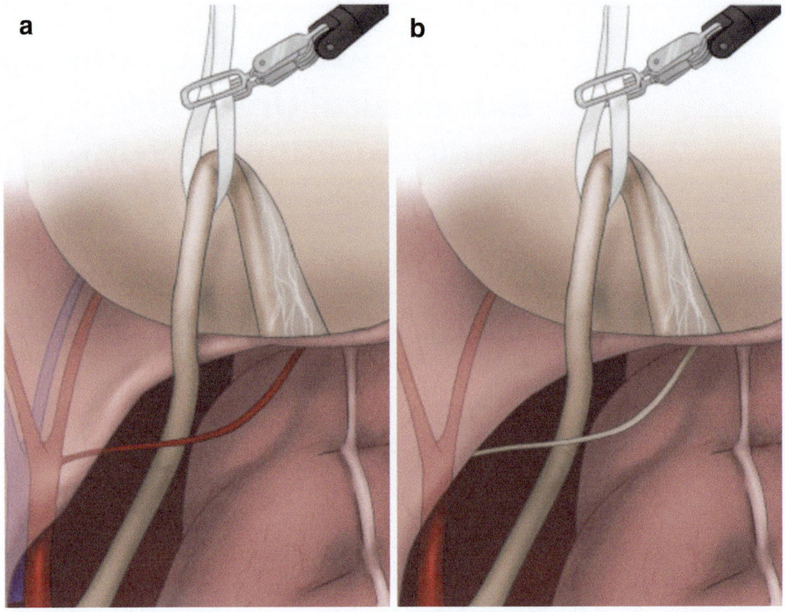

Fig. 1 Ureteral dissection in a female patient (**a**) and male patient (**b**)

2 Patient Positioning and Planning

The patient is placed in a low dorsal lithotomy with pediatric stirrups (Fig. 1). The face and chest are padded. A safety strap is applied to the patient's chest. A Foley catheter is placed before preparing the sterile field. We prepare the patient with betadine solution from the xiphoid to the upper thighs. Sterile towels and drapes are then applied. The surgical field includes the entire abdomen and the pelvis. We do not routinely perform any endoscopic procedures before docking the robot. We do not utilize ureteral stents during REVUR as we have found that they interfere with the flexibility of the ureter, which impedes ureteral dissection and detrusor tunnel creation.

3 Incision and Port Placement

Port placement begins with placement of a 12-mm balloon port at the umbilicus via open Hassan technique. The ideal distance from the pubis to the umbilicus should be at least 10–12 cm to allow for enough working space. We utilize a balloon port to prevent the port from slipping out of the patient given that pediatric patients have thinner abdominal walls. The abdomen is then insufflated at a pressure of 12 mm Hg and then later reduced to 10 mm Hg after all ports are placed. We then place two 8-mm trocars at the midclavicular lines bilaterally and then place a 5-mm assistant port at the right or left upper quadrant, depending on the surgeon and bedside assistant's preference (Fig. 1). All ports are placed under direct vision. We utilize a bedside assistant for easy insertion and removal of suture, assisting with retraction, and suctioning.

4 Robot Positioning

The robot is then positioned between the child's legs, and the second arm is docked to the umbilical port. A camera with a 0-degree lens is inserted into the umbilical port, and the robotic arms are targeted toward the pelvis. The first and third robotic arms are then docked to the 8-mm midclavicular ports. We utilize an 8-mm monopolar scissor in the third robotic arm and an 8-mm bipolar Maryland forceps in the first robotic arm. We do not utilize the fourth robotic arm.

5 Procedural Steps

5.1 Step 1: Identify and Dissect the Ureter

Identification of the ureter begins at the pelvic brim. Beginning the ureteral dissection at the pelvic brim allows for increased ureteral length and easier identification of the plane between the ureter and uterine vessels or vas deferens. The peritoneum overlying the ureter is incised, and a window around the ureter is created. The ureter must not be handled directly to avoid injury to the ureter. The space around the ureter is made large enough for a piece of umbilical tape to be passed underneath the ureter into a loop. The loop of umbilical tape around the ureter is then used to handle the ureter atraumatically [13].

The ureter is then mobilized to the level of the uterine artery in females or the vas deferens in males (Fig. 2). Another peritoneal window is incised distally to these structures in order to preserve them, and then the ureter is mobilized distally to them. The umbilical tape is passed through this second window to allow for handling of the distal ureter. The ureteral dissection then continues distally to the ureterovesical junction (UVJ). Care must be taken to avoid dissection at the dorsomedial ureterovesical junction to avoid damaging any neurovascular tissue at this location.

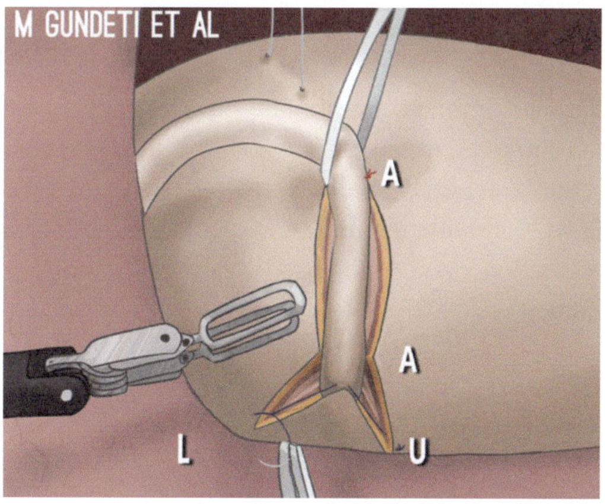

Fig. 2 Illustration of the detrusor tunnel inverted Y shape and the placement of the U-stitch and apical alignment stitch. The bladder hitch stitch and umbilical tape handle are also depicted

5.2 Step 2: Hitch the Bladder

Once the ureteral dissection is completed, the bladder is distended with sterile saline instilled through the Foley catheter. The bladder can be hitched anteriorly with a 2–0 Vicryl suture inserted through the abdominal wall near the pubis with a straightened needle. The suture is passed by the bedside assistant through the abdominal wall. The surgeon then passes the needle through the posterior bladder wall serosa and then up to the abdominal wall on the contralateral side of insertion. The ends of the suture are clamped by the bedside assistant with the desired amount of tension to elevate the bladder, which then improves the exposure of the UVJ.

5.3 Step 3: Create the Detrusor Tunnel

Once the bladder is hitched, we then begin to create the detrusor tunnel. The detrusor tunnel must be carefully planned to create an ideal ureteral reimplantation. The shape of the detrusor tunnel is an inverted Y, where the stem of the inverted Y extends anteriorly to become the length of the detrusor tunnel and the arms of the inverted Y extend from the ureter posteriorly (Fig. 3). The tunnel length we utilize is 4 cm. This can be measured with a measuring tape. The angle of the tunnel must be in alignment with the natural lie of the ureter to avoid excessive angulation and subsequent obstruction.

The tunnel is incised with the monopolar scissors, continuing the depth of the tunnel through the detrusor muscle until the bladder mucosa is reached. Care should also be taken to avoid the dorsomedial UVJ at this step as well.

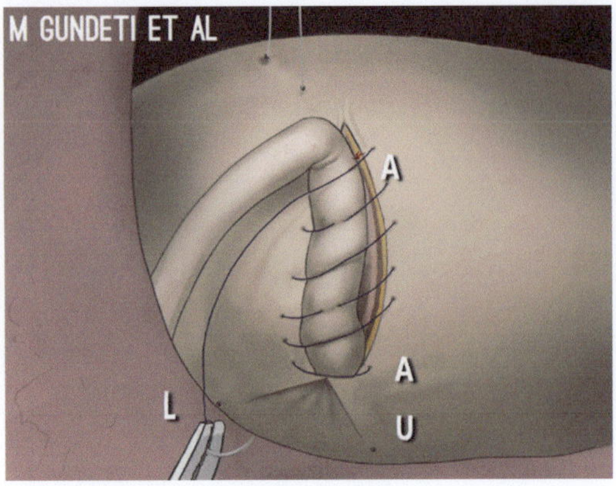

Fig. 3 Illustration of the detrusorrhaphy

5.4 Step 3: Create the Detrusorrhaphy

Once the detrusor tunnel is made, the ureter is then placed into the tunnel. We then utilize several suture techniques to optimally anchor the ureter into the tunnel. We use 5–0 PDS (polydiaxonone) suture for the detrusorrhaphy. This begins with the U-stitch at the distal portion of the detrusor tunnel near the UVJ. The U-stitch is formed by stitching together the most distal and posterior ureteral adventitia to the detrusor muscle at the ends of the arms of the inverted Y. This serves as a distal anchor of the ureter in the tunnel.

Then the apical alignment stitch is performed at the apex of the detrusor tunnel in the same fashion, incorporating the more proximal ureteral adventitia. This stitch will not only anchor the ureter proximally but also stabilize the alignment of the detrusorrhaphy. The detrusorrhaphy is then completed from distal to proximal with every other throw incorporating the ureteral adventitia. While the detrusorrhaphy is formed, bedside assistant keeps the ureter elevated by retracting the umbilical tape anteriorly. The ideal tightness of the detrusor tunnel causes capillary blanching of the ureteral adventitia but still allows for adequate mobility of the ureter in the tunnel.

Once the detrusorrhaphy is completed, that concludes the ureteral reimplant. The robot is undocked, and all ports removed. We close the fascia on all ports to prevent port hernia.

6 Postoperative Period

The patient is admitted for postoperative observation. Their normal diet is resumed. We do not routinely order postoperative labs. The Foley catheter is left to drainage overnight and removed the following morning. We obtain a post-void residual bladder scan as there is a low risk of urinary retention especially after bilateral ureteral reimplant.

Most patients are discharged the following morning after surgery. The postoperative follow-up includes a renal bladder ultrasound 4–8 weeks after surgery and then a VCUG 4–6 months after surgery.

Tips and tricks	
Tip #1	Begin mobilization of the ureter above the pelvic brim
Tip #2	Keep the adventitia and vasculature intact around the ureter
Tip #3	Use a loop of umbilical tape around the ureter to handle the ureter
Tip #4	Use careful dissection around the dorsomedial UVJ
Tip #5	Align the detrusor tunnel with the natural lie of the ureter
Tip #6	Create detrusor flaps in proportion to the ureteral diameter to create an adequate tunnel

7 Conclusion

REVUR remains a minimally invasive option for the surgical treatment of VUR, although open reimplantation remains the gold standard. We have found that the robotic system allows for fine dissection and increased ease of suturing intraoperatively.

References

1. Blais AS, Bolduc S, Moore K. Vesicoureteral reflux: from prophylaxis to surgery. Can Urol Assoc J [Internet]. 2017;11(1-2Suppl1):S13–8. Available from: https://www.ncbi.nlm.nih.gov/pmc/articles/PMC5332225/
2. Mattoo TK, Mohammad D. Primary vesicoureteral reflux and renal scarring. Pediatr Clin N Am. 2022;69(6):1115–29.

3. Arant BS. Vesicoureteric reflux and renal injury. Am J Kidney Dis. 1991;17(5):491–511.
4. Edwards D, Normand IC, Prescod N, Smellie JM. Disappearance of vesicoureteric reflux during long-term prophylaxis of urinary tract infection in children. BMJ. 1977;2(6082):285–8.
5. Lich R, Howerton LW, Davis LA. Recurrent Urosepsis in children. J Urol. 1961;86(5):554–8.
6. Smellie JM, Poulton A, Prescod NP. Retrospective study of children with renal scarring associated with reflux and urinary infection. BMJ [Internet]. 1994;
7. Politano VA, Leadbetter WF. An operative technique for the correction of vesicoureteral reflux. J Urol. 1958;79(6):932–41.
8. Gregoir W. The surgical treatment of congenital vesico-ureteral reflux. Acta Chirurgica Belgica [Internet]. 1964 Apr 1 [cited 2024 Apr 14];63:431–9. Available from: https://pubmed.ncbi.nlm.nih.gov/14197630/
9. Zaontz MR, Maizels M, Sugar EC, Firlit CF. Detrusorrhaphy: extravesical ureteral advancement to correct vesicoureteral reflux in children. J Urol [Internet] 1987 Oct 1 [cited 2021 Dec 28];138(4 Pt 2):947–9. Available from: https://pubmed.ncbi.nlm.nih.gov/3656576/
10. Eckstein HB, Hohenfellner R, Williams DI. Surgical pediatric urology. 1977.
11. Grimsby GM, Dwyer ME, Jacobs MA, Ost MC, Schneck FX, Cannon GM, et al. Multi-institutional review of outcomes of robot-assisted laparoscopic extravesical ureteral reimplantation. Multicenter Study. 2015;193(5S):1791–5.
12. Sforza S, Marco BB, Haid B, Baydilli N, Donmez MI, Spinoit A-F, et al. A multi-institutional European comparative study of open versus robotic-assisted laparoscopic ureteral reimplantation in children with high grade (IV-V) vesicoureteral reflux. J Pediatr Urol. 2023;
13. Gundeti MS, Boysen WR, Shah A. Robot-assisted laparoscopic extravesical ureteral reimplantation: technique modifications contribute to optimized outcomes. Eur Urol. 2016;70(5):818–23.

Robotic Bladder Neck Procedures

Alfredo Berrettini, Michele Gnech, and Dario Guido Minoli

1 Introduction

In recent years, minimally invasive surgery has become a fundamental tool in pediatric urology. Complex reconstructive procedures, as Mitrofanoff appendico-vesicostomy and enterocystoplasty, can be faced with a laparoscopic or, even better, robotic approach.

Among these, procedures to correct urinary incontinence due to an absent or incompetent bladder neck/sphincteric mechanism, are challenging and tough.

The choice of the surgical approach depends on whether to aim for voiding continence or simply secure dryness through bladder neck closure that will require lifelong intermittent catheterization. This chapter will focus on the construction/reconstruction of a functional bladder neck preserving the capacity of a voiding continence, without considering other many alternatives such as slings, artificial urinary sphincters, and bladder neck closure with a continent diversion.

The functional bladder neck reconstruction finds its ideal application in the exstrophy/epispadias complex and cloaca/urogenital sinus groups of abnormalities. Patients must be carefully selected for this approach with a video-urodynamic assessment of a weak outflow and a compliant bladder capacity of the order of at least 50% of the expected capacity for age.

The possibility to obtain an optimal 3D robotic exposure of the bladder neck region has been achieved, thanks to the experience gained by adult urologists performing radical prostatectomy. This innovative approach to pediatric bladder neck reconstructive surgery opens fascinating and stimulating therapeutic paths compared to the traditional frustrating and very demanding open surgery.

The aim of this chapter is to report and describe our experience in robotic bladder neck construction techniques for voiding continence in children with bladder neck plication (BNP) and keel bladder neck construction (KBNC).

2 Patient Positioning and Planning

2.1 Preoperative Preparation

Simple enema given the evening before the surgery should be enough, while a standard extensive intestinal preparation is not necessary. Perioperative antibacterial prophylaxis (usually with a second-generation cephalosporin) should be administered.

A. Berrettini (✉) · M. Gnech · D. G. Minoli
Department of Pediatric Urology, Fondazione IRCCS Ca' Granda, Ospedale Maggiore Policlinico, Milan, Italy
e-mail: alfredo.berrettini@policlinico.mi.it; michele.gnech@policlinico.mi.it; darioguido.minoli@policlinico.mi.it

C. Esposito et al. (eds.), *Pediatric Robotic Assisted Surgery*,
https://doi.org/10.1007/978-3-031-99532-3_17

General anesthesia with endotracheal intubation and muscle relaxation is applied, and a nasogastric tube is placed to keep empty the stomach during the procedure.

2.2 Preoperative Endoscopy

With the patient in frog leg position a preliminary, an endoscopy (endoscope size 8–9.5 Fr is adequate in most of the cases) is performed to identify the anatomy of the urethra and bladder neck.

When the KBNC procedure is planned, bilateral ureteral catheters (JJ stents) are placed to allow a secure identification of the ureteral orifices during the procedure.

A Foley catheter is initially positioned into the bladder, and it will be used to fill the bladder to help identification and preparation of the bladder neck area. Then, it will be removed, especially in bladder neck plication to permit the insertion of the endoscope that will control the tightening of the urethra. At the end of the procedure, the Foley catheter will be repositioned and left in place.

The procedure generally starts with an endoscopy. With the patient in frog leg position, an endoscope of suitable size (a size between 8 and 9.5 Fr is adequate in most of the cases) is introduced into the urethra and the anatomy identified.

2.3 Positioning

The patient is placed supine, and the legs are opened wide, as in frog leg position: In bladder neck construction procedures, it is compulsory to have simultaneous endoscopical access to the urethra and bladder neck to confirm and to monitor the progression of the reconstructive procedure. The patient is secured to the bed with wide adhesive tape and strips. All pressure points, including the heels, must be carefully padded and protected to prevent pressure lesions. We generally use a depression mattress to move and keep the patient into the desired position easily. A memory foam mat is placed under the patient to offer a controlled compression of the body during the procedure (Fig. 1).

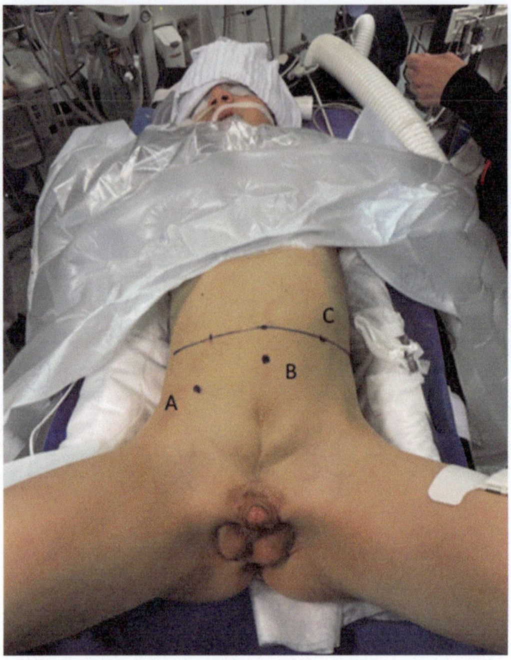

Fig. 1 Patient positioning in bladder exstrophy patient (**a**) Site for 10-mm port and Mitrofanoff stoma (**b**) umbilicus site (absent in bladder exstrophy patient). (**c**) Line marked for robotic ports positioning

The patient is then prepared and draped. The operating table is inclined in the Trendelenburg position moving the bowel cranially by gravity and facilitating exposure of the bladder and the pelvic region.

3 Incision, Port Placement, and Robot Positioning

Compared to the Si model, the DaVinci Xi model has a different structure with a boom-mounted architecture of the patient cart that provides flexible and accurate deployment of the four arms. The Xi model cart is placed at the patient side, while the four arms are latched deriving from a remote center and deployed perpendicularly to the patient. Compared to the SI model, the port siting is different: An angled linear port configuration is used to align the ports from the right lower quadrant toward the left costal margin, and the robot is side docked on the patient's side. The first trocar is an 8 mm used for camera access: It is placed in the midline, through a supraumbilical incision. The trocar is positioned with an open access and direct view of the peritoneum to reduce the risk of bowel lesion. We generally position a square knot to fix the peritoneum to the trocar: This stitch will be very useful to close to peritoneum, when the trocar will be removed at the end of procedure. After an initial overview of the abdominal cavity, the other 8-mm robotic ports are positioned. Depending on the procedures, two or three trocars are positioned: one to two in the left flank and one in the right one. A four-arm configuration is used for KBNC, while three arms could be enough for BNP. Approximately 7–8 cm is respected between the robotic ports. In cases where, together with bladder neck surgery, the creation of a catheterization conduit is performed, one of the trocars is positioned in the right iliac fossa exactly at the point where the Mitrofanoff stoma will be placed. In these cases, a 12-mm port is also used to introduce clips and hemolocks inside the abdomen (Fig. 2).

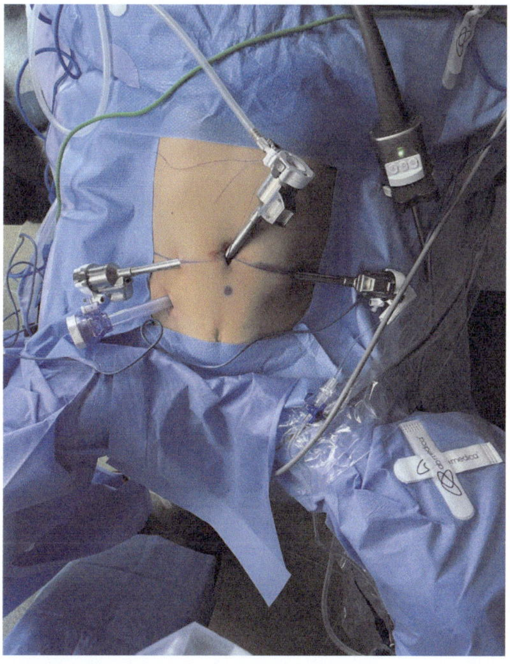

Fig. 2 Port placement

After completing the port placement, the robot can be docked and the instrumentation placed. Usually, we use a 30° down camera in the supraumbilical port even if in specific time of the procedure, a 30° up camera (that can be obtained only with the pressure of a single button on the XI console without removing the camera itself) or a 0° camera could be very helpful. We generally use monopolar scissors and needle holder on the right arm, while a bipolar Maryland forceps is connected to the left. When the fourth robotic arm is active, a Maryland or a needle driver is used.

4 Procedure Steps

In our institute, we typically employ two distinct surgical techniques for constructing a voiding bladder neck: BNP and KBNC. After completing the docking and instrument insertion into the abdomen, the procedure begins with the opening of the pelvic peritoneum via a broad transverse incision. The movement of the catheter and visualization of the balloon, or the use of combined endoscopic-robotic maneuvers, can aid in identifying the bladder neck region. Initial dissection is carried out retropubically and laterally, with particular caution to avoid venous bleeding in males and vaginal injury in females. Complete posterior urethral dissection, as performed for sling placement, is unnecessary.

In BNP, following the isolation of the bladder neck, a gradual plication of the proximal urethra is achieved using multiple interrupted braided polyester (polyethylene terephthalate) 2/0 sutures. Simultaneous endoscopic control, allowing direct visualization of the lumen caliber reduction, is very beneficial.

The Da Vinci Xi system features the Firefly vision mode, an integrated fluorescence capability that employs near-infrared technology. Even without the injection of a fluorescent dye, activating the Firefly mode during a combined endoscopic/laparoscopic approach enhances the definition of the urethral channel, allowing for precise isolation and plication [6].

In the KBNC procedure, the bladder neck is prepared, and the anterior bladder wall is opened along the midline. Two everting holding stitches can help to better expose and stabilize the bladder neck region. The Foley catheter is withdrawn, and the position of the new bladder neck is identified as the midpoint between the veru montanum and the ureteral orifices in males, or the midpoint between the external urethral meatus and the ureteral orifices in females. Starting from this point and extending caudally, two mucosal triangles are outlined, and the mucosa is excised, leaving only a midline mucosal strip of adequate width, depending on the patient's age, which will constitute the "new" posterior urethra and bladder neck. Only the mucosal layer is excised, without damaging or incising the muscular component (Fig. 3).

The intact midline mucosal strip is measured and folded over a Nelaton catheter of appropriate size (usually 8 Fr) and tubularized with interrupted 5/0 polyglyconate (Maxon) stitches. A second and third layer, above the newly constructed bladder neck, are created by approximating the detrusor muscle with interrupted 4/0–3/0 polyglactin (Vicryl) stitches. This anatomical reconstruction results in a funnel with a "keel" configuration (Fig. 4) [7].

A percutaneous suprapubic cystostomy and a transurethral catheter are mandatory to ensure optimal postoperative bladder drainage. All instruments and ports are removed, and the fascia is closed with 2–0 polyglactin (Vicryl). The skin is closed with a subcuticular suture using 5–0 poliglecaprone (Monocryl), and skin adhesive is applied to cover the incisions.

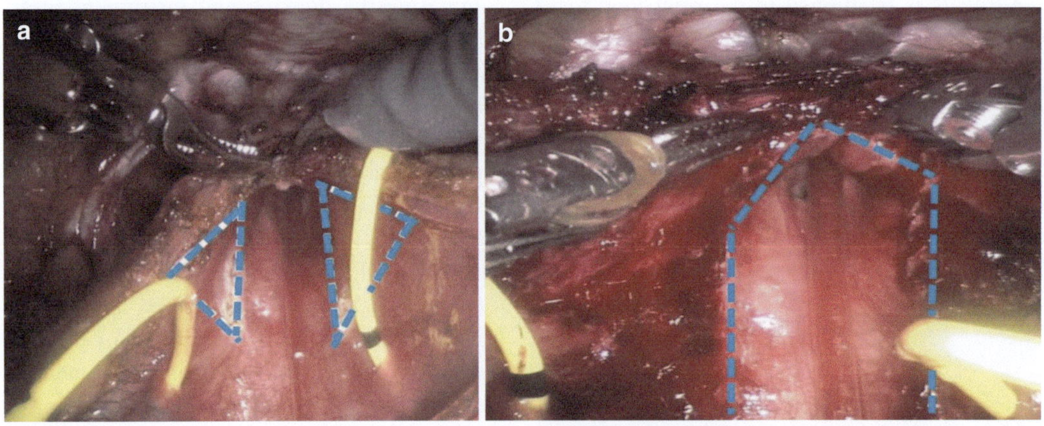

Fig. 3 KBNC (**a**) Outline of mucosal triangles. (**b**) Post-excision. Blue dots define in the middle mucosal strip to be tubularized, outside the demucosalized triangles

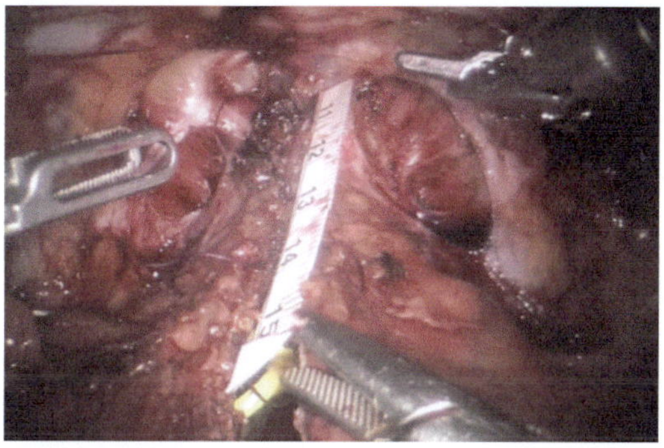

Fig. 4 KBNC final appearance. (Video: See references [6, 7])

5 Postoperative Period

Patients begin oral feeding a few hours postoperatively. Analgesic therapy is based on paracetamol (15 mg/kg at 8-hour intervals) and ketorolac (0.3 mg/kg at 8-hour intervals, if necessary) typically administered within the first 12–24 postoperative hours. Antibiotic therapy with the same agent used perioperatively continued for the next 72 hours. Patients are usually discharged from the hospital on the fourth or fifth postoperative day with both the transurethral and suprapubic catheters on constant free drainage (day and night). The first postoperative clinical checkup is scheduled after 1 week.

After 4 weeks, the transurethral catheter is removed, and the first suprapubic micturating cystourethrogram (MCUG) is performed. Depending on the results, a safe removal of the suprapubic cystostomy can be carried out. If the patient is not fully ready for regular spontaneous micturition, the suprapubic cystostomy is maintained with a clamp-void-release training program. Following the removal of the suprapubic catheter, regular renal and bladder ultrasounds (US) are scheduled to monitor the upper urinary tracts and post-void residuals. Minor urinary leakages observed during follow-up can be effectively managed with endoscopic bladder neck injections of bulking agents.

6 Tips and Tricks

It is mandatory to perform a preliminary cystoscopy to gather all necessary information regarding urethral length, ureteral orifices, and, in male patients, the position of the veru montanum. This step is crucial for understanding the anatomy to correctly position the newly constructed bladder neck and posterior urethra.

- During cystoscopy, if KBNC is planned, bilateral ureteral stents should always be placed to maintain complete control of the ureteral orifices during intravesical surgery. Ureteral reimplantation for additional length is usually unnecessary.
- A transurethral Foley catheter with the balloon inflated is useful for identifying the bladder neck.
- During the BNP procedure, a simultaneous endoscopic view is very helpful and important for confirming the correct position of the plication sutures.
- During the KBNC procedure, using a Nelaton catheter (8 Fr) is preferable to a Foley catheter. If a Foley catheter is used, the balloon should be deflated at the end to avoid any subsequent risk of bladder neck breakdown. It is important to suture the urethral strip close to its edges to ensure the lumen remains uniform in caliber and to use interrupted sutures for security. The transurethral catheter is left in place and fixed both internally and externally.
- The use of suprapubic diversion is mandatory to guarantee complete bladder drainage and maintain total control until regular and safe bladder emptying, with spontaneous voiding, is eventually achieved. The suprapubic clamp-and-release process is normally started 3 weeks after the bladder neck procedure is performed.

7 Discussion and Conclusion

Robotic-assisted laparoscopic bladder surgery in children has gained widespread acceptance for complex reconstructive procedures over the last two decades. The use of robotic systems is particularly advantageous for procedures that necessitate suturing in areas with limited access, such as bladder neck construction techniques for achieving voiding continence.

Patient selection is crucial, and our primary indications for voiding continence procedures have been quite stringent, limited only to cases of epispadias or cloaca/urogenital sinus anomalies. Even within this limited patient group, numerous surgical techniques for bladder neck repair have been proposed, but there is no consensus on the best option, and no standardized protocols exist [1, 2]. Adequate bladder capacity with normal compliance is mandatory prerequisite for considering a robotic procedure aimed at voiding continence.

As confirmed in the literature, laparoscopic bladder neck plication has proven to be successful [3, 4, 5]. Therefore, robotic-assisted BNP appears to be a logical option for achieving voiding continence, with preliminary experience being very encouraging.

In addition to the benefit of working in a confined space with excellent 3D vision, other significant advantages of robotic versus open reconstruction include the following:

- A minimally invasive approach with better cosmetic results
- Lower intraoperative blood loss due to more precise dissection
- Reduced postoperative narcotic use and shorter hospital stays

Take-Home Points

1. Robotic-assisted laparoscopic surgery represents a minimally invasive solution for some of the most severe reconstructive challenges in pediatric urology.
2. Robotic-assisted laparoscopic surgery allows excellent vision within the pelvis and the retropubic region, facilitating any type of bladder neck repair.
3. Preliminary experience with KBNC or BNP performed robotically are encouraging and opening new horizons.

References

1. Gargollo PC, Manzoni G, Rocco B. Robotic bladder outlet procedures. In: Mattioli G, Petralia P, editors. Pediatric robotic surgery. Springer; 2017. p. 109–20. https://doi.org/10.1007/978-3-319-41863-6.
2. Bagrodia A, Gargollo P. Robot-assisted bladder neck reconstruction, bladder neck sling and appendicovesicostomy in children: description of technique and initial results. J Endourol. 2011;25(8):1299–305. https://doi.org/10.1089/end.2011.0031.
3. Kajabfzadeh AM, Talab SS, Elmi A, Tourchi A. Single-stage subsymphyseal cystoscopic-guided bladder neck plication and urethra-genitoplasty in female epispadias: presentation of long-term follow-up. BJUInt. 2011;108(7):1200–7. https://doi.org/10.1111/j.1464-410X.2010.10022.x.
4. Lazarus J, Van Den Heever A, Kotekaas B, Alexander A. Female epispadias management by bladder neck plication via a perineal approach. J Pediatr Urol. 2012;8:244–8. https://doi.org/10.1016/j.jpurol.2011.06.006.
5. Yadav SS, Agarwal N, Kumar S, Tomar V, Vyas N, Teli R, et al. Single-stage female epispadias repair by combined infra-symphyseal bladder neck plication and urethrogenitoplasty: a novel technique. Urology. 2017;100:240–5. https://doi.org/10.1016/j.urology.2016.09.002.
6. Minoli DG, Albo G, De Marco EA, Gnech M, Montanari E, Manzoni G, et al. Robotic bladder neck plication for incontinence treatment. Cent European J Urol. 2021;74(2):274–5. https://doi.org/10.5173/ceju.2021.0355.R3.
7. Minoli DG, De Marco EA, Gnech M, Rocco B, Manzoni G, Berrettini A. Laparoscopic robotic-assisted "keel" bladder neck construction. J Pediatr Urol. 2020;16:857–8. https://doi.org/10.1016/j.jpurol.2020.09.027.

Robotic-Assisted Ileocystoplasty in Children

Amane-Allah Lachkar, Annabel Paye,
Matthieu Peycelon, and Alaa El-Ghoneimi

1 Introduction

Robotic-assisted laparoscopic surgeries gained in popularity in pediatric urology during the last decade [1]. Among these, ileocystoplasty stands out as a particular complex procedure often associated with continent catheterizable channels (CCC), bladder neck reconstruction (BNR), or closure, as well as ureteral reimplantation.

While open surgery remains the gold standard, few surgical teams have pioneered minimally invasive approaches utilizing robotics in recent years [2]. Robot-assisted laparoscopic ileocystoplasty has emerged as a feasible alternative, exhibiting reduced hospital length of stay compared to the traditional open approach [3]. However, the adoption of these procedures is limited, primarily attributed to a steep learning curve that requires advanced robotic skills and extensive surgical experience.

As the W configuration has been our preferred method in open surgery [4], we have decided to adapt the technique described in adult done by Robotic approach [5].

A.-A. Lachkar · A. Paye · M. Peycelon ·
A. El-Ghoneimi (✉)
Department of Pediatric Surgery and Urology, National Reference center for Rare Urinary Tract Malformations (MARVU), University Hospital Robert Debré, APHP, University Paris-Cité, Paris, France
e-mail: amane-allah.lachkar@aphp.fr; annabel.paye@aphp.fr; matthieu.peycelon@aphp.fr; alaa.elghoneimi@aphp.fr

2 Patient Preoperative Preparation, Positioning, and Planning

- We do not routinely do preoperative bowel preparation; patients with chronic constipation of fecal incontinence (myelomeningocele patients, anorectal malformation, etc.) have their routine bowel management program to follow with evacuation enema the day before surgery.
- Urine analysis and culture is done systematically, and any pathogenic urine microbe is treated to have sterile urine during surgery.
- Antibiotic prophylaxis: The local protocol for antibiotic administration is followed; in our institution, antibiotic prophylaxis was cefotaxime and metronidazole. Vancomycin was added in case of ventriculoperitoneal diversion.
- The patient is positioned in supine position; lower limbs are in abduction to allow an access to the urethra if needed. Upper limbs are positioned parallel to the body.
- General endotracheal anesthesia, muscle relaxants, warming table, nasogastric tube, protection of all pressure points with jelly pads. Locoregional anesthesia is applied routinely, for preference epidural anesthesia, in the absence of any contraindication. The

C. Esposito et al. (eds.), *Pediatric Robotic Assisted Surgery*,
https://doi.org/10.1007/978-3-031-99532-3_18

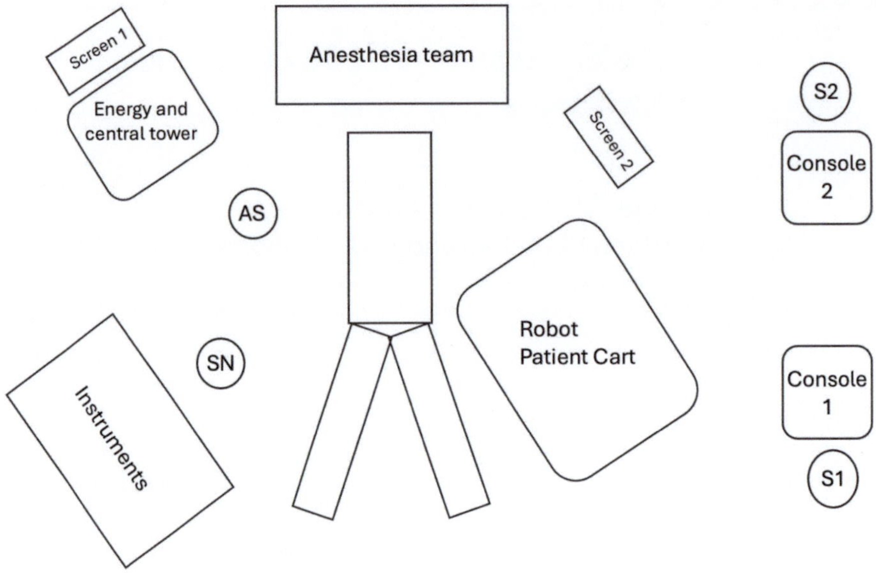

Fig. 1 Operating theater organization for robotic-assisted bladder augmentation. AS, assistant surgeon; SN, scrub nurse; S1, first surgeon; S2, second surgeon

anesthesia plan is discussed with the senior anesthesiologist beforehand.

- If cystoscopy is needed, it is done before docking the robot. An indwelling catheter is inserted in the bladder.
- The table is positioned in Trendelenburg position at 12°. The best option is to have a special table synchronized with the Da Vinci system to be able to change the position if needed without undocking. Otherwise, the position is done definitively after trocars' insertion and before docking.
- The room planning is demonstrated in Fig. 1.
- We routinely do this surgery by at least two senior robotic surgeons using the double console, because of the long duration of the surgery.

3 Incision and Port Placement

All robotic trocars are inserted in the upper abdominal quadrants on a horizontal line (Fig. 2).

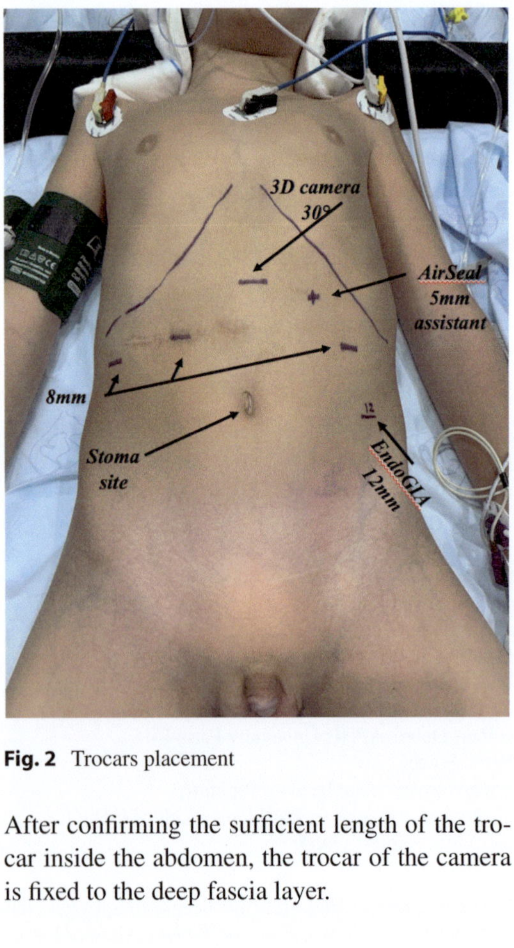

Fig. 2 Trocars placement

Fist trocar is for the camera: halfway between the umbilicus and the xiphoid, through open approach to insert the first robotic trocar of 8 mm. After confirming the sufficient length of the trocar inside the abdomen, the trocar of the camera is fixed to the deep fascia layer.

Further robotic ports are inserted under laparoscopic control on the same horizontal line; local anesthesia is injected at each trocar site before incision.

We use the four arms of the Da Vinci Xi© Robot: one for camera and three for operating robotic ports.

An accessory port on the left hypochondrium is inserted at the end for 5-mm air seal© trocar.

A second accessory trocar is inserted in the left iliac fossa for 12-mm port (endo GIA©).

The umbilicus is left free from any port placement to be used for the Mitrofanoff channel anastomosis, as it is our preferred site for stoma.

4 Robot Positioning

We use Da Vinci Xi©, double consol.

The robot is positioned on the left lower side of the patient (Fig. 1).

5 Procedure Steps

The operative steps of the open procedure were replicated laparoscopically using robotic assistance. In summary, we use the W configuration ileocystoplasty (Ref).

1. Laparoscopic abdominal cavity exploration: Lysis of adhesions is frequently needed during the ports' placement to have free movement of instruments and optimal position of the ports.
2. Appendix preparation: (if Mitrofanoff conduit is indicated)

   The appendix is identified; mesentery window is created at the base. Then an endocorporal ligature of the base is done, we use sharp cutting of the appendix, and the appendix is kept closed by a ligature. The apex is sutured by traction suture. Choice of the appendix orientation is done in situ, apex or the proximal part to the skin according to the mesentery orientation.
3. Bladder preparation: The bladder is filled with sterile saline, and then midline incision is done on the posterior wall tell 2 cm. from the trigone and anterior wall tell 2 cm. from the bladder neck (bivalved bladder) (Fig. 3).
4. Traction sutures on the bivalved bladder, fixed to the lateral abdominal wall, insertion of both ureteral catheters by robotic instruments (Fig. 3).
5. UV reimplantation: When needed, the technique used is according to the bladder pathology; for bladder exstrophy, a Jeff technique is used (cranial submucosal tunnel). The catheters are reinserted through the abdominal wall, bladder wall, and secured by fine 5/0 stitches to the bladder mucosa.
6. Bladder neck surgery: When needed, reconstruction can be done as in open surgery according to the underlying pathology. Our preference is Mitchel bladder neck reconstruction for bladder exstrophy or progressive tailoring technique for other pathology.

   Bladder neck closure: Rarely indicated. When needed, after opening of the bladder, the posterior wall is incised 2 cm from the ureteral orifices and then dissected for at least 2 cm to have a free edge. We do not close the urethra. We use the free edge of the detubularized intestinal segment to be

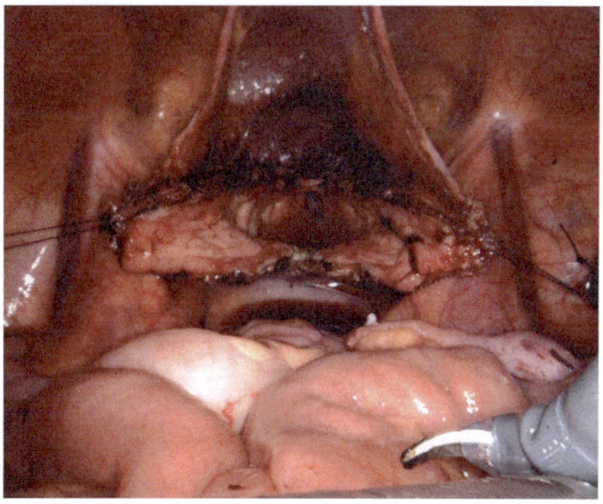

Fig. 3 The bladder is opened to have a bivalve figure; each half is pulled by a retraction suture and fixed to the iliac fossa

sutured tightly with the posterior wall of the bladder neck.

7. Ileal Segment Preparation.

   The terminal ileum is identified, and a traction suture is done at 20 cm from the ileocecal junction. The ileal segment is then identified, and the length is between 20 and 30 cm according to age and size of the bladder. The mesenteric window is opened with the help of bipolar coagulation and scissors or vessel sealer©. Endo-GIA© is introduced by the 12-mm port, and the ileal segment is isolated. A side-to-side anastomosis is done using one endoGia© stapler. The remaining opening of the anastomosis is closed using running 4/0 absorbable suture. The mesenteric base of the isolated segment is kept wide to avoid any torsion. The mesenteric window is closed routinely.

8. Ileal Segment W Configuration.

   We use the W configuration as already described in open surgery (ref Alliot). Traction sutures are stitched on the apex of the W. Small antimesenteric opening is done at this site, and a 4/0 resorbable stiches (Vilock© or PDS ©) is sutured to the posterior bladder wall to stabilize the W segment configuration (Fig. 4).

9. Demutualization.

   The W segment is detubularized by incising the antimesenteric border using the monopolar robotic scissors, cutting energy, and one blade is used (Fig. 5). The middle parts of the W are sutured together by running sutures.

10. Anastomosis of the appendix with the ileal segment:

    The right limbs of the W are left opened to prepare the anastomosis with the appendix. Extra serosal tunnel is done as described (ref). Two lines of fairy cuts in the serosa are done by diathermy. The proximal or distal end of the appendix is chosen according to the disposition of the mesentery. We spatulate the appendix without coagulation, only sharp scissors, and then anastomosis full thickness between the appendix and the ileal wall by two running stiches of PDS 5/0. We do not rinse the appendix, and we do not do the anastomosis around a stent.

    The extra serosal tunnel is done by interrupted sutures between the two limbs of the W at the coagulated fairy cuts already incised (Fig. 6). We use 5/0 PDS for these stitches, but recently we have decided to use nonresorbable sutures to avoid disruption of the tunnel. If the mesentery is on the way, multiple small windows are done to suture together the two ileal walls. The minimal length of the tunnel should be 4 cm, and then the free edges of the ileal segments are

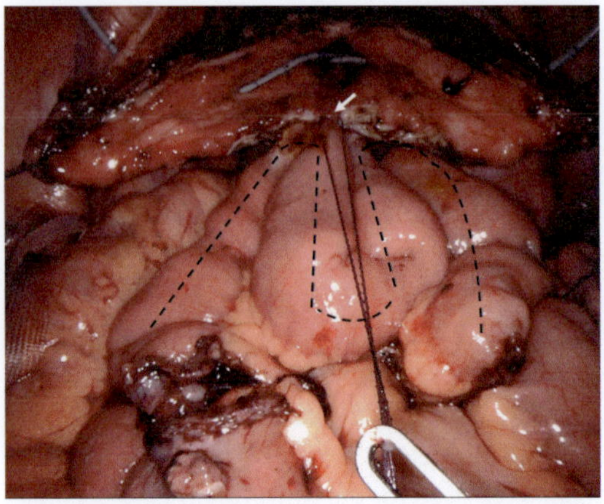

Fig. 4 W configuration of the ileal segment. The two angles of the W are sutured at the midline (white arrow) before tubularization

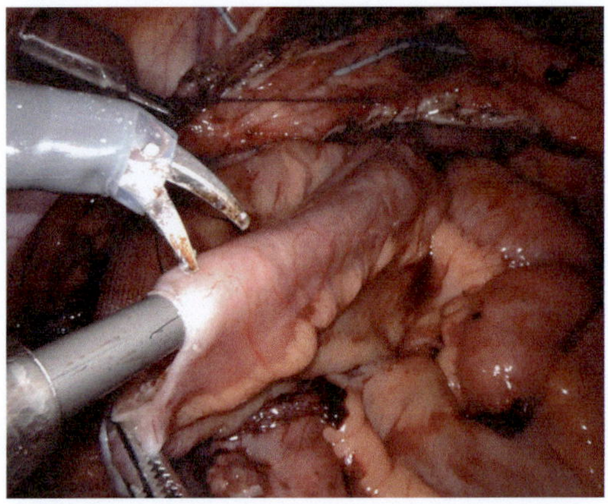

Fig. 5 Detubularization of the W, the ileal segment is incised at the antimesenteric bord by monopolar scissors, using one blade and helped by the suction tube to have a regular cut

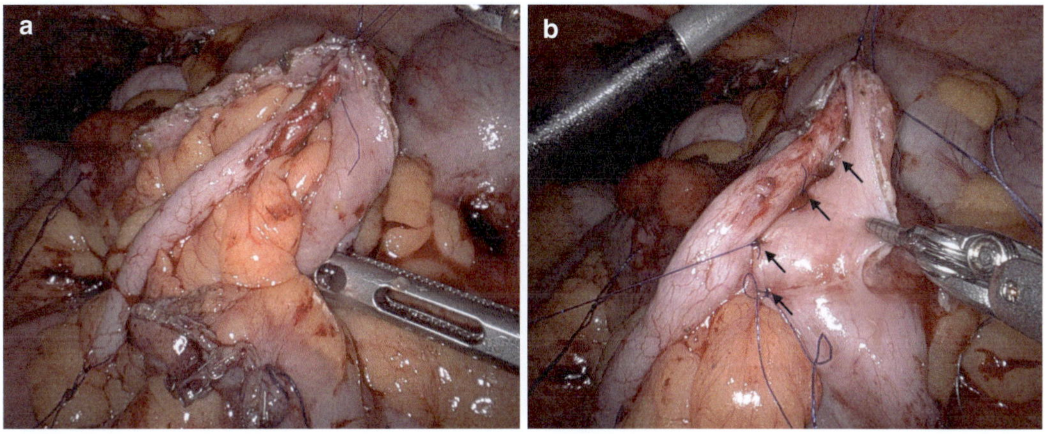

Fig. 6 Extraserosal reimplantation of the appendix. (**a**) The appendix is anastomosed to the angle of the W. (**b**) The two arms of the detubularized W are sutured at the serosal level by multiple sutures (black arrows), transmesenteric to fit the appendix between the line of sutures, and the edges of the ileal segments

sutured together around the appendix, passing through the appendix serosa at each suture. The other end of the appendix remains closed to be externalized at the end of the procedure through the umbilicus.

11. Suturing the posterior wall

    The free edge of the detubularized segment is sutured with multiple running stiches using absorbable sutures to the posterior and lateral wall of the bivalved bladder.

12. Supra pubic tube insertion

    The suprapubic is inserted under vision through the abdominal wall and in preference through the ileal segment, especially if the bladder is small and fragile. We use Ch 12 without balloon. A purse string is securing the hole of insertion.

13. Suturing the anterior wall

    The anterior wall anastomosis between the ileal segment and the bladder starts by the midline then gradually advanced retrograde; the running sutures are full thickness bladder and extra-mucosal of the intestinal segment to reduce mucosal secretions specially in the region of the bladder neck.

    The water tightness of the sutures is controlled by injecting saline through the suprapubic.

14. Drainage

    We routinely drain the retropubic area by a multi-tubulated small caliber silastic drain, externalized through the 12-mm port.

15. Undocking

    Undocking is proceeded, but the ports remain in the patient to make the final check of the Mitrofanoff channel after skin anastomosis.

16. Externalization of the appendix to the umbilicus, anastomosis with the umbilicus (or neo-umbilicus if bladder exstrophy case): sharp incision arciform at the lower edge of the umbilicus, the flap is prepared carefully without traumatizing the skin. An artery forceps is introduced through the fibrous ring under laparoscopic control. The forceps handling the traction suture will exteriorize the appendix, and the mesentery is checked for any torsion through laparoscopic vision.

    The appendix is spatulated for at least 1 cm, sutured full thickness to the skin flap, and interrupted 5/0 PDS ©.

    At the end of anastomosis, the bladder is filled with 100 ml of saline; pneumoperitoneum is exsufflated; and only then we introduce the Silastic Ch12 dry multiperforated catheter, if any difficulty is encountered, a laparoscopic control is proceeded with removal of obstructing stiches.

The Mitrofanoff catheter is sutured to the skin away from the flap.

6 Postoperative Period

We have kept the same protocol as for open surgery.

1. Nasogastric tube is removed on day 1 postoperative; oral fluids and meal are progressively given.
2. Pelvic free drainage: It is removed when it decreases in volume < 20 ml.
3. Ureteral stents: They are flushed with 2 ml saline if they are not productive and then removed at fifth postoperative day.
4. Suprapubic catheter is left on free drainage and flushed with 30 ml of saline twice per day.
5. Antibioprophylaxy is continued for 48 h00, and then no antibiotics are given.
6. Mitrofanoff indwelling catheter: irrigation routinely twice per day with 30 ml of saline and every time if the urine output is less than expected for weight of the patient.
7. The child is discharged with both Mitrofanoff catheter and suprapubic. Then the child is scheduled to come back at the outpatient clinic at 15th postoperative day.
8. Outpatient management:

   The parents are trained to flush the suprapubic and the Mitrofanoff once per day for each catheter with 30 ml of saline. They are instructed to come to emergency if there is no urine output by the catheters, fever, abdominal pain, and vomiting.

   Starting the intermittent catheterization:

   - 15th postoperative day: The Mitrofanoff catheter is removed, the suprapubic is closed, and first catheterization is done by the pediatric urology outpatient nurse. The suprapubic catheter is kept closed, and CIC is done by the parents or the child every 2 hours; the first 2 days are done at the outpatient clinic and then at home. Suprapubic free drainage is left for the night.
   - 21st postoperative day: The suprapubic catheter is removed. If the night drainage is more than 500, indwelling catheter in the Mitrofanoff is left for the night, until the daily CIC drains at least 300 ml of bladder capacity.
9. Bladder augment irrigation: For the first year, the family does an irrigation of the bladder augment with 60 ml of saline or water to rinse the mucus filaments. Then the irrigation is only on demand if the catheter has increased to CH 14; otherwise, if it remains Ch12, irrigation is done routinely.
10. Midterm and long-term follow-up is mandatory, during the first year at least every 3 months, the child is also seen by the urotherapist nurse at the clinic and then every 6 months and then annually. Follow-up by pediatric nephrologist is routinely done at least annually. Renal ultrasound is done at 3 months and then yearly. Video urodynamic study is done routinely at 1 year and then repeated if any clinical or ultrasound changes.

7 Tips and Tricks

1. Preoperative intensive preparation of the patient for bladder augmentation and intermittent catheterization. The time-consuming education of the patient and the family is mandatory to be sure that the child is ready for such strict CIC discipline. The role of specialized nurse and psychologist is the key for success of postoperative acceptance of rigorous discipline.
2. Start by preparing the appendix as a first step of the procedure to be able to planify the next steps in case the appendix is not suitable.
3. To avoid ischemia of the channel or stricture at the skin or the bladder anastomosis: minimal use of diathermy at the sites of the skin or the bladder anastomosis. Use irrigation to see it's better than coagulation; avoid using the stoma site as trocar site to reduce skin trauma.

4. To have regular incision of the intestinal segment, use the suction tube as tutor to open the intestinal wall with the monopolar scissors.
5. At the beginning of the W configuration, suture the two apexes of the W to the posterior bladder wall to stabilize the intestinal segment.
6. The use of objective measures by a thread to measure the appendix, length of the intestinal segment, and the length of anti-reflux tough.
7. Long surgery needs experienced teamwork; do not hesitate to ask for help specially during the long time consuming of suturing.
8. Keep the intraperitoneal pressure as low as it is needed according to the anatomy of the patient.
9. Insert the free drainage lame without suction in a dependent position, and keep it long to connect it to a drainage bag in a dependent position.

8 Discussion and Conclusion

Bladder augmentation associated or not with a CCC is a complex procedure requiring expertise and significantly affects patients' quality of life. The robotic approach was recently adopted in children and is still limited to few centers [2]. Gundetti et al. report the first case of complete intracorporeally robotic-assisted augmentation ileocystoplasty associated with APV [2].

Our experience is still limited to eight pediatric cases with different underlying pathologies (multiple operated bladder exstrophy, neurogenic bladder, operated bladder rhabdomyosarcoma). 62.5% of our patients had various abdominal surgeries before bladder augmentation. We believe that the robotic approach is feasible and spares the abdominal wall.

Robotic surgery showed promising results despite a steep learning curve and a long operative time. The approach described by Gundetti et al. results in a significantly longer operative time (623 vs. 287 minutes; $p < 0.01$) compared to open surgery. There were no significant differences in length of stay or complication rates [3].

In our series, the median operative time was 625 min (450–905); the variation of operative time was depending on associated procedures to bladder augmentation.

We have observed 37.5% rate of leakage through the appendicular Mitrofanoff, compared to 19.2% in our open surgery series (4). Before leakage, three patients experienced bladder retention ($N = 2$) and bladder perforation ($N = 1$). El Schal et al. described stoma-related complications in five patients (8.4%), stomal stenosis in six (10%), and parastomal hernia in two (3.3%) in a cohort of 55 pediatric patients who had W configuration ileocystoplasty in open surgery [6]. The leakage rate observed in our study could be attributed to several factors such as the use of absorbable suture, an overestimation of anti-reflux channel length, or an infrequent catheterization regimen, which may have resulted in an overdistended bladder and subsequent weakening of the anti-reflux channel. The use of nonabsorbable suture, as extra-serosal sutures, can be an improvement in the future.

No stenosis was reported in our series.

We encountered two CIC difficulties requiring endoscopic treatment. Adamic et al. reported two CIC difficulties and one false passage [7]. Such complications can be attributed to an overfilled bladder, which may result in a narrowed APV and consequently impede the catheter's passage.

We also encountered a case of stone formation on staples which remains at the end of the reconfigured segment. This is one of the specific complications of RALAWI compared to open surgery in our experience as we do not use staples in open surgery. Webster et al. reported a similar case of stone formation on staples with ureteral obstruction following ileal conduit construction, and they recommended to remove the staple line and to close with absorbable sutures [8]. In the future, we will remove the staples lines at the end of the detubularized segment.

We had observed a case of perforation that was successfully repaired laparoscopically. Thanks to the robotic approach, minimal adhesions were observed, facilitating the laparoscopic approach.

In conclusion, our limited experience shows that robotic-assisted bladder augmentation is feasible in children. Meanwhile, the number of cases remains limited to have an efficient progression in the learning curve. Improvements are expected to decrease the operative time and to reduce the postoperative complications to a level at least as after open surgery. The robotic approach seems to us potentially of benefits in cases of multiple abdominal wall surgery (bladder exstrophy).

References

1. Chen CJ, Peters CA. Robotic assisted surgery in pediatric urology: current status and future directions. Front Pediatr. 2019;7:7. https://doi.org/10.3389/fped.2019.00090.
2. Gundeti MS, Eng MK, Reynolds WS, Zagaja GP. Pediatric robotic-assisted laparoscopic augmentation ileocystoplasty and mitrofanoff appendicovesicostomy: complete intracorporeal—initial case report. Urology. 2008;72:1144–7; discussion 1147. https://doi.org/10.1016/j.urology.2008.06.070.
3. Murthy P, Cohn JA, Selig RB, Gundeti MS. Robot-assisted laparoscopic augmentation ileocystoplasty and mitrofanoff appendicovesicostomy in children: updated interim results. Eur Urol. 2015;68:1069–75. https://doi.org/10.1016/j.eururo.2015.05.047.
4. Alliot H, Tapsoba T, Paye-Jaouen A, Ashkanani Y, Josset-Raffet E, Natio L, et al. A catheterizable serous-lined urinary outlet associated with the ileal bladder augmentation Abol-Enein and Ghoneim procedure: a safe and reliable procedure in children. Front Pediatr. 2024;12:1273505. https://doi.org/10.3389/fped.2024.1273505.
5. Grilo N, Chartier-Kastler E, Grande P, Crettenand F, Parra J, Phé V. Robot-assisted supratrigonal cystectomy and augmentation cystoplasty with totally intracorporeal reconstruction in neurourological patients: technique description and preliminary results. Eur Urol. 2021;79:858–65. https://doi.org/10.1016/j.eururo.2020.08.005.
6. Elshal AM, Abol-Enein H, Sarhan O, Hafez AT, Mosbah A, Abdel-Latif M, et al. Catheterizable serous lined urinary outlet in children and adolescents: a choice when other treatments fail. J Urol. 2011;185:1083–7. https://doi.org/10.1016/j.juro.2010.10.041.
7. Adamic B, Kirkire L, Andolfi C, Labbate C, Aizen J, Gundeti M. Robot-assisted laparoscopic augmentation ileocystoplasty and mitrofanoff appendicovesicostomy in children: step-by-step and modifications to UChicago technique. BJUI Compass. 2020;1:32–40. https://doi.org/10.1002/bco2.7.
8. Webster GD, Henry HH, Tomlin EM. Calculus formation and ureteral obstruction after ileal conduit construction using autosuture stapling device. Urology. 1987;30:571–3. https://doi.org/10.1016/0090-4295(87)90439-0.

Robotic Mitrofanoff Procedure in Children

A. Paye Jaouen and A. El Ghoneimi

1 Introduction

The Mitrofanoff principle involves the creation of a conduit going into a low-pressure reservoir, which can be emptied with clean intermittent catheterization through an easily accessible stoma. The trans-appendicular continent cystostomy was first described by Mitrofanoff [1] in 1980, using the appendix as a conduit between the bladder and the skin. Currently, the appendix remains the conduit of choice, and the most common second option is the transverse ileal (Yang-Monti) tube [2].

Advances in surgical technique have seen the development of both laparoscopic [3] and robotic Mitrofanoff procedures [4] as the robotic-assisted laparoscopic Mitrofanoff appendicovesicostomy RALMA.

2 Patients Positioning and Planning

The operation was performed in a Trendelenburg position. Preoperative intravenous antibiotics of *Cefazolin* 50 mg/kg were administered. A urinary catheter was inserted under aseptic conditions.

3 Incision and Port Placement

A 8-mm 30-degree camera robotic port was placed in the supraumbilical position between umbilicus and epigastric area. Three 8-mm working ports were placed, one at the left upper quadrant, one on the lower right quadrant, and the last on the right upper quadrant. An 8-mm Airseal assistant port was placed in the epigastric area, mainly for bowel retraction and passing sutures (Fig. 1).

A. Paye Jaouen (✉) · A. El Ghoneimi (✉)
Chirurgie viscérale et urologie pédiatriques, Hôpital Robert-Debré, Paris, France
e-mail: annabel.paye-jaouen@aphp.fr

C. Esposito et al. (eds.), *Pediatric Robotic Assisted Surgery*,
https://doi.org/10.1007/978-3-031-99532-3_19

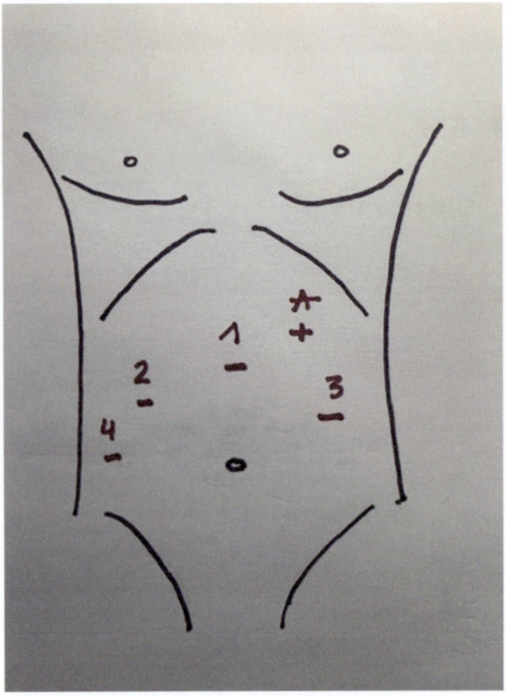

Fig. 1 Port placement. 8-mm robotic ports (2–4); optic 30 degree (1). 8-mm *airseal* assistant trocar (A)

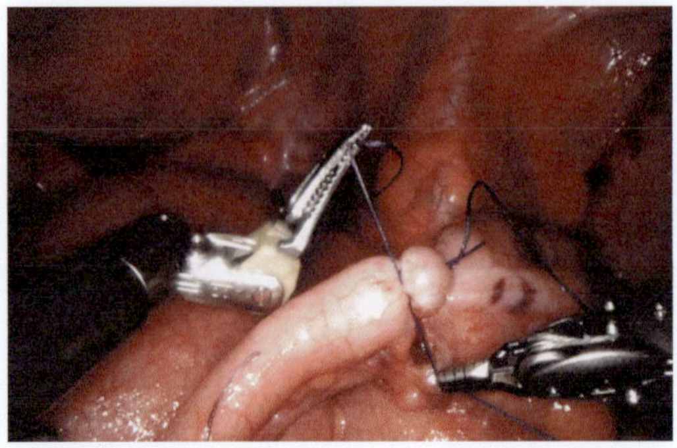

Fig. 2 Appendix

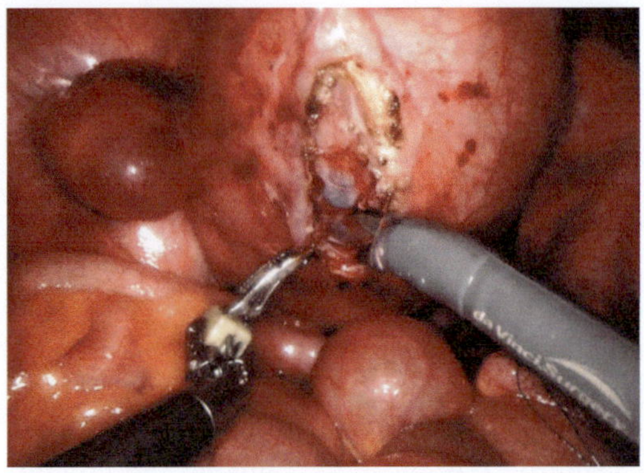

Fig. 3 Detrusorotomy

4 Robot Positioning

The robotic system was docked on the right side of the patient.

5 Procedure Steps

The appendix is identified; a stay suture is placed at the appendicular end for later manipulation. It should be sufficiently mobile to reach the bladder and the umbilicus on the anterior abdominal wall without tension (Fig. 2). The appendix is mobilized with its mesentery near its base and is disconnected from the cecum between two sutures; the mesentery has to be carefully preserved. The appendix is spatulated to prepare the anastomosis with the bladder. An additional mobilization of the cecum and the right colon can be performed if necessary.

The bladder is partially infused with normal saline via the urinary catheter.

A stay suture is placed on the dome of the bladder for retraction and is manipulated using the fourth robotic arm. The site of conduit implantation into the bladder is posterior in our practice.

With the bladder partially filled, a detrusorotomy is made to create a submucosal tunnel (Fig. 3).

The detrusor muscle was incised and opened by electrocautery at the posterior wall of the bladder, and the bladder mucosa is carefully exposed with the scissors. A minimum tunnel length of 4 cm is done. Once the submucosal tunnel is created, the tip of the appendix is spatuled, and the bladder mucosal is opened at the lower side of the tunnel. It is anchored to the bladder with two 5/0 PDS sutures on each side (Fig. 4).

The anterior wall of the appendix is matured to the bladder mucosa with interrupted 6/0 PDS sutures. The appendicovesicostomy was per-

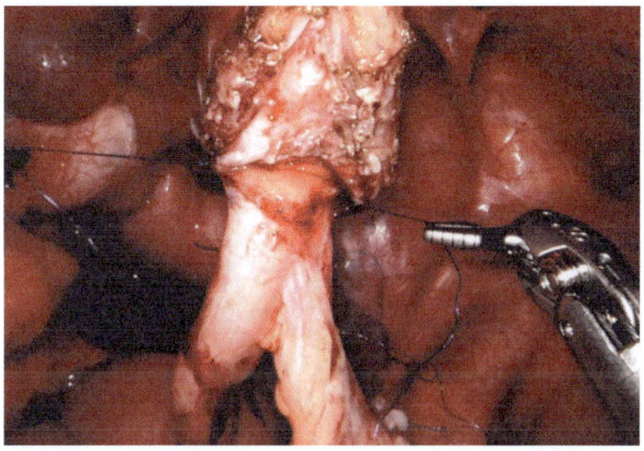

Fig. 4 Appendico-vesicostomy

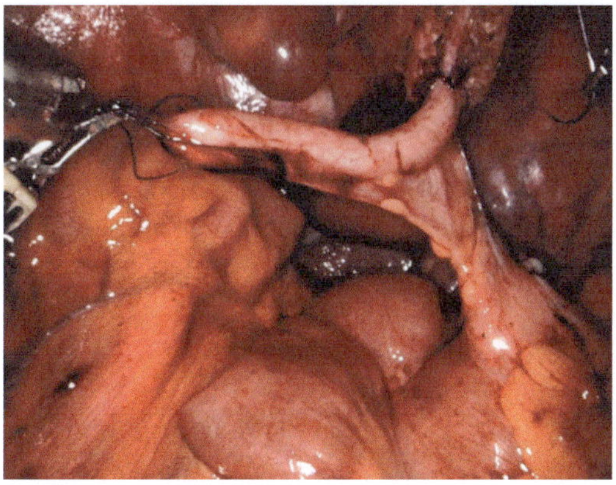

Fig. 5 End of the anastomosis

formed with 6/0 *PDS* in an interrupted manner (Fig. 5). The detrusor layer is reapproximated over the appendix with a running 4/0 polyglactin suture after making fenestrations in the appendix mesentery to create an anti-reflux channel (Fig. 6).

The end of the appendix is next brought through the umbilical area and spatulated, allowing the flap to be placed into a more proximal portion of the umbilical site. The rest of the skin is approximated with interrupted 6/0 PDS sutures. An 12 Fr feeding tube is placed inside and secured with a stitch (Fig. 7).

We use the simplest technique for stoma formation, a direct anastomosis of the intestinal conduit to the skin. This site should be easily accessible by the patient like umbilicus.

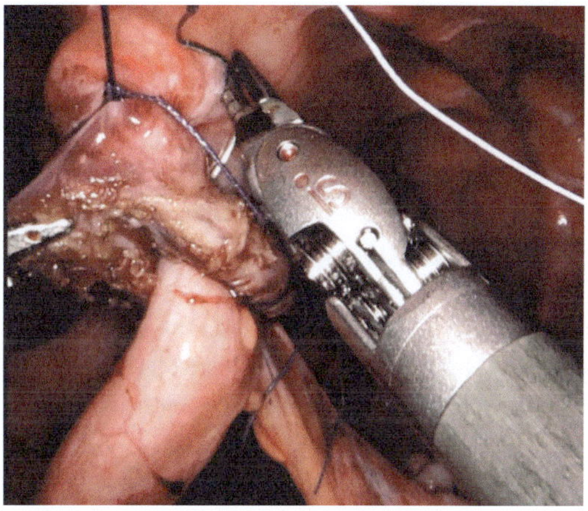

Fig. 6 Antireflux channel

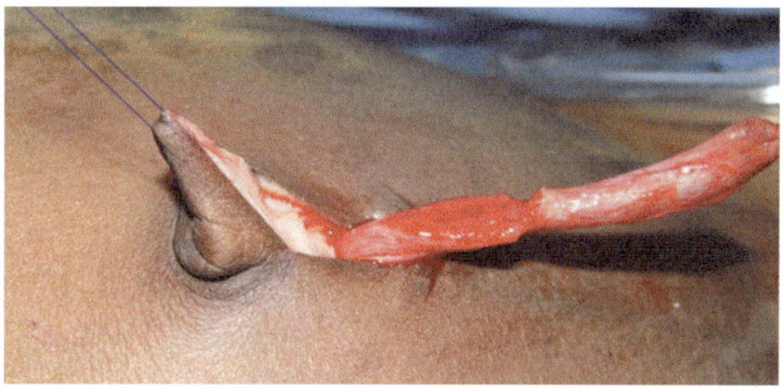

Fig. 7 Umbilical stoma

The port sites are closed with 2/0 Vicryl. Subcutaneous tissues are approximated with 4/0 Vicryl, and the skin is approximated with subcuticular 5/0 PDS sutures.

6 Postoperative Period

Patients were allowed to eat a regular diet immediately. They were discharged once their pain was controlled with oral medications, and they were tolerating a regular diet. The appendicovesicostomy catheter was left in place for 2 weeks. Patients were taught how to perform CIC and instructed to begin CIC with a 12 F straight catheter through the appendicovesicostomy.

7 Tips and Tricks

A stay suture is placed on the dome of the bladder for retraction.

8 Conclusions

Minimally invasive complex bladder reconstruction has become a viable surgical option in pediatric patients since the introduction of the robot [5, 6]. The surgical robot offers three-dimensional visualization and increases degrees of freedom of the instruments [7]. The benefits of applying robotic technology for this procedure are greatest at two stages: first when dissecting the appendiceal blood supply and second when recreating a sealed anastomosis joining the appendix and the bladder mucosa [8]. This anastomosis is easier and faster to perform with the surgical robot, and this procedure is more comfortable for the surgeon too. Robotics can be safely performed in children, especially if surgeon has a previous laparoscopic background [9].

A first multicenter study (Gundetti) reporting the outcomes of RALMA which was performed in a pediatric patient population of 88 patients at 5 centers [10]: Regarding functional outcomes, 75 (85.2%) patients were initially continent, and after additional procedures, 81 (92.0%) patients were continent at last follow-up. The mean operative time was more favorable at 309 min (5.2 h). Short-term results are encouraging, but longer follow-up reports are required.

References

1. Mitrofanoff P. Trans-appendicular continent cystostomy in the management of the neurogenic bladder. Chir Pédiatrique. 1980;21:297e305.
2. Storm DW, Fulmer BR, Sumfest JM. Laparoscopic robot-assisted appendicovesicostomy: an initial experience. J Endourol. 2007;21:1015–7.
3. Blanc T, Muller C, Pons M, Pashootan P, Paye-Jaouen A, El Ghoneimi A. Laparoscopic Mitrofanoff procedure in children: critical analysis of difficulties and benefits. J Pediatr Urol. 2015 Feb;11(1):28.e1–8.
4. Nguyen HT, Passerotti CC, Penna FJ, Retik AB, Peters CA. Robotic assisted laparoscopic Mitrofanoff appendicovesicostomy: preliminary experience in a pediatric population. J Urol. 2009;182:1528–34.
5. Gundeti MS, Acharya SS, Zagaja GP, Shalhav AL. Paediatric robotic- assisted laparoscopic augmentation ileocystoplasty and Mitrofanoff appendicovesicostomy (RALIMA): feasibility of and initial experience with the University of Chicago technique. BJU Int. 2011;107:962–9.
6. Rodriguez MV, Wallace A, Gundeti MS. Robotic bladder neck reconstruction with mitrofanoff appendicovesicostomy in a neurogenic bladder patient. Urology. 2020;137:206–7.
7. Fuchs M, DaJusta DG. Robotics in pediatric urology. IBJU. 2020;46(3):322–7.
8. Chan IHY, Li FHQ, Lan LCL, Wong KKY, Yip PKF, Tam PKH. Use of robotic-assisted laparoscopic Mitrofanoff appendicovesicostomy in a paediatric patient: problem encountered. Hong Kong Med J. 2015;21:468–70.
9. Esposito C, Autorino G, Castagnetti M, Cerulo M, Coppola V, Cardone R, Esposito G, Borgogni R, Escolino M. Robotics and future technical developments in pediatric urology. Semin Pediatr Surg. 2021;30:151082.
10. Gundeti MS, Petravick ME, Pariser JJ, Pearce SM, Anderson BB, Grimsby GM, et al. A multi-institutional study of perioperative and functional outcomes for pediatric robotic-assisted laparoscopic Mitrofanoff appendicovesicostomy. J Pediatr Urol. 2016;12(386):e1–386.e5.

Robotic Retroperitoneal Approach

Kiarash Taghavi, Aline Broch, Fabrizio Vatta, Nathalie Botto, and Thomas Blanc

1 Introduction

The retroperitoneal approach in pediatric urology, when part of a surgeon's armamentarium, has many possible applications and benefits. The parietal peritoneum is covered in a dense network of nerves sensitive to pain, pressure, touch, friction, cutting, and temperature. Noxious stimuli are perceived as a localized, sharp pain [1]. Causes of pain after transperitoneal laparoscopy include (in varying degrees): distension-induced neuropraxia of the phrenic nerves, acid intraperitoneal milieu, residual intra-abdominal gas after laparoscopy, humidity of the insufflated gas, and volume of insufflated gas [2]. Therefore, it is not surprising that the retroperitoneal approach is associated with less postoperative pain when compared to transperitoneal in patients undergoing adrenal or kidney surgery [3–5].

Avoiding violation of the peritoneal approach also avoids potential organ injury, ileus, and formation of intraperitoneal adhesions. Return of bowel function has been confirmed to be reduced when a retroperitoneal approach is utilized for adrenal or kidney surgery [3, 5]. Furthermore, in the unlikely event of urinary leak, limiting this to perirenal space is advantageous. Benefits in postoperative pain and return of bowel function translate to the frequently reported reduced hospital stay for retroperitoneal surgery in comparative studies [6]. In pediatrics, this has led to retroperitoneal robot-assisted laparoscopic pyeloplasty being performed as a day procedure in selected cases [7]. The rate of admission for small bowel obstruction over the first 5 years in children following abdominal surgery is 1.1% [5]. This also has significant implications when considering the lifelong risk in children. Furthermore, in redo-surgery, application of ability to utilize either approach allows surgery to be performed through virgin planes.

There are further benefits of retroperitoneoscopy when applied to oncology surgery. A retroperitoneal approach provides better access for nephron-sparing surgery in posterior tumors and a more direct approach to small adrenal tumors [8]. It also limits radiotherapy to the tumor bed in the unlikely event of Wilms tumor rupture or breach [9] in nephron-sparing surgery. It can also

K. Taghavi
Department of Paediatric Urology, Monash Children's Hospital, Melbourne, VIC, Australia

Department of Paediatrics, Monash University, Monash Children's Hospital Level 5, Melbourne, VIC, Australia

A. Broch · N. Botto
Service de Chirurgie Viscérale, Urologie et Transplantation Pédiatrique, Hôpital Necker-Enfants Malades, APHP, Paris, France

F. Vatta · T. Blanc (✉)
Service de Chirurgie Viscérale, Urologie et Transplantation Pédiatrique, Hôpital Necker-Enfants Malades, APHP, Paris, France

Université Paris Cité, Paris, France
e-mail: thomas.blanc@aphp.fr

C. Esposito et al. (eds.), *Pediatric Robotic Assisted Surgery*,
https://doi.org/10.1007/978-3-031-99532-3_20

be applied to retroperitoneal lymph node dissection.

The selective use of retroperitoneal robotic surgery requires deliberate development and maintenance of experience in both retroperitoneal surgery and robotics. Challenges to achieving this include technical challenges, limited case numbers, restricted training time, and a steep learning curve [10]. The multidisciplinary robotic program at Hôpital Necker-Enfants Malades has applied robotic retroperitoneal surgery in children undergoing pyeloplasty, nephron-sparing surgery, adrenal surgery, and lymph node dissection with safety and efficacy [9, 11, 12]. These results have been reproduced in other pediatric contexts [13]. A meticulous and systematic approach is required at every step to ensure safe and effective application.

2 Patient Positioning and Planning

The patient is placed in the lateral position with their back close to the edge of the table (Fig. 1). Small lumbar padding is placed underneath them to widen the costo-iliac distance. The arms are placed above the shoulders while maintaining pressure cares. The patient is secured with tape to prevent displacement.

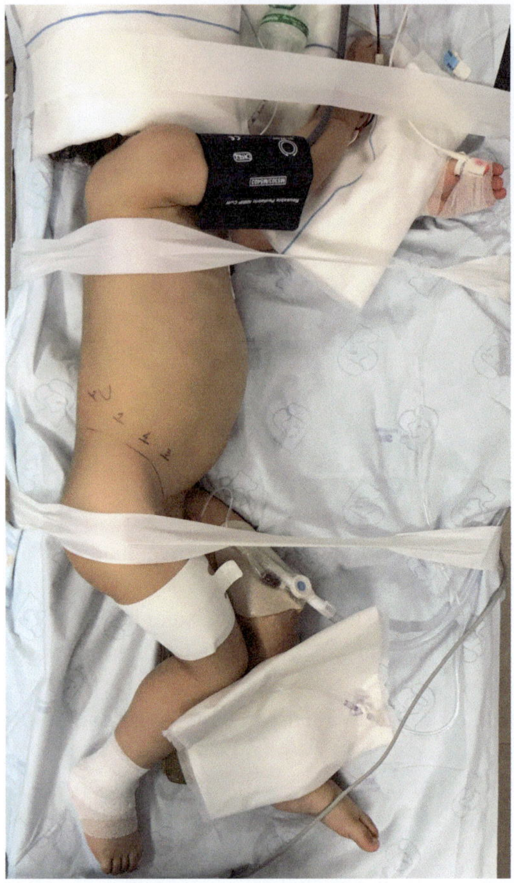

Fig. 1 Patient positioning and port placement for robotic retroperitoneal surgery

3 Incision and Port Placement

Surface landmarks are marked: the iliac crest, the 12th rib, and the costovertebral angle (Fig. 2). Three 8-mm robotic ports and one 5-mm assistant port are placed in an imaginary line drawn from the iliovertebral angle to the iliac fossa. Port placement is identical for all cases and ages.

4 Robot Positioning

The patient cart is placed on the side of the operating table anterior to the patient (Fig. 3).

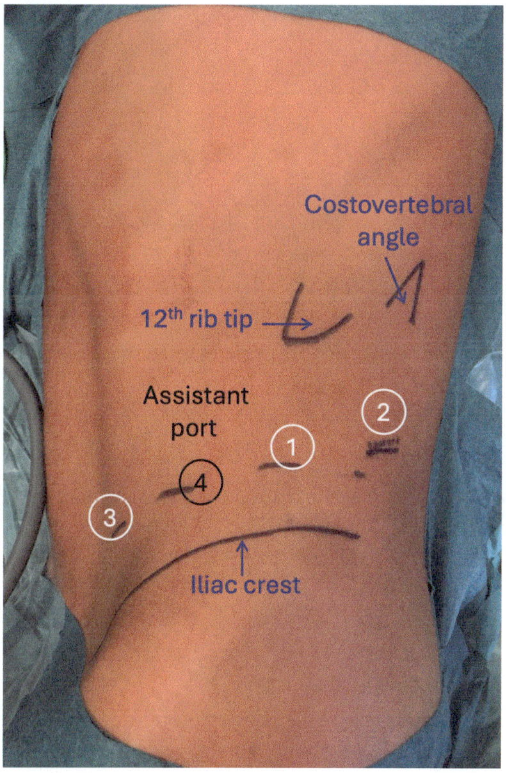

Fig. 2 Details of key surface landmarks and port placement

Fig. 3 Illustration of room setup

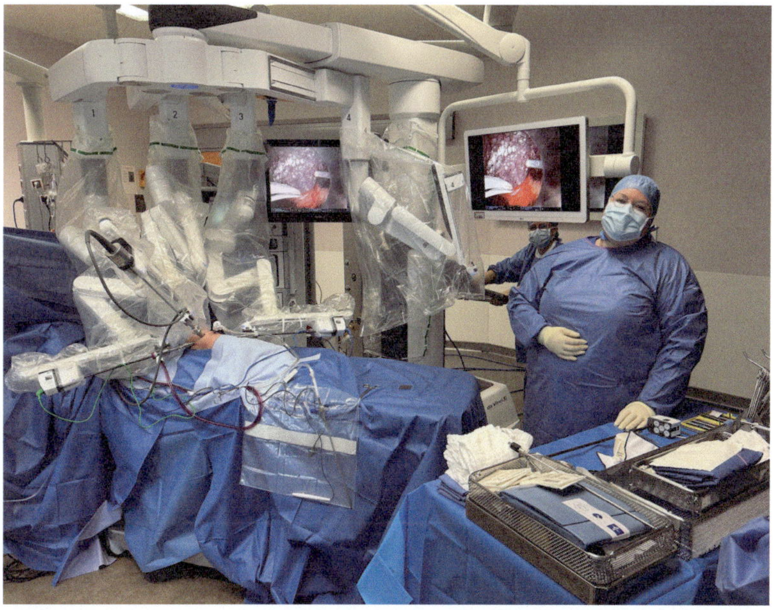

5 Procedure Steps

- An initial 15-mm incision is made for the camera port in the midaxillary line, between the iliac crest to the 12th rib, and retroperitoneal access is achieved with a muscle splitting blunt dissection. For ease of insertion of the 8-mm robotic trocar port, blunt dissection is completed with a straight Halsted mosquito forceps.
- Expansion of the retroperitoneal space is commenced under direct vision with the flat tip of the 0-degree camera (no need for finger or balloon dissection).
- The second port is inserted under direct vision at the angle of the iliac crest and the lateral border of the paraspinal muscles. An 23G needle is used to visualize port placement to ensure the location as optimal and safe. Working space is further expanded with the 0-degree camera.
- A third 8-mm port is inserted in the iliac fossa (at the edge of rectus abdominis muscle).
- The 0-degree optical system is now used and when turning it with the laparoscope just parallel to the inner layer of the abdominal wall, the peritoneal reflection is easily identified.
- The camera is moved to the costovertebral angle to optimize the view for the insertion of the optional assistant port (between the camera and the iliac fossa port). Again, the needle is used to ensure optimal port placement.
- The ports are placed linearly from the iliovertebral angle to the iliac fossa. The robotic Airseal system is plugged onto the posterior trocar and insufflation onto the assistant port. Carbon dioxide insufflation pressure does not exceed 12 mmHg, and the flow rate is 5 L/min.
- After docking, due to the limited working space, the first instrument inserted in the tunnel created with the camera is the monopolar curved scissors (left port).
- The retroperitoneal space is further developed with the two robotic instruments in a caudocranial manner, close to the quadratus lumborum muscle. Gerota's fascia is identified and widely opened with the monopolar curved scissors. With the scissors in the left hand, adhesions between the posterior aspect of the kidney and the psoas muscle are divided. It is very important to maintain meticulous hemostasis to maintain clear vision.
- The two robotic instruments are swapped to have the scissors in the right hand. The scissors must stay parallel to the psoas muscle (1 cm above), maintaining distance from the vena cava on the right or the aorta on the left.
- Insufflation and gravity displace the kidney superomedially, which correspondingly appears on the upper portion of the screen. The left hand (with micro bipolar forceps) is crucial in lifting the kidney up and freeing it from the psoas. The insufflation pressure also facilitates creation evolution of this space. The lower pole of the kidney, the renal pelvis, the ureter, and the renal pedicle are systematically defined.

6 Postoperative Period

In the context of a multidisciplinary pathway, we have performed retroperitoneal pyeloplasty as day surgery in selected cases [7]. This can be considered once the robotic program is well-established, and surgical team is comfortable with the retroperitoneal approach. The defined criteria were the following:

- Preoperative criteria: parental informed consent, family home within 150 km of the hospital, child over 2 years of age, primary pelviureteric junction obstruction (e.g., not redo cases).
- Intraoperative criteria: first case on a morning list, robotic surgery completed by 1:00 PM, uneventful intraoperative course, no urinary catheter, no perirenal drainage tube required.
- Postoperative criteria: no immediate postoperative complications, hemodynamically stable in recovery, ambulating without significant difficulty, tolerating oral fluids, pain controlled on oral analgesics, void prior to discharge.

7 Tips and Tricks

- The first trocar is fixed with a 0 PDS purse-string suture to ensure an airtight seal and to allow traction with the Hasson cone in order to maximize working space.
- To avoid inadvertent transperitoneal insertion/breach, the retroperitoneal working space is fully developed with the 0-degree camera by identifying the deep surface of the anterior wall muscles and pushing the peritoneum medially with a laparoscopic bipolar forceps. The objective is to create a tunnel (mirroring the line of port insertion externally) in which the robotic instruments can be inserted safely for docking.
- The camera is moved in the iliac fossa to reduce the depth of insertion of the two first trocars and maximize working space for the procedure. The Hasson cone is advantageous in maintaining stability to the depth of insertion selected.
- A major limitation lies in the depth needed to operate the robotic instrument in the small retroperitoneal space in children. Insertion of the robotic instruments has to be carefully performed.
- It is very important to keep orientation in the retroperitoneal space with the psoas muscle being a major landmark which has to be always kept on the lower part of the screen. The camera is orientated to have the psoas muscle parallel to the screen.

8 Discussion and Conclusion

Retroperitoneal kidney and adrenal surgery is safe and effective in children and presents significant potential benefits. Implementation must be staged, with careful case selection in the context of a multidisciplinary team setting. Surgical technique should follow a meticulous step-by-step pathway with attention to patient positioning, port placement, surgical orientation, and careful systematic dissection.

References

1. Struller F, Weinreich F-J, Horvath P, Kokkalis M-K, Beckert S, Königsrainer A, Reymond MA. Peritoneal innervation: embryology and functional anatomy. Pleura Peritoneum. 2017;2(4):153–61.
2. Mouton W, Bessell J, Otten K, Maddern G. Pain after laparoscopy. Surg Endosc. 1999;13:445–8.
3. Lee CR, Walz MK, Park S, Park JH, Jeong JS, Lee SH, Kang S-W, Jeong JJ, Nam K-H, Chung WY. A comparative study of the transperitoneal and posterior retroperitoneal approaches for laparoscopic adrenalectomy for adrenal tumors. Ann Surg Oncol. 2012;19:2629–34.
4. Rassweiler J, Frede T, Henkel TO, Stock C, Alken P. Nephrectomy: a comparative study between the transperitoneal and retroperitoneal laparoscopic versus the open approach. Eur Urol. 1998;33(5):489–96.
5. Chua ME, Ming JM, Kim JK, Milford KL, Silangcruz JM, Ren L, Rickard M, Lorenzo AJ. Meta-analysis of retroperitoneal vs transperitoneal laparoscopic and robot-assisted pyeloplasty for the management of pelvi-ureteric junction obstruction. BJU Int. 2021;127(6):687–702.
6. Blanc T, Abbo O, Vatta F, Grosman J, Marquant F, Elie C, Juricic M, Laraqui S, Broch A, Arnaud A. Transperitoneal versus retroperitoneal robotic-assisted laparoscopic pyeloplasty for ureteropelvic junction obstruction in children. A multicentre, prospective study. Eur Urol Open Sci. 2022;41:134–40.
7. Broch A, Paye-Jaouen A, Bruneau B, Glenisson M, Taghavi K, Botto N, Goulin J, Lopez P, Querciagrossa S, El Ghoneimi A, Dahmani S, Hidalgo M, Blanc T. Day surgery in children undergoing retroperitoneal robot-assisted laparoscopic pyeloplasty: is it safe and feasible? Eur Urol Open Sci. 2023;51:55–61.
8. Taghavi K, Glenisson M, Loiselet K, Fiorenza V, Cornet M, Capito C, Vinit N, Pire A, Sarnacki S, Blanc T. Robot-assisted laparoscopic adrenalectomy: Extended application in children. Eur J Surg Oncol. 2024;50(12):108627.
9. Blanc T, Taghavi K, Glenisson M, Capito C, Couloigner V, Vinit N, Sarnacki S. Robotic surgery in paediatric oncology: expanding boundaries and defining relevant indications. J Pediatr Surg. 2024;60:162017.
10. Andolfi C, Adamic B, Oommen J, Gundeti MS. Robot-assisted laparoscopic pyeloplasty in infants and children: is it superior to conventional laparoscopy? World J Urol. 2019;38(8):1827–33.
11. Blanc T, Kohaut J, Elie C, Clermidi P, Pio L, Harte C, Brönnimann E, Botto N, Rousseau V, Sonigo P, Vaessen C, Lottmann H, Aigrain Y. Retroperitoneal approach for ureteropelvic junction obstruction: encouraging

preliminary results with robot-assisted laparoscopic repair. Front Pediatr. 2019;7.
12. Franzini S, Querciagrossa S, Brebion M, Consonni D, Blanc T, Orliaguet G. Effect of retropneumoperitoneum on cerebral and renal oxygen saturation during retroperitoneal robotic-assisted laparoscopic pyeloplasty (R-RALP) in a pediatric population: Preliminary results of a prospective observational study using a dedicated anesthetic protocol and Near-InfraRed Spectroscopy. Anaesth Crit Care Pain Med. 2023;42(5):101234.
13. Li P, Ma Y, Jin X, Xiang L, Li H, Wang K. Comparative efficacy and safety of different minimal invasive pyeloplasty in treating patients with ureteropelvic junction obstruction: a network meta-analysis. World J Urol. 2023;41(10):2659–69.

Robot-Assisted Kidney Transplantation in Children

Inge Van de Caveye, Joris Vangeneugden, Mauro Van den Ende, Eva Donck, Charles van Praet, Karel Decaestecker, and Anne-Françoise Spinoit

1 Introduction

Kidney transplantation is universally acknowledged as the golden standard treatment for both adults and children with end-stage renal disease (ESRD) [1]. Kidney transplant recipients, who are immunocompromised, may face a higher risk of perioperative surgical complications, adding to the challenges in their management. Utilizing minimally invasive surgical techniques may help to improve clinical outcomes and reduce morbidity in this fragile patient population.

Although robot-assisted kidney transplantation (RAKT) is more and more studied in the adult population [2], reports describing RAKT in children are scarce.

Pediatric RAKT brings additional challenges to both the surgical and anesthesiology team, due to specific characteristics in this population such as a small abdominal cavity and a smaller circulating blood volume. Initial data prove RAKT in children to be safe and feasible resulting in excellent graft function when performed by an experienced team [3].

Bansal et al. were one of the first to compare RAKT versus open kidney transplantation (OKT) in a pediatric population. Their results revealed comparable outcomes in terms of graft function and a significantly lower analgesic requirement for the RAKT group [4]. Moreover, robotic procedures offer the advantage of almost no surgical site infections, shorter drain removal time, shorter hospital stay, and better cosmetic results [2, 3]. It seems that we can extend these perceptions to the pediatric population but, as already cited, the scientific evidence on this is limited. Patients undergoing kidney transplantation, regardless of the technique used, are usually fragile and immunocompromised state and might be at a higher risk for developing perioperative complications compared to renal donors. These complications impact not only short-term patient recovery but also compromise long-term graft and patient survival. It seems that we can extend these perceptions on RAKT to the pediatric population, but the scientific evidence on this is limited.

In the literature, various techniques for RAKT have been described in adults. These techniques differ in patient positioning, graft placement, and the method of ureteral reimplantation. In this

I. Van de Caveye · J. Vangeneugden · M. Van den Ende · E. Donck · C. van Praet · A.-F. Spinoit (✉)
Department of Urology, ERN eUROGEN Accredited Centre, Ghent University Hospital, Ghent, Belgium
e-mail: Inge.VandeCaveye@uzgent.be; Joris.vangeneugden@uzgent.be; Mauro.vandenende@uzgent.be; Eva.donck@uzgent.be; Charles.vanpraet@uzgent.be

K. Decaestecker
Department of Urology, Maria-Middelares Hospital, Ghent Belgium & Department of Urology, ERN eUROGEN Accredited Centre, Ghent University Hospital, Ghent, Belgium
e-mail: Karel.decaestecker@uzgent.be

C. Esposito et al. (eds.), *Pediatric Robotic Assisted Surgery*,
https://doi.org/10.1007/978-3-031-99532-3_21

chapter, we elaborate on the surgical steps of pediatric RAKT and provide tips and tricks for optimizing results in this fragile patient population.

2 Patient Positioning and Planning

The patient is positioned in a dorsal decubitus position. The challenge in this pediatric population compared to the adult one is port placement, as the space is usually limited. Padding is essential and cannot be standardized as needs to be adapted according to the child's weight and height.

The required robotic instruments include monopolar curved scissors, bipolar forceps, Maryland bipolar forceps, needle driver, prograsp forceps, and robotic bulldog clamps.

When possible, two operating rooms will work simultaneously, one for harvesting the kidney in the donor and the second one for preparation of the recipient's side. If this can be performed simultaneously, it allows for minimal ischemia time between the harvesting and the placement in the recipient.

In the first room, the donor kidney is harvested using robot-assisted techniques as well described. This can either be performed laparoscopically or robotically. When two robots are available like in our department, we prefer to use both robots. The organ is defatted and when need further preparted, while perfused with cold Ringer's lactate, as is standard in conventional kidney transplantation, starting the cold ischemia time. The graft is then encased in a gauze jacket filled with ice slush, leaving an opening for the hilar structures. A long silk tie is used to mark the upper pole of the kidney. This ice jacket serves dual purposes: cooling the kidney and enabling atraumatic handling during anastomoses [4] (Fig. 1).

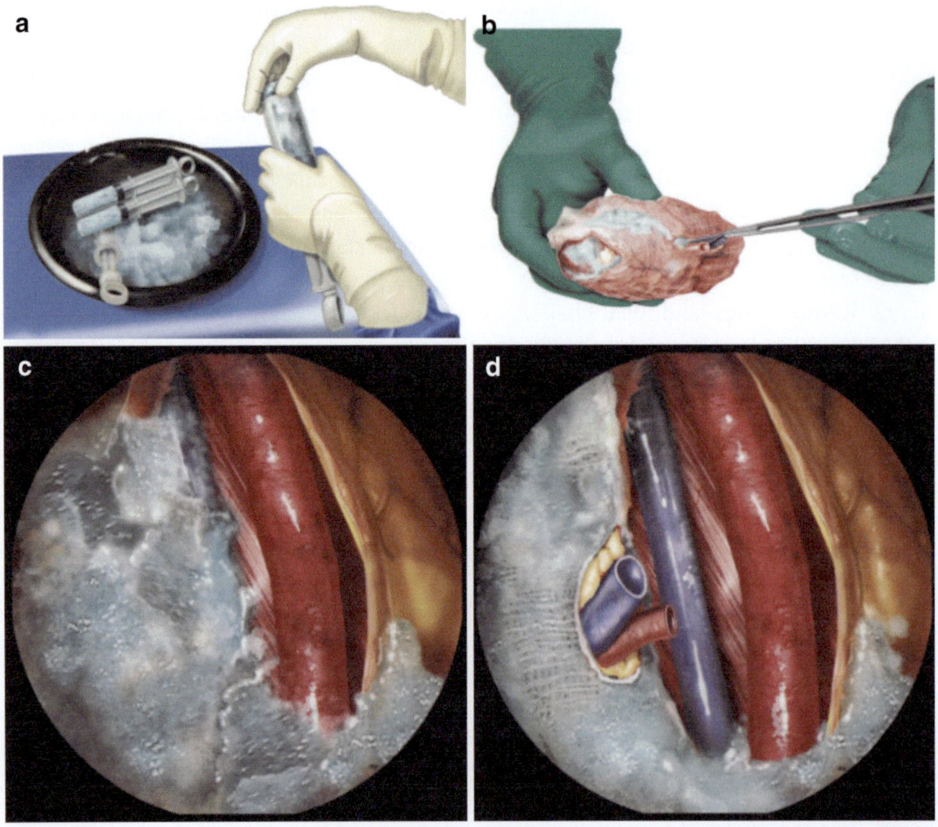

Fig. 1 (**a**) Multiple modified Toomey syringes being readied for rapid delivery of ice slush. (**b**) Graft kidney wrapped in a gauze jacket filled with ice slush. (**c**) Pelvic bed lined with ice slush to achieve pelvic-bed cooling before introduction of the graft kidney. (**d**) Additional ice slush delivered onto the graft kidney immediately after its introduction to achieve uniform cooling. (Adapted from Menon et al. [4])

3 Incision and Port Placement

A median supraumbilical incision of 5 cm is used to place the GelPOINT device. The GelPOINT device (Applied Medical Resources Corp, Rancho Santa Margarita, CA, USA), a hand-access platform, allows easy introduction of the ice slush and the graft. The GelPOINT device consists of two parts: a GelSeal cap and an access port. A robotic camera port and a 12-mm assistant port are placed into the GelSeal cap.

The AirSeal system is used to maintain a stable and low-pressure pneumoperitoneum of 8 mmHg. Three extra robotic ports of 8 mm are placed under direct vision, 2 in the left fossa and 1 in the right iliac fossa (Fig. 2). Optimal positioning of ports is of high importance in pediatric patients. After the ports are placed, this is followed by a transition to a lithotomy position and shift to 15–20 degree Trendelenburg tilt.

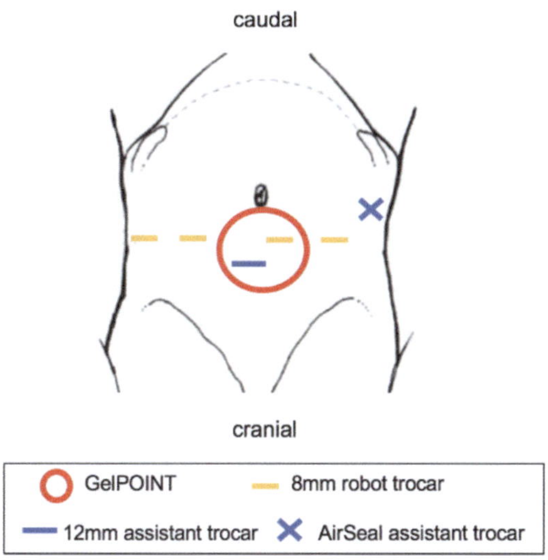

Fig. 2 Port positioning in pediatric RAKT

4 Robot Positioning

For this procedure, the Da Vinci robot is side-docked at the left side.

5 Procedure Steps

An overview of the different steps (Fig. 3):

Step 1: Preparing iliac vessels and bladder for anastomosis
Step 2: Creating retroperitoneal pocket
Step 3: Graft introduction
Step 4: Venous anastomosis
Step 5: Arterial anastomosis
Step 6: Flipping and retroperitonealization
Step 7: Ureteroneocystostomy (Lich-Gregoir)

The procedure starts with the identification and skeletonization of the right external iliac vessels. The bladder is dissected laterodorsally on the right side (if right-sided graft implantation). An incision is made in the peritoneum laterally, approximately 2 cm from the colonic flexure of the ascending colon to create a peritoneal flap. Slushed ice is introduced into the abdomen, and the donor kidney is placed inside, wrapped in a compress with slushed ice. Bulldog clamps are placed proximally and distally on the common iliac vein, followed by a longitudinal venotomy. The site is rinsed with heparinized saline. An end-to-side anastomosis is performed using a Gore-Tex 8-0 continuous suture. Flushing with heparinized saline via a 5F catheter is conducted before completing the suture. The renal vein is clamped with a Bulldog clamp. The clamps on the external iliac vein are released, and new

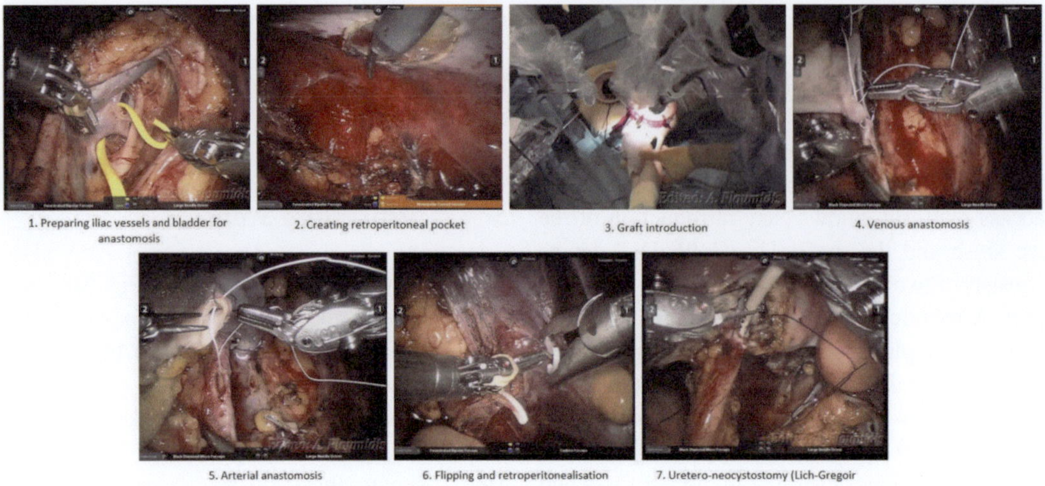

Fig. 3 Overview of the different surgical steps in pediatric RAKT

clamps are placed on the external iliac artery proximally and distally. The kidney is recovered with slushed ice. An incision is made in the common iliac artery and extended with an aortic punch. An end-to-side anastomosis is then performed with the donor artery, which has been spatulated, using a Gore-Tex 8-0 continuous suture. Flushing is conducted before completing the suture. Clamps are released, allowing for kidney reperfusion. The kidney is checked for coloration, turgor, and diuresis. The kidney is retroperitonealized, and the peritoneum is closed with two Hem-o-Lock clips. The bladder is inflated, and incision of the detrusor is performed for a modified Lich-Gregoir ureteroneocystostomy with dissection down to the mucosa. The ureter is tunneled under the spermatic cord or round ligament depending on sex. The ureter is trimmed to the appropriate length and spatulated. An incision is made in the bladder mucosa, and a corner stitch is placed with PDS 5.0 caudally for the vesicoureteral anastomosis. A continuous suture is performed. A double J stent is placed, and the suture is completed. The detrusor muscle is approximated with a V-lock 3.0 continuous suture. We check for adequate hemostasis. A 21 silicone drain is placed. The trocars are removed under direct vision. The median laparotomy is closed with PDS 2.0 for the fascia, Vicryl 2.0 for the subcutaneous tissue, and Monocryl 4.0 using an intradermal technique for the skin. The trocar incisions are closed with Vicryl 1 and Monocryl 4.0, followed by application of skin adhesive.

6 Postoperative Period

Postoperative care for robot-assisted kidney transplantation does not significantly differ from that of open kidney transplantation, with the primary difference being faster recovery and mobilization.

Immediately posttransplantation, most children are cared for in the pediatric intensive care unit to ensure close monitoring of hemodynamic stability, fluid balance, and graft perfusion optimization. Thus, pediatric intensivists should be well-versed in immediate postoperative management [5].

6.1 Postoperative Monitoring

Frequent hemodynamic evaluation is crucial, with vital signs checked every hour for 24 hours, every 2 hours for the next 8 hours, and then every 4 hours for stable patients. Blood pressure should be kept above 90 mmHg for adequate graft perfusion, and urinary catheter patency maintained for at least 72 hours. Urine output must be monitored every 30–60 minutes initially, and central venous pressures assessed to guide fluid management. Abdominal drains should be monitored for at least 48 hours to detect complications such as urinary fistula, lymphorrhea, or bleeding. Signs of infection, which may not include elevated temperature, should be closely watched, including changes in consciousness, cloudy or foul-smelling urine, or purulent wound drainage [6, 7].

6.2 Postoperative Laboratory Orders and Investigations

Upon arrival in the PICU, a CBC, serum creatinine, and liver function tests should be obtained and then repeated daily. Electrolytes need to be monitored two to three times daily for the first few postoperative days. Additional investigations include a Doppler ultrasound of the renal arteries to assess vascular integrity and graft perfusion [8]. Coagulation parameters should be obtained, and low-molecular-weight heparin is administered to target an APTT of 60 seconds, and acetylsalicylic acid is started. Creatinine levels in drainage liquid are monitored on the first postoperative day.

6.3 Sedation and Pain Control

As morphine is contraindicated in impaired renal function, postoperative analgesia may be provided with fentanyl and paracetamol. Fentanyl synthetic opioid may be used in renal failure as continuous infusion. It provides good postoperative analgesia without respiratory depression [6].

6.4 Immunosuppression

Immunosuppression induction therapy during the perioperative period typically involves high-dose corticosteroids and either anti-IL2 receptor antibodies (basiliximab) or antilymphocyte antibodies, depending on the risk of graft loss. Maintenance immunosuppression includes corticosteroids, antimetabolites (azathioprine or mycophenolate), and calcineurin inhibitors (cyclosporine or tacrolimus) [9].

6.5 Infection in Renal Transplant

For perioperative antibacterial prophylaxis, cefazolin (or vancomycin/clindamycin for allergies) is used for 24 hours. Ganciclovir or valganciclovir is administered for CMV prophylaxis in at-risk patients, while oral nystatin and cotrimoxazole prevent fungal and pneumocystis carinii infections. Posttransplant infection risks are categorized into three time frames: the first month, the second to sixth months, and beyond the sixth month. Due to immunosuppression masking typical infection signs like fever and leukocytosis, diagnosing infections requires high clinical suspicion and prompt empiric antimicrobial therapy based on the infection site. Several diseases can recur [10, 11].

6.6 Double J Stent

Double J stent remains in situ for 3 weeks and may subsequently be removed under targeted antibiotic therapy based on previous urine culture.

6.7 Complications

Delayed graft function (DGF), indicated by the need for dialysis within the first week posttransplant or persistently elevated serum creatinine, often involves acute tubular necrosis and is signaled by declining urine output [9]. Acute rejection, typically occurring 5–7 days posttransplant, is suspected with rising serum creatinine levels. Monitoring for drug toxicity (leucopenia, neutropenia, high blood sugar, nephrotoxicity, hyperkalemia, hypomagnesemia) is essential. Hypertension, commonly due to intravascular volume expansion, high-dose steroids, and calcineurin inhibitors, can be managed with long-acting agents like amlodipine [12–14].

7 Tips and Tricks

7.1 Specifics Requiring Special Attention for Kidney Transplantation in Children

Warm ischemia time has been recognized as a negative predictive factor for long-term patient and graft survival outcomes. In adult RAKT series, a broad range of ischemia times has been documented, but no correlation has been found between rewarming time and graft function. To mitigate potential damage from prolonged warm ischemia, Menon et al. introduced a technique involving regional hypothermia with ice slush during vascular anastomosis. Unlike the adult RAKT procedure, in pediatric RAKT, the graft renal vessels are anastomosed to the common iliac vessels rather than the external iliac vessels. This adjustment accommodates the size discrepancy between the donor's adult-sized renal vessels and the recipient's pediatric-sized iliac vessels [4].

It should be noted that, according to the literature, renal blood flow and function are reduced in the presence of pneumoperitoneum, potentially leading to graft impairment. The potential damage to the graft as a result of pneumoperitoneum is not yet fully understood, and no correlation between operative time (and thus exposure to pneumoperitoneum) and graft function in adult RAKT has been identified. Besides the anesthetic concerns regarding intra-abdominal pressure, this may be another reason to keep intra-abdominal pressure around 10 mmHg or lower. We prefer a stable low pneumoperitoneum pressure of 8 mmHg for both the (RA) laparoscopic living donor nephrectomy and RAKT from the moment of reperfusion to mitigate any potential adverse effects of higher pneumoperitoneum pressures on the donor and/or recipient [3].

7.2 Surgical Challenges of RALS in Children

The relatively small size of the abdominal cavity of a child presents multiple operative challenges. This decreased workspace in pediatric abdominal surgeries makes trocar placement a critical procedural component as it can impact desufflation risk, bleeding risk, and organ damage. Poorly positioned trocars may generate a gas leak, provoking rapid desufflation and further decreasing the small workspace. The use of the AirSeal system can help to maintain a stable working space with a very low pneumoperitoneum pressure. Bleeding can be particularly dangerous in children, as their already limited circulating volume causes any unrecognized or uncontrolled bleeding to be hazardous to cardiovascular function. Pediatric abdominal cavities typically contain adjacent organs in tight proximity to each other, increasing the risk for damage to surrounding organs during surgical procedures. Therefore, surgeons should be aware that open placement of the first trocar under direct vision (Hasson technique) is the preferred method for the pediatric population. Trocar positioning is also important for maximization of robot dexterity within the already restricted pediatric abdominal cavity. The recommended 8-cm gap for collision avoidance between the robot arms in adult RALS cases is often impossible in children due to workspace space limitations. Contrary to some adult procedures, there is no standardized trocar placement in robotic pediatric procedures due to broad variations in weight and height which are dependent on patient age. Trocar positioning should therefore be individually adjusted to allow optimal workspace. It is also worth to mention that the later generation robots (such as Da Vinci Xi and X) facilitate the docking procedure related to easy connection of instruments and the increased movement ability of the patient cart. Additionally, while most robotic adult procedures involve four robot arms, the limited workspace in pediatric patients commonly only allows usage of three out of four robot arms (camera port and two robotic ports) without any additional 5-mm assisting port. In our initial phase of RAKT in children, our team opted for four robot arms with two assisting ports (the standardized adult port position) to limit operative time and more specifically to limit the (re) warm(ing) ischemia time, as these factors are potentially associated with adverse long-term patient and graft survival outcomes [3].

7.3 Anesthetic Considerations for RALS

Anesthetists should consider the following challenges in robotic surgical case: increased abdominal pressure, hypothermia, increased CO2 absorption, and the physiologic effects of Trendelenburg position. These may impair cardiovascular function and ventilation, induce cerebral vasodilatation, and negatively affect urine output. Anesthetists should take note that intra-abdominal pressures lower than 10 mmHg do not appear to induce any significant clinical hemodynamic effects, and pressures up to 12 mmHg seem to be well-tolerated [3].

8 Discussion and Conclusion

Performing RAKT in children with ESRD is a safe and feasible procedure. The procedure and outcomes are comparable with RAKT in an adult population, but nevertheless there are some non-negligible differences.

References

1. Collins AJ, Foley RN, Gilbertson DT, Chen SC. United States Renal Data System public health surveillance of chronic kidney disease and end-stage renal disease. Kidney Int Suppl. 2015;5(1):2–7.
2. Breda A, Territo A, Gausa L, Tuğcu V, Alcaraz A, Musquera M, Decaestecker K, Desender L, Stockle M, Janssen M, Fornara P. Robot-assisted kidney transplantation: the European experience. Eur Urol. 2018;73(2):273–81.
3. Grammens J, Schechter M, Desender L, Claeys T, Sinatti C, VandeWalle J, Vermassen F, Raes A, Vanpeteghem C, Prytula A, Silay M, Breda A, Decaestecker K, Spinoit AF. Pediatric challenges in robot-assisted kidney transplantation. Front Surg. 2021;8:649418. https://doi.org/10.3389/fsurg.2021.649418.
4. Menon M, et al. Robotic kidney transplantation with regional hypothermia: a step-by-step description of the Vattikuti Urology Institute–Medanta technique (IDEAL phase 2a). Eur Urol. 2014;65(5):991–1000.
5. Decaestecker K, Territo A, Campi R, Van Parys B, Bevilacqua G, Desender L, Breda A. Robot-assisted kidney transplantation. 2020. https://doi.org/10.5772/intechopen.90276.
6. Sumithra S, Lalitha AV, Pais P, Shubha AM. Post-operative challenges in pediatric renal transplant: nephro-intensivist perspective. J Pediatr Crit Care. 2018;5(3):67–71. https://doi.org/10.21304/2018.0503.00392.
7. Torricelli FCM, Watanabe A, Neto ED, Nahas WC. Current management issues of immediate post-operative care in pediatric kidney transplantation. Clinics (Sao Paulo). 2014;69(S1):39–41.
8. Naesens M, Kuypers D, Sarwal M. Calcineurin inhibitor nephrotoxicity. Clin J Am Soc Nephrol. 2009;4:481–508.
9. Morris P, Knechtle S. Kidney transplantation. 7th ed. Elsevier, Saunders; 2014. Chapter 14, p. 37. ISBN: 9781455774050.
10. Moudgil A. Primer on renal transplantation. Indian J Pediatr. 2012;79(8):1076–83.
11. Dharnidharka V, Fiorina P, Harmon W. Kidney transplantation in children. N Engl J Med. 2014;371(6):549–58.
12. Avner E, Harmon W, Emma F. Chapter 73: Pediatric renal transplantation. In: Pediatric nephrology. 7th ed. Springer; 2016. ISBN 978-3-662-43596-0.
13. Trachtman R, Sran S, Trachtman H. Recurrent focal segmental glomerulosclerosis after kidney transplantation. Pediatr Nephrol. 2015;30(10):1793–802.
14. Rubin RH. Infectious disease complications of renal transplantation. Kidney Int. 1993;44:221–36.

Robotic Management of Urinary Stones

Ciro Esposito, Fulvia Del Conte, Roberto Cardone, Mariapina Cerulo, Francesco Tedesco, Claudia Di Mento, Louise Montalva, Annalisa Chiodi, Roberta Guglielmini, Benedetta Cesaro, Marialuisa Pirone, and Maria Escolino

1 Introduction

Pediatric stone disease is uncommon in developed countries.

In general, nonsurgical management is used for the treatment of the majority of cases of kidney, ureteral, and bladder stones disease in children.

Nonsurgical treatment using medical therapy eventually associated with the positioning of a JJ stent is the first-line treatment for the majority of small stones in symptomatic children [1]. However alternative techniques are also described [2, 3].

In older children extracorporeal shock wave lithotripsy (ESWL) is largely adopted as a second option with good results.

If extraction is necessary, the majority of the urinary stones are accessible to percutaneous nephrolithotomy (PCNL) and ureterorenoscopy (rigid and flexible).

C. Esposito (✉) · F. Del Conte · R. Cardone · M. Cerulo · F. Tedesco · C. Di Mento · A. Chiodi · R. Guglielmini · B. Cesaro · M. Pirone · M. Escolino
Paediatric Surgery Unit, Federico II University of Naples, Naples, Italy
e-mail: ciroespo@unina.it; fulvia.delconte@unina.it; mariapina.cerulo@unina.it; claudia.dimento@unina.it; maria.escolino@unina.it

L. Montalva
Pediatric Surgery Unit, University Hospital of Paris Robert Debré, Paris, France
e-mail: louise.montalva@aphp.fr

About 10–15% of urinary stones in children require a traditional surgical approach. When surgery is needed, robotic-assisted surgery (RAS) seems the preferable way adopted from the majority of the pediatric urologists [3].

Children with urinary stones disease should be referred in high-volume centers with a strong experience in robotics, owning all the material and devices necessary for the management of urinary stones.

In general, a combination of different techniques requires robotics, cystoscopy, ureteroscopy, and endourology [4].

The best approach will depend on the available material and the experience of the urological team.

The international literature shows that the use of a robot may increase stone clearance with fewer auxiliary procedures in those difficult cases [1, 5].

2 Patients Positioning and Planning

In general, preoperative workup should include ultrasonography and renal scintigraphy. All children with urinary tract stones should undergo a complete metabolic evaluation.

Before surgery, to better clarify the anatomy of the entire urinary tract, a magnetic resonance (MR) urogram and eventually a contrast-enhanced

C. Esposito et al. (eds.), *Pediatric Robotic Assisted Surgery*,
https://doi.org/10.1007/978-3-031-99532-3_22

CT can be performed. Preoperative broad-spectrum antibiotic prophylaxis is recommended [1–3].

The parents have to sign an informed consent before the surgical procedure.

All the procedures are performed in general anesthesia.

Before positioning the patient on the operative table, a cystoscopy with placement of a JJ stent is performed. After positioning the patient, room has to be prepared for fluoroscopic material. The use of a multimedia integrated multiscreens operating room is strongly recommended.

For pelvic stones, the patient is positioned in a semilateral decubitus posture, with the surgical side up by 45° using silicone pads beneath them (Fig. 1a). In case of bladder stones, the patient is positioned in supine position (Fig. 2a). A bladder catheter suitable for the patient's age is inserted preoperatively.

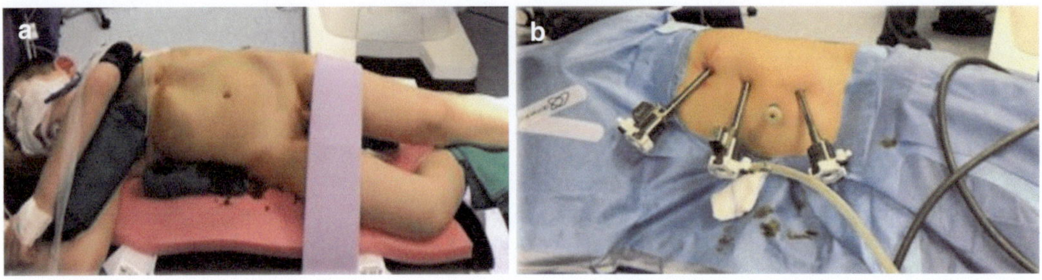

Fig. 1 (**a**) Patient position for upper urinary tract stones, (**b**) trocars position for upper urinary tract stones

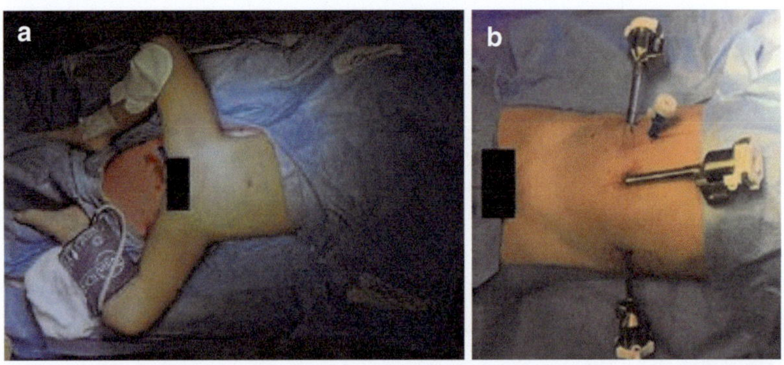

Fig. 2 (**a**) Patient position for lower urinary tract stones, (**b**) trocars position for lower urinary tract stones

3 Incision and Port Placement

The 8-mm robotic trocars are placed in line with the optical trocar positioned in the umbilicus, orientated to the target point (Figs. 1b and 2b).

The main concern is to be sure that the trocars are separated at least 8–9 cm which is sometimes difficult to obtain in pediatric patients under 15–20 kg.

We usually place three robotic 8-mm trocars and one 5-mm assistant port which should be positioned to allow the assistant to use the instruments effectively, aligning with a monitor while remaining clear of the robotic arms' range of motion.

Docking and dedocking take few minutes in experienced hands.

Cystoscopes, flexible ureteroscope, and JJ stents from different sizes (depending of the age of the patient) are always required. This material has to be checked before the beginning of the surgery.

In addition, a variety of flat-wire baskets can be useful as dye or holmium YAG laser may be necessary for fragmentation or vaporization of large stones.

As for robotic instruments, we prefer to adopt: a 30° optic, a Maryland forceps, a fenestrated forceps, a needle holder, a robotic hook, a curved scissors, and the sealing device.

4 Robot Positioning

For renal and upper ureteral stones, the robot is docked from the upper side.

The chart advances at an almost perpendicular angle to the operative table, although allowance of a few degrees of angulation toward the head allows for the slightly superior position of the renal pelvis above the transumbilical plane.

For bladder stones and for lower ureteral stones, the Da Vinci robot should be adjusted to pelvic setting and should be positioned contralaterally to the stone position, so that the bedside surgeon can have more mobility assisting the console surgeon.

5 Procedure Steps

5.1 Renal Stones

First step is to open the retroperitoneum reflecting the colon along the white line of Toldt. Sealing devices make this part easier. Once the renal pelvis is free, the ureter (identified by the indwelling stent) and the main vessels are recognized, and the stone is identified by the bulge, by palpating it with forceps or, if needed, using intraoperative ultrasound. In case of renal stones without associated UPJO, pelvis is incised longitudinally parallel to the renal parenchyma (Fig. 3b). It is preferable to insert an endobag, because the stones are fragile, and they can break, and in this way, you can put the stones easily in the endobag and removed them safely (Fig. 4). Then if there is the suspect of other stones located in the calices, you can introduce thorough one of the trocars a flexible ureteroscope to remove the residual stones

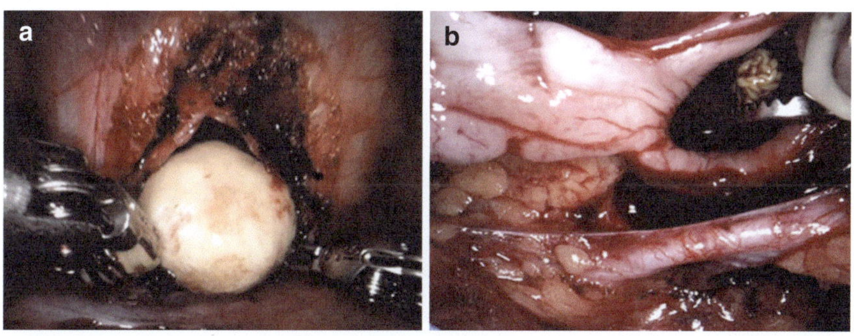

Fig. 3 (**a**) Extraction of bladder stone, (**b**) extraction of pelvic stone

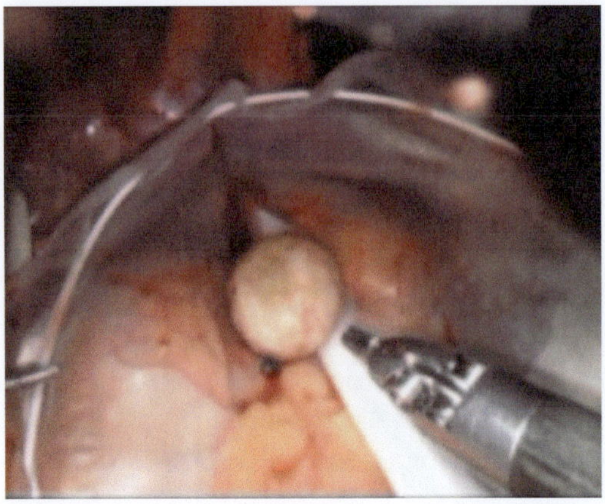

Fig. 4 Retrieval bag

(Fig. 5a, b). At the end of the procedure, the pelvis is closed with a running suture.

In case of concomitant stone and UPJ obstruction, the operation begins with a «V-shaped» incision made closer to the UPJ. Once the surgeon has dealt with the stones, a transcutaneous threat will fix the pelvis to the anterior abdominal wall before beginning with the ureteral incision and spatulation. Further steps depend on surgeon's preference. Best option is mostly not to separate completely the ureter from the pelvis before beginning the first running suture. Some teams put a second transcutaneous threat on the ureter. Perhaps a good advertising in the begin-

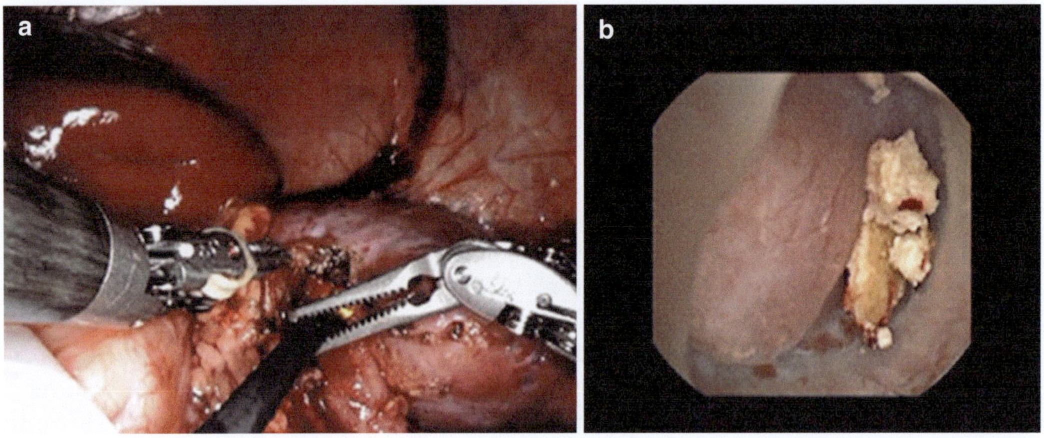

Fig. 5 (**a**) Introduction of ureteroscope into the renal pelvis, (**b**) visualization of residual fragments into the calix

ning because things are better stabilized. Generally, there are only two running sutures required if the incision of the pelvis was not too far from the UPJ. This will also depend on the size of the delivered stone. In case of larger pelvic resection, a third running suture is conducted in order to close the pelvis. Some authors use interrupted sutures for the anastomosis part.

5.2 Bladder Stones

The bladder was suspended using two-stay sutures that were introduced intracorporeally through the abdominal wall. After filling the bladder with normal saline, a 3.5-cm longitudinal incision of the detrusor muscle was performed in the midline using monopolar scissors, till the mucosa was seen pouting out. The bladder mucosa was also incised, and the bladder cavity was inspected. Once identified the stone, it is grasped using the robotic fenestrated grasper and put into a retrieval bag that was extracted through the umbilical port at the end of the procedure (Figs. 3a and 4). The bladder was then flushed with normal saline in order to ensure removal of all stone fragments, and the bladder wall was finally reconstructed using a two-layer running 3-0 polyglactin suture, first closing the mucosa and thereafter the detrusor muscle.

6 Postoperative Period

At the end of the operation, all trocar incisions are closed, even the 5-mm ones in little children, at the level of the fascia. Patients start oral feeding once they are discharged from the recovery room, beginning mostly with liquids. Pain medication is given according to hospital protocols. Generally, level 2 or 3 analgesics are not required after the first night. Antibiotics are administrated for 48–72 hours. Bladder catheter is removed in the first or second postoperative day. Antibioprophylaxis during JJ stenting is not recommended. Patients are discharged on the second to third postoperative day.

JJ stent is removed between 2 and 4 weeks postoperatively.

Follow-up will depend on the type of operation and the chemical analysis of the calculus.

In the last few years, there are more and more results about a robotic approach of stones in adults and children. Results are globally good. Robot-assisted surgery seems to increase the number of complete, one-time, stone management [5–8].

7 Tips and Tricks

Clearly define operative strategy as a key point for a successful management of patients affected by urinary stones [10].

Before beginning, robotic stone surgery is essential to own all instrumentations and materials required. Having a good flushing system is important (suction/irrigation).

Positioning accurately the patient is of main importance [10–11].

Blue dye or ICG may be interesting to use in order to control if the sutures are « water tied ». Stenting before beginning surgery helps during dissection and in order to find the stone (opacification just before beginning surgery) [12].

It is mandatory to add always 5-mm trocars for the bedside surgeon, extremely important in this type of surgery [9].

8 Conclusions

The management of urinary tract stones, in pediatric population, may be challenging and require multiple procedures. In the last 10 years, robot-assisted approaches have been reported as viable treatment options in selected patients with large stones, anomalies of collecting system, and complex stone burdens [1, 13].

Robotic-assisted surgery (RAS) overcomes the potential technical challenges of the laparoscopic approach, related to intracorporeal dissection and suturing, due to its demonstrated advantages of improved dexterity and three-dimensional visualization [11–15].

However, there is still limited evidence regarding the role of RALS in the management of pediatric urolithiasis. Analyzing the pediatric literature, the first study focused on the robot-assisted management of stone disease in the pediatric population was published in 2007 by Lee et al. [11] who reported a safe and effective use of robot-assisted pyelolithotomy in five adolescent patients with large stone burdens. The second [12] and last [14] published study confirmed that endoscopic-assisted robotic pyelolithotomy is a reasonable alternative to endourological and percutaneous approaches for selected pediatric patients with concomitant ureteropelvic junction obstruction and nephrolithiasis or with stones inaccessible by standard methods.

Probably, the main indications for RAS in pediatric urolithiasis should include patients with large stones or bilateral stones; patients who underwent previous failed endourological procedures; and patients with concomitant anomaly of collecting system, such as ureteropelvic junction obstruction, requiring simultaneous reconstruction [15].

The major indications for RAS are patients with large stones, impossibility to perform percutaneous nephrolithotomy due to lack of surgical expertise, or failure of other minimally invasive procedures [13, 15].

It is important to know some tips and tricks of the technique in order to achieve high stone clearance rate. It is very useful to perform in all kidney stones an intraoperative nephroscopy through the pyelolithotomy incision to explore the entire pelvicalyceal system, regardless of stone location in the upper collecting system. We always adopted a flexible ureteroscope that was easily introduced through the assistant port or through a robotic port after one of the arms was undocked. The use of flexible ureteroscope was very useful in case of multiple stones or stones in a difficult location, such as a lower pole calyx, allowing to reposition the stone into a more convenient position or to use stone baskets in order to maximize the stone clearance. The stone was retrieved using the robotic graspers, if it lied within the renal pelvis and was easily visible, or using endoscopic graspers or baskets. Another important trick was to flush the calices and the renal pelvis using normal saline at the end of the procedure in order to wash all cavities and ensure the removal of all fragments. Furthermore, for removal of stones from the abdominal cavity, although they can be directly extracted through the assistant port or through a robotic port, we suggest to put all fragments into a retrieval bag or a homemade bag, using the index finger of a sterile glove, and extract it through the umbilical port. Using this trick, we avoided the potential risk of fragment loss into the peritoneal cavity.

In conclusion, based on our experience, RAS seems to be a safe and effective treatment option for urinary tract stones in pediatric patients. The possibility to perform an intraoperative nephroscopy using flexible ureteroscope in order to localize and extract stone burden allowed to achieve a high stone-free rate. RAS should be considered the first choice of treatment in selected cases such as complex urinary tract stones, huge bladder stones in patients with neurogenic bladder, bilateral kidney stones, prior failed endoscopic procedures, or concomitant urinary anomalies such as UPJO requiring simultaneous pyeloplasty.

References

1. Jobs K, Rakowska M, Paturej A. Urolithiasis in the pediatric population - current opinion on epidemiology, pathophysiology, diagnostic evaluation and treatment. Dev Period Med. 2018;22(2):201–8.
2. Aydogdu O, Karakose A, Celik O, Atesci YZ. Recent management of urinary stone disease in a pediatric population. World J Clin Pediatr. 2014;3(1):1–5.
3. Esposito C, Masieri L, Bagnara V, Tokar B, Golebiewski A, Escolino M. Ureteroscopic lithotripsy for ureteral stones in children using holmium: yag laser energy: results of a multicentric survey. J Pediatr Urol. 2019;15(4):391.e1–7.
4. Simforoosh N, Aminsharifi A. Laparoscopic management in stone disease. Curr Opin Urol. 2013;23:169–74.
5. Ballesteros N, Snow ZA, Moscardi PRM, Ransford GA, Gomez P, Castellan M. Robotic management of urolithiasis in the pediatric population. Front Pediatr. 2019;7:351.
6. Suntharasivam T, Mukherjee A, Luk A, Aboumarzouk O, Somani B, Rai BP. The role of robotic surgery in the management of renal tract calculi. Transl Androl Urol. 2019;8(Suppl 4):S457–60.

7. Spinoit AF, Nguyen H, Subramaniam R. Role of robotics in children: a brave New World! Eur Urol Focus. 2017;3(2–3):172–80.
8. Andolfi C, Kumar R, Boysen WR, Gundeti MS. Current status of robotic surgery in pediatric urology. J Laparoendosc Adv Surg Tech A. 2019;29(2):159–66.
9. Atug F, Castle EP, Burgess SV, Thomas R. Concomitant management of renal calculi and pelvi-ureteric junction obstruction with robotic laparoscopic surgery. BJU Int. 2005;96(9):1365–8.
10. Siddiqui KM, Albala DM. Robotic-assisted surgery and treatment of urolithiasis. Int J Surg. 2016;36(Pt D):673–5.
11. Lee RS, Passerotti CC, Cendron M, Estrada CR, Borer JG, Peters CA. Early results of robot assisted laparoscopic lithotomy in adolescents. J Urol. 2007;177(6):2306–10.
12. Roth JD, Gargollo PC, DaJusta DG, et al. Endoscopic-assisted robotic pyelolithotomy: a viable treatment option for complex pediatric nephrolithiasis. J Pediatr Urol. 2019;S1477-5131(19):30431. https://doi.org/10.1016/j.jpurol.2019.12.007.
13. Kumar R, Yadav R, Kolla SB. Simultaneous bilateral robot-assisted dismembered pyeloplasties for bilateral ureteropelvic junction obstruction: technique and literature review. J Endourol. 2007;21(7):750–3.
14. Zheng J, Yan J, Zhou Z, Chen Z, Li X, Pan J, Li W. Concomitant treatment of ureteropelvic junction obstruction and renal calculi with robotic laparoscopic surgery and rigid nephroscopy. Urology. 2014;83(1):237–42.
15. Esposito C, Masieri L, Blanc T, Lendvay T, Escolino M. Robot-assisted laparoscopic surgery for treatment of urinary tract stones in children: report of a multicenter international experience. Urolithiasis. 2021;49:575–83.

Robotic Management of Retrovesical Structures in Children

Alexandra M. C. Carolan and Craig A. Peters

1 Introduction

The retrovesical space can harbor a variety of entities that may need to be addressed surgically, including prostatic utricles, seminal vesicle cysts, and ectopic ureteral stumps. This space is challenging to approach with open surgery. Robot-assisted laparoscopy offers excellent visualization of this space, with improved surgeon ergonomics and patient recovery relative to open surgery, as well as improved 3D visualization and dexterity relative to traditional laparoscopy [1, 2].

Indications for surgical intervention vary depending on the particular structure. Prostatic utricles are Mullerian duct remnants which are outpouchings that communicate with the prostatic urethra (Fig. 1) [3]. They occur in 11–50% of patients with hypospadias, with higher incidence reported with increasing severity of hypospadias, as well as in patients with other disorders of sexual differentiation [4]. Surgical excision is most commonly considered when symptoms arise secondary to urine trapping in the outpouching, which can manifest as recurrent urinary tract infections, pseudoincontinence (dribbling of trapped urine), or stone formation [2]. There are also reports of malignancy formation in prostatic utricles and other persistent Mullerian duct structures [5, 6]. Successful excision of prostatic utricles with robotic or laparoscopic approaches has been described in case reports and series of children and adults [1, 2, 4, 7–9].

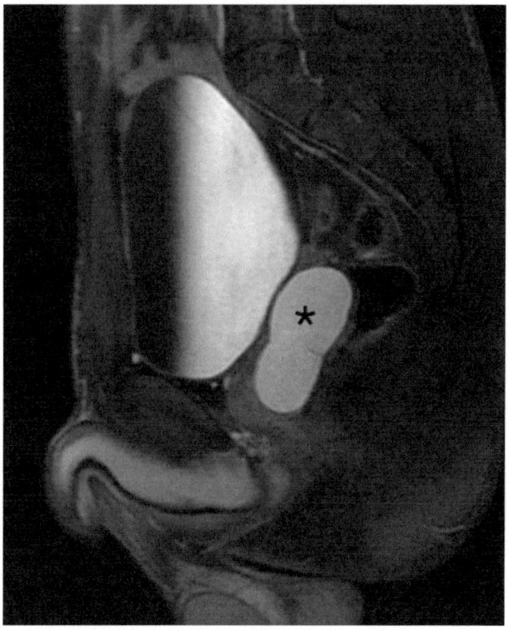

Fig. 1 MRI T2 weighted image. Prostatic utricle (*) posterior to bladder

Supplementary Information The online version contains supplementary material available at https://doi.org/10.1007/978-3-031-99532-3_23.

A. M. C. Carolan · C. A. Peters (✉)
University of Texas Southwestern Medical Center, Dallas, TX, USA
e-mail: alexandra.carolan@utsouthwestern.edu; craig.peters@utsouthwestern.edu

C. Esposito et al. (eds.), *Pediatric Robotic Assisted Surgery*,
https://doi.org/10.1007/978-3-031-99532-3_23

Seminal vesicle cysts can vary in size, and the mass effect on surrounding structures may result in symptoms including lower urinary tract symptoms, pelvic pain, or abdominal pain. They can cause upper tract obstruction, epididymitis, and prostatitis [10]. Zinner syndrome is the association of seminal vesicle cyst, ipsilateral ejaculatory duct obstruction, and ipsilateral renal agenesis. It may be diagnosed as early as infancy [11]. Robotic and laparoscopic approaches to seminal vesicle cyst excision have been performed with success in adult and pediatric patients [2, 10, 12].

Ureteral stumps are the distal remnants of ureters left behind after surgical intervention such as nephroureterectomy, heminephrectomy, ureteroureterostomy, or ureteral reimplant. These stumps are commonly clinically insignificant, but rates of "ureteral stump syndrome" have been reported in 0.8–9.5% of patients [13–15]. For these patients, urine and bacterial trapping within the stump may lead to recurrent urinary tract infections, hematuria, lower quadrant abdominal pain, or abscess [14]. We have found the robotic approach to ureteral stump excision to be viable even for ectopic ureteral stumps inserting into the urethra.

Here, we present the robotic approach to excision of structures in the retrovesical space, which can be applied to any of these entities.

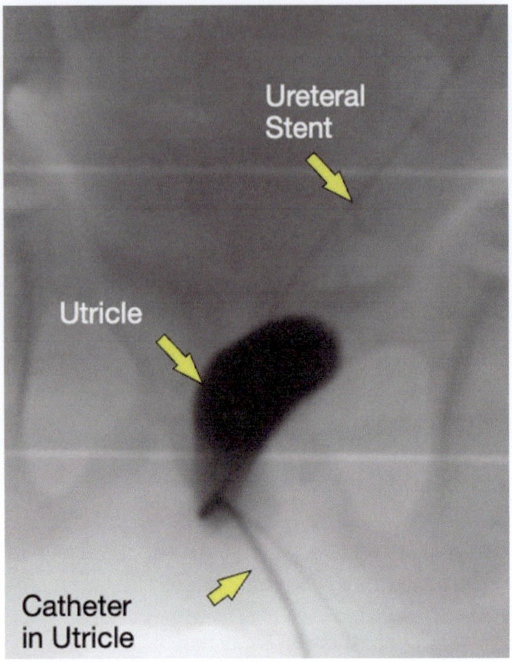

Fig. 2 Placement of catheter into prostatic utricle and ureteral stent into adjacent ureter to be used for intraoperative identification. Utricle opacificed with contrast

2 Patient Positioning and Planning

The patient is positioned supine. In many instances, it is useful to have the patient in dorsal lithotomy or supine split leg, so that the case may begin with a cystoscopy and the bladder may be easily accessed throughout the case. The patient is secured to the table with tape at the level of the chest in preparation for Trendelenburg positioning. A tilt test is performed. The operative field is prepped from xiphoid to the perineum and thighs.

Cystoscopy at the beginning of the case may be performed for identification of anatomy. For prostatic utricles and ectopic ureteral stumps, it is often helpful to place a catheter (such as a 10F council tip Foley catheter, a 3-5F open ended ureteral catheter, or a Fogarty catheter) over a wire into the structure. Through this, retrograde fluorography can be performed (Fig. 2). The catheter is left in place, so that during the robotic procedure, the structure can be filled with saline, methylene blue, or indocyanine green for assistance with identification and dissection. If a small caliber ureteral catheter is used, a Foley catheter may be placed next to this to allow bladder drainage and filling. It may also be helpful to place a ureteral stent or externalized ureteral catheter in any nearby ureter (such as the lower pole ureter of an ectopic upper pole ureteral stump to be removed) (Fig. 2).

3 Incision and Port Placement

After cystoscopy, the robotic ports are placed (Fig. 3). Access is gained at the umbilicus. We prefer a subumbilical incision, with the camera port placed with an open technique. Insufflation is achieved. Two lateral working ports are then

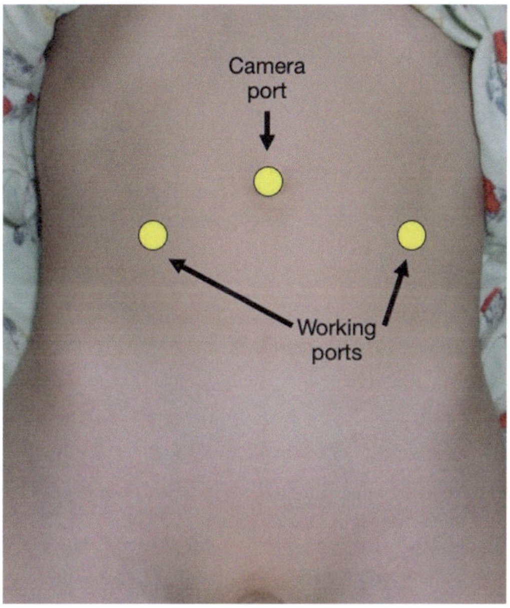

Fig. 3 Robotic port placement

placed under laparoscopic vision along the midclavicular line. These ports are typically at the level of the umbilicus or a couple of centimeters caudal. It is important to avoid the inferior epigastric vessels. We typically do not use the fourth robotic arm for cases of this type and typically do not use an additional assistant port, though these can be added as needed.

After port placement, the patient is placed in enough Trendelenburg to allow the bowels to retract out of the pelvis with gravity.

4 Robot Positioning

The robot is brought in from the side, and the boom is rotated to allow targeting to the pelvis, posterior to the bladder. The camera is placed, followed by targeting and placement of working instruments. Our preferred dissection tools are a Maryland bipolar in the left hand and a monopolar hook in the right.

5 Procedure Steps (Describe Step by Step the Procedure) (See Video 1)

Step 1: Incision of peritoneum The peritoneum is incised sharply over the structure of interest. If the structure cannot be identified initially after filling through the retrograde catheter, proceed with incision of the peritoneum over the posterior aspect of the bladder and dissect distally until the structure is identified.

Step 2: Bladder hitch In many instances, it is useful to hitch the bladder anteriorly to gain better exposure to the retrovesical space. We use a 3-0 PDS on a CT-2 needle, with the needle somewhat straightened. The bedside assistant passes the needle through the suprapubic abdominal wall. The console surgeon passes the needle through the bladder wall at one to two locations and then back through the abdominal wall. The tension on the suture can be adjusted by the beside assistant.

Step 3: Further dissection and excision of the structure of interest The structure is then further dissected to its neck or os. Dissection should remain as close to midline as possible to avoid lateral structures. Ensure that the ureters are visible and avoided. For seminal vesicle cysts, it may be helpful to drain the cyst to better identify the caudal anatomy. Pay careful attention to the course of the vas deferens. To protect the vas, a strip of the cystic wall can be left on the vas and lightly fulgurated. At times, the vas may enter the structure needing to be excised, and preservation may not be possible.

As dissection is carried down to the neck or os, take care not to avulse the structure. At the confluence with the urethra or prostate, a stay suture can be placed after partially transecting the neck to allow for exposure. There is no need to dissect too close to the urethra, as this can produce stricture. The structure may then be transected, followed by oversewing the area with an absorbable suture in a figure of eight fashion. A second layer closure is sometimes possible.

Step 4: Closure of the peritoneum We typically reapproximate the peritoneum back over the retrovesical space with a running suture such as 3-0 Vicryl or V-loc.

The procedure is then concluded with port site closure. We do not routinely leave a drain.

6 Postoperative Period

Patients are typically admitted overnight for observation and advanced to a regular diet after tolerating clear liquids on postoperative day 0 or 1.

The Foley catheter duration is dependent on the entity. After seminal vesicle cyst excision, a catheter is optional. After prostatic utricle excision or excision of an ectopic ureteral stump to the urethra, we typically leave a Foley catheter for 1–5 days.

Patients are discharged home on postoperative day 1–2 and follow-up with a pelvic ultrasound in 6 to 8 weeks.

7 Tips and Tricks

For all robotic procedures, we prefer to place 3-0 Vicryl fascial stitches in a box configuration around the port sites at the beginning of the procedure. The first at the umbilicus is placed after open access is gained to the peritoneum. The others are placed after incising skin but before placing the port. These sutures aid in placement of the ports, providing countertraction when pushing the port against the abdominal wall and peritoneum. They are then fixed to the port with a Tegaderm to prevent port dislodgement during the case. At the conclusion of the case, the box stitch is cinched to close the fascia.

At times, identification of the retrovesical structure is challenging with dissection and retrograde filling of the structure through the preplaced catheters alone. It may be helpful to have a bedside surgeon drive a cystoscope or ureteroscope into the structure. The light of the scope may then be visible to the surgeon at the robot console.

8 Conclusions

In conclusion, the robotic approach is well suited for managing retrovesical structures including excision of ureteral stumps, prostatic utricles, and seminal vesicle cysts.

References

1. Able C, Srinivasan A, Alzweri L. Robotic management of a large mullerian duct cyst: a case report and review of surgical options. Transl Androl Urol. 2022;11:1354.
2. Hong YK, Onal B, Diamond DA, et al. Robot-assisted laparoscopic excision of symptomatic retrovesical cysts in boys and young adults. J Urol. 2011;186:2372.
3. Shebel HM, Farg HM, Kolokythas O, El-Diasty T. Cysts of the lower male genitourinary tract: embryologic and anatomic considerations and differential diagnosis. Radiographics. 2013;33:1125.
4. Goruppi I, Avolio L, Romano P, et al. Robotic-assisted surgery for excision of an enlarged prostatic utricle. Int J Surg Case Rep. 2015;10:94.
5. Farikullah J, Ehtisham S, Nappo S, et al. Persistent Müllerian duct syndrome: lessons learned from managing a series of eight patients over a 10-year period and review of literature regarding malignant risk from the Müllerian remnants. BJU Int. 2012;110:E1084.
6. Gualco G, Ortega V, Ardao G, Cravioto F. Clear cell adenocarcinoma of the prostatic utricle in an adolescent. Ann Diagn Pathol. 2005;9:153.
7. Lima M, Maffi M, Di Salvo N, et al. Robotic removal of Müllerian duct remnants in pediatric patients: our experience and a review of the literature. Pediatr Med Chir. 2018;40:27.
8. Passerotti C, Cendron M, Gargollo P, et al. Minimally invasive surgical approaches to retrovesical structures. Int J Med Robot. 2007;3:307.
9. Yeung CK, Sihoe JD, Tam YH, Lee KH. Laparoscopic excision of prostatic utricles in children. BJU Int. 2001;87:505.

10. Moore CD, Erhard MJ, Dahm P. Robot-assisted excision of seminal vesicle cyst associated with ipsilateral renal agenesis. J Endourol. 2007;21:776.
11. Shashi KK, Garg H, Yu RN, Chow JS. Zinner syndrome in pediatric age group: an underdiagnosed entity. J Pediatr Urol. 2024;20:705.e1.
12. Kulkarni K, Dhua AK, Goel P, et al. Successful laparoscopic management of Zinner syndrome in a pediatric patient. J Indian Assoc Pediatr Surg. 2024;29:180.
13. Androulakakis PA, Stephanidis A, Antoniou A, Christophoridis C. Outcome of the distal ureteric stump after (hemi)nephrectomy and subtotal ureterectomy for reflux or obstruction. BJU Int. 2001;88:586.
14. Biswas K, Singh AG, Ganpule AP, et al. Clinical features and management of ureteric stump syndrome: single-centre experience and contemporary literature review. Asian J Urol. 2022;9:193.
15. Escolino M, Farina A, Turrà F, et al. Evaluation and outcome of the distal ureteral stump after nephroureterectomy in children. A comparison between laparoscopy and retroperitoneoscopy. J Pediatr Urol. 2016;12:119.e1.

Thorax

Robotic Resection of Mediastinal Masses and Other Anomalies

John J. Meehan

1 Introduction

The mediastinum is a challenging surgical field due to complex anatomy in a relatively small space with important structures including the heart, great vessels, phrenic and recurrent laryngeal nerves, and the thoracic duct. A clear understanding of the patient's anatomy and complete knowledge of the pathology of the mass is crucial to reduce for a safe surgical resection and reduce the risk of potentially formidable intraoperative or postoperative complications. With the three-dimensional imaging, increased degrees of freedom, and improved dexterity and precision control afforded to robotic instruments, robotic technology is ideally suited for the mediastinum in both adult and pediatric patients when compared to traditional minimally invasive instrumentation. In this chapter, we will discuss the wide variety of mediastinal pathology and suggest strategies for robotic surgery.

1.1 Mediastinal Anatomy

Understanding the anatomy of the mediastinum is crucial for the surgeon. The mediastinum is split at the level of T4 into the superior mediastinum and the inferior mediastinum [1]. The inferior mediastinum is further subdivided into anterior, middle, and posterior mediastinum. These locations are important in helping to determine the potential origin of a given mediastinal mass (Table 1) [1, 2, 3]. The differential diagnosis of a given mass can be narrowed based on recognizing the likely originating location. Patient age, symptoms, and radiographic characteristics can help narrow down the diagnosis further directing therapy and potential interventions. Due to the expansive nature of some of these masses and large potential space in the mediastinum and nearby thoracic cavities, a mass may originate in one zone but extend into others or laterally into either hemithorax.

1.2 Tips and Tricks for Mediastinal Anomalies and Masses

A primary goal of this chapter is to create a simplified algorithm, so the surgeon can plan a resection for any potentially resectable mediastinal mass or anomaly by following a few basic principles and strategies. Step 1 is to determine the optimal approach for a given mass or anomaly in regards to left chest or right chest approach. It may be a straightforward decision in some cases but less clear in others. For example, if the majority of a tumor is on the right, then a right approach should be taken. Some masses may be central,

J. J. Meehan (✉)
Seattle Children's Hospital, Seattle, WA, USA
e-mail: john.meehan@seattlechildrens.org

C. Esposito et al. (eds.), *Pediatric Robotic Assisted Surgery*,
https://doi.org/10.1007/978-3-031-99532-3_24

Table 1 Topographic anatomy, normative structures, and disease associations within the mediastinal compartments [1, 2]

Mediastinum zone	Boundaries	Normal structures	Potential pathology
Superior	Anteriorly: Sternum Posteriorly: T1-T4 Laterally: Sides of the pleura Inferiorly: Imaginary line joining sternal angle to lower border of T4	Aortic arch Innominate vein Superior vena cava Left common carotid Left subclavian artery Trachea Proximal esophagus Thoracic duct, thymus Vagus nerve Left recurrent laryngeal nerve Phrenic nerve Lymphatics	Lymphangioma (cystic hygroma)
Anterior	Anterior: sternum Posterior: pericardium Superior: imaginary line from sternal angle to bottom of T4 Inferior: diaphragm Lateral: mediastinal pleura	Thymus Lymph nodes Fat	Lymphangioma (cystic hygroma) Thymic cyst Teratoma Seminoma Germ cell tumor Thymoma Hodgkin's lymphoma Non-Hodgkin's lymphoma
Middle	Anterior: posterior surface of sternum Posterior: esophagus, descending aorta Superior: imaginary line from sternal angle to T4 Inferiorly: diaphragm Laterally: mediastinal pleura	Heart Ascending aorta Pulmonary trunk with left and right branches SVC Bifurcation of trachea	Bronchogenic cyst Teratoma Hodgkin's lymphoma Non-Hodgkin's lymphoma
Posterior	Anteriorly: pericardium Posteriorly T5 to T12 Superiorly imaginary line from sternal angle to T4 Inferiorly diaphragm Laterally: mediastinal pleura	Mid and distal esophagus Descending aorta and vertebral branches Azygous Hemiazygous Vagus Thoracic duct Splanchnic nerves	Esophageal duplication Lipoma Neuroblastoma Ganglioneuroma Ganglioneuroblastoma Leiomyoma Sarcoma Liposarcoma

and it becomes a matter of surgeon's preference. For example, the best approach for a thymectomy or thymic mass is a common debate among surgeons. The left approach allows an excellent visualization of the aortopulmonary window and the clearest view of the left phrenic nerve, while the right approach gives better visualization of the junction between the superior vena cava and innominate vein, so these structures can be visualized more easily recognized. There may be no correct answer as there are advantages to and disadvantages to both. However there are anatomic nuances that may favor one side over the other based on the specific location within the anatomy of a structure. An esophageal duplication which is distal may best be approached from the left, while a mid-esophageal duplication is better approached from the right. A CT or MRI will help the surgeon decide which approach (left vs. right) is best in addition to giving clues as to the potential underlying pathology based on location.

The patient is intubated and positioned. A modified lateral decubitus position is helpful for posterior masses. We recommend rolling the patient forward slightly to help roll the lung out of the way. Anterior mediastinal masses can be accessed with the patient supine and a bump under the shoulder (see thymectomy section later in this chapter). Single lung ventilation is recommended and can be accomplished with either dual lumen endotracheal tube for older patients or a bronchial blocker for smaller patients.

Deciding the optimal robot cart location is next. This can be simplified by remembering the following basic principle: The robot cart goes wherever the mass is located. If the mass is superior and anterior, the robot arms will have the best advantage if they are also are pointing in an anterior and superior direction, i.e., pointing back to the robot cart itself. Therefore, the robot cart should be placed superior and anterior (Fig. 1). If the mass is inferior and posterior, the robot cart should be placed inferior and posterior (Fig. 2). Remembering this recommendation will optimize the dissection and simplify planning any mediastinal mass regardless of the size, location, or etiology.

The next step is optimizing port location. The camera port is selected first and usually placed in a location such that the camera port, the target tissue, and the center column of the robot are all in a straight line. The port locations should be on a slight arc also demonstrated in Fig. 3. The important principle for port placement is to remember the angles of the robot arms to each other are the key parameter to measure and not

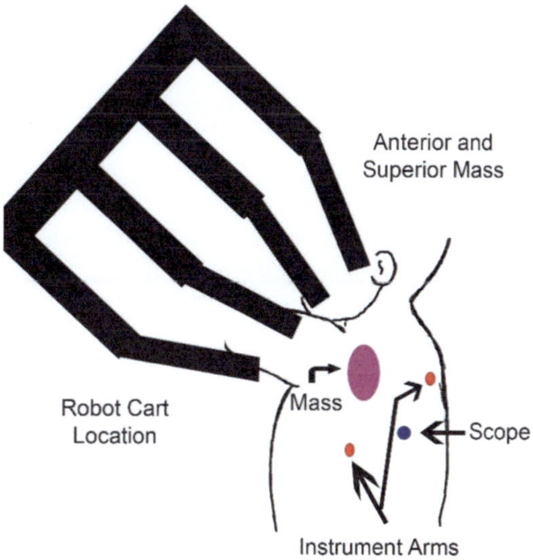

Fig. 1 Example—Robot cart placement for an anterior and superior mass, the cart should be anterior and superior

Fig. 2 Example—Robot cart placement for a posterior and inferior mass, the cart should be posterior and inferior

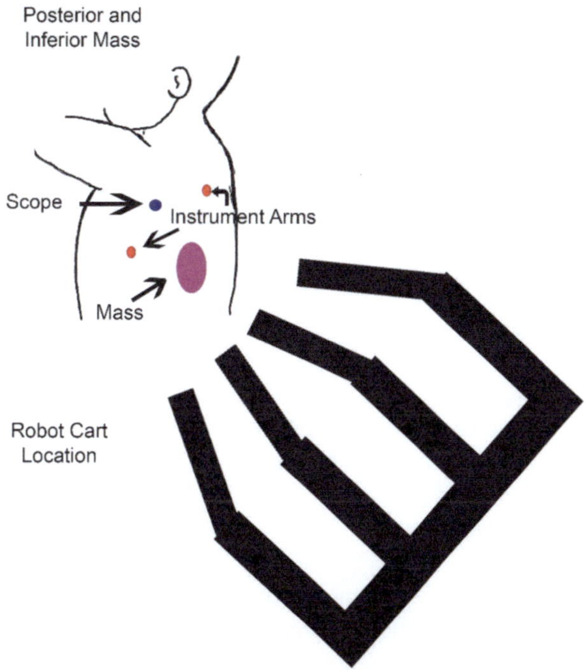

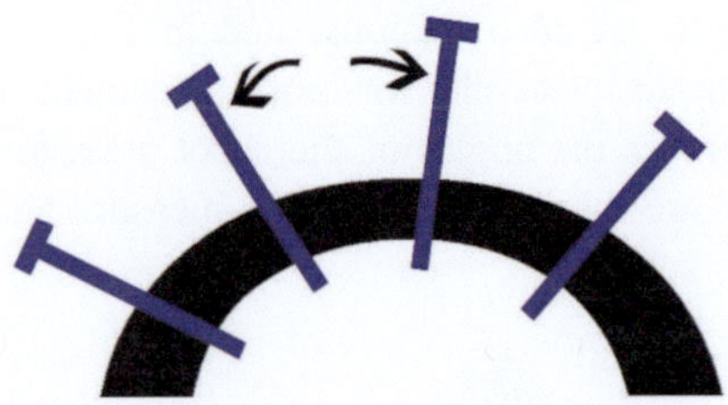

Fig. 3 The ideal robotic port angle from one port to the next neighboring port is 45–60 degrees. Using this principle instead of distance will help optimize port placement even for small patients

distance between ports. When each port is pointed directly at the center of the target tissue, the left and right hand ports closest to the camera port should create a 45–60-degree angle from each other. Any closer will result in external collisions, and any further apart may limit instrument mobility or cause collisions with the OR table. A fourth arm can be added laterally to either the left or right hand as space allows following the same principle of 45–60-degree angle from the nearest adjacent port. Alternatively a non-robotic bedside assistant port can be added at the same fourth port site or halfway between any other two robotic ports. We recommend to recess the port slightly back about 1–2 cm from an imaginary line between the two robotic ports on whichever side seems to be the easiest to access.

The robotic endoscope provides outstanding 3 D vision. In general, we prefer a 30-degree scope for nearly all resections. But since mediastinal masses may be quite large and the view seems can get difficult as the procedure progresses, we do not hesitate to switch between the 30-degree up and 30-degree down views to optimize the visibility.

2 Examples of Anterior Mediastinal Masses

2.1 Teratoma

The word teratoma comes from the Greek word *teras* meaning monster. These interesting tumors can occur in a multiple gonadal and extragonadal locations including the ovary, testes, neck, mediastinum, and sacrococcygeal region. They arise from postmeiotic germ cells and by definition contain all three cell embryonic cell layers: ectoderm, endoderm, and mesoderm [4]. Teratomas can be benign (mature) or malignant (immature). The malignant teratomas produce markers that can be serologically assessed by checking serum alpha fetoprotein and beta human choriogonadotropin hormone. If these markers are positive, a search for potential metastatic disease should be taken, and consideration for chemotherapy may be required preoperatively. Benign teratomas will have normal levels of these markers and can go straight to resection with no need for biopsy. The classic feature on CT scan to help differentiate these tumors from others is the finding of fat within the mass which is diagnostic. While these tumors often contain calcium deposit such as teeth or bone, the finding of calcium is common but not unique to teratomas, as some neurogenic tumors may have calcium as well. The symptoms are often mild for most teratomas, and the size of the mass may eventually be the culprit which generates a mild symptom such as cough or mild dysphagia. The mass is often discovered on plane film radiograph and confirmed by CT scan. The majority of teratomas are benign. Biopsy is not often necessary unless malignancy is suspected. The risk of recurrence following resection is linked to degree of immaturity.

Since teratomas arise in the anterior compartment, a more anterior location of the robot would help optimize the resection. A 16-year-old girl presented with a chronic cough, and a chest X-ray revealed a mediastinal mass. Figure 4a shows the CT scan of this anterior and somewhat superior mass. The classic features of a teratoma were noted including fat and calcifications. Serum markers were normal. Because the majority of this mass is on the left, we will obviously select a left approach.

By CT scan, the mass is in the anterior mediastinum and is also somewhat superior. Therefore, the robot cart is strategically placed in an anterior and superior location in relation to the patient and the port locations (Fig. 4b). Dissection is carried

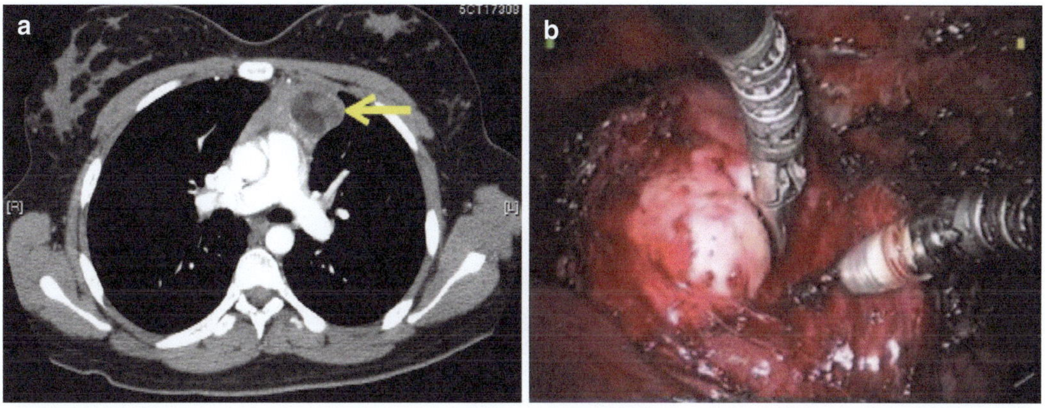

Fig. 4 Anterior mediastinum—teratoma resection. (**a**) CT scan demonstrating classic features of fat and calcifications in a mediastinal teratoma in the anterior mediastinum. (**b**) Robot cart location and port placement. (**c**) Dissecting the teratoma off the adhered lung and pleural adhesions

out beginning with hook cautery to free the mass from the adhered lung, as teratomas often create significant inflammatory adhesions to the pleural or lung. Eventually, the mass is freed from other mediastinal structures using blunt dissection and electrocautery (Fig. 4c).

Thymic tumors also arise in the anterior mediastinum. The thymus is located in the anterior mediastinum and develops from the third pharyngeal pouch. In a relative sense, it is quite large in newborns and infants but involutes in adults. The arterial blood supply is from small branches off the internal mammary. The important vessel to recognize is the thymic vein (sometimes referred to as the great vein of Keynes). This vessel drains into the innominate. Additional smaller internal thoracic veins may exist as well.

Germ cell tumors can be quite large and originate in the thymus [5]. These masses can get quite large before they are detected. Figure 5a shows the MRI of a large 10-cm right-sided germ cell tumor that developed in an 11-year-old boy. This is a right-sided mass, so we will plan a right approach. This mass is so large that a central orientation of our robot is ideal as shown in Fig. 5b. Dissection began by first freeing the mass from the adhered pleura of the lung followed by careful dissection off the pericardium (Fig. 5c, d).

Although the thymus may not qualify as a mass in myasthenia gravis, the resection of the thymus should also be considered in this mediastinal chapter as the same principles apply. Patients may present with a long history of neurological symptoms and weakness. Thymectomy may be required for patients that do not respond to medical management or have progressive symptoms [8]. It should be noted that many of these patients are quite weak and may have postoperative ventilation challenges. We plan a post ICU stay regardless of how straightforward and uneventful a thymectomy may be.

For the thymectomy, we prefer a left-sided approach. The patient's left arm is placed at their side with a slight roll under the left shoulder Fig. 6a. Following the principles discussed earlier in this chapter, the robot cart is placed superiorly and over the right shoulder. Our typical three-port placement is shown in Fig. 6b with the optional fourth port also depicted. We start with the camera in a 30-degree down orientation knowing we may need to flip the camera to the 30-degree up position periodically, particularly when we follow the thymus up the right neck near the conclusion of the procedure. We use the hook cautery throughout the entire case as our preferred method of dissection and prefer the Cadiere forceps to hold the thymus. It's important to identify the left phrenic nerve early and stay clear of this structure by at least 1 cm throughout the remainder of the case. The pleura overlying the thymus is opened 1 cm anterior to the left phrenic nerve (Fig. 6c). Carry the dissec-

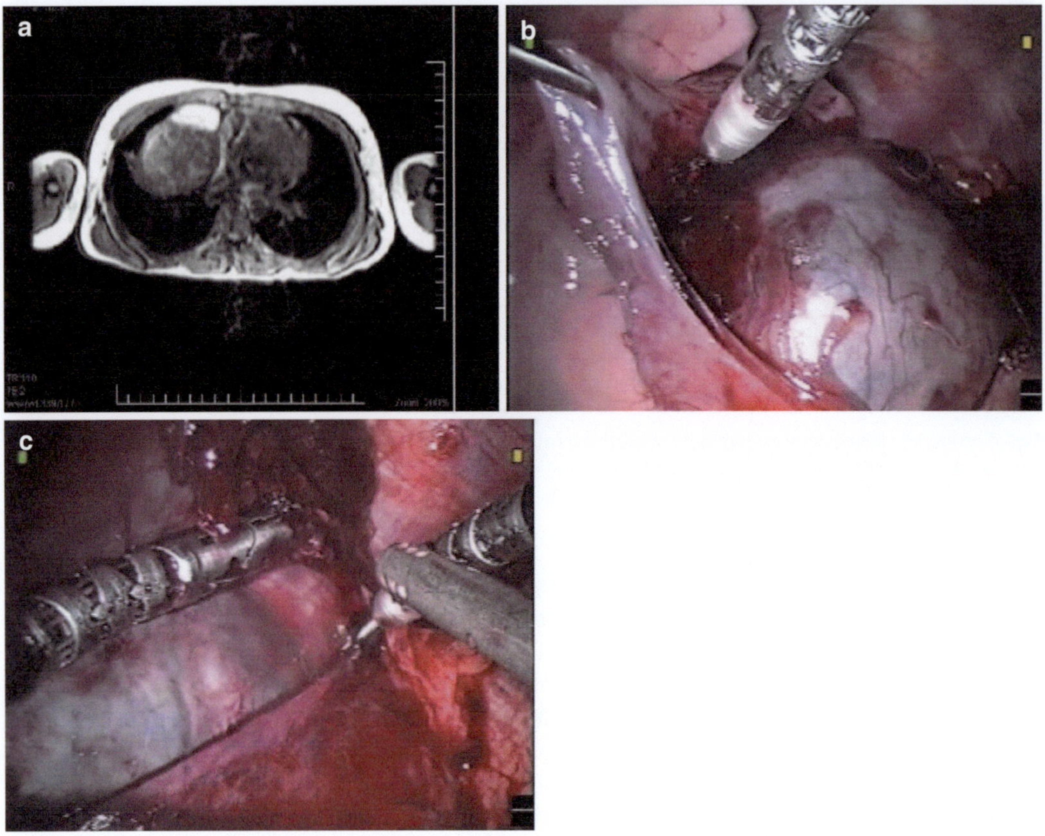

Fig. 5 Anterior mediastinum—germ cell tumor. (**a**) MRI of the large 10-cm germ cell tumor. (**b**) Robot cart location and port placement. (**c**) Taking down pulmonary adhesions to the mass. (**d**) Resecting the mass off the pericardium

tion superiorly and inferiorly in a path parallel to the phrenic. Use blunt dissection over electrocautery whenever possible when close to the phrenic. We prefer to follow the thymus inferiorly to mobilize and reflect the lower pole of the thymus and then follow it superiorly along the left lateral edge. Be cautious of the vascular structures at the superior extent. Dissect the thymus off the mediastinal pericardium posteriorly and off the chest wall anteriorly. The thymus may have thin sections or may be lobular. Be cautious not to inadvertently split the thymus into additional pieces. Next, we return to the inferior pole and reflect the thymus off the pericardium as we travel cranially. The thymic vein is often generous and will eventually be encountered as we approach the superior mediastinum. This vessel should be clipped and divided. As the dissection traverses the mediastinum and approaches the right thoracic cavity, the right lung will be visible as it billows under the right pleura. Ideally, the surgeon should avoid entering the contralateral pleura on the right if possible. Once the thymus has been freed from the patient's mediastinum posteriorly and right pleura, the remaining portion will be up the right neck. Follow the finger like extension of the thymus up into the right neck using blunt dissection and traction (Fig. 6d). The articulating robotic instruments are particularly very useful here. Once the specimen is free, undock the robot, and extend one of the port incisions as necessary to retrieve the specimen. Temporarily place a chest tube or red rubber tube through one of the port sites, and leave on suction while closing. This can be removed before the end of the case, and a chest tube is rarely needed postoperatively.

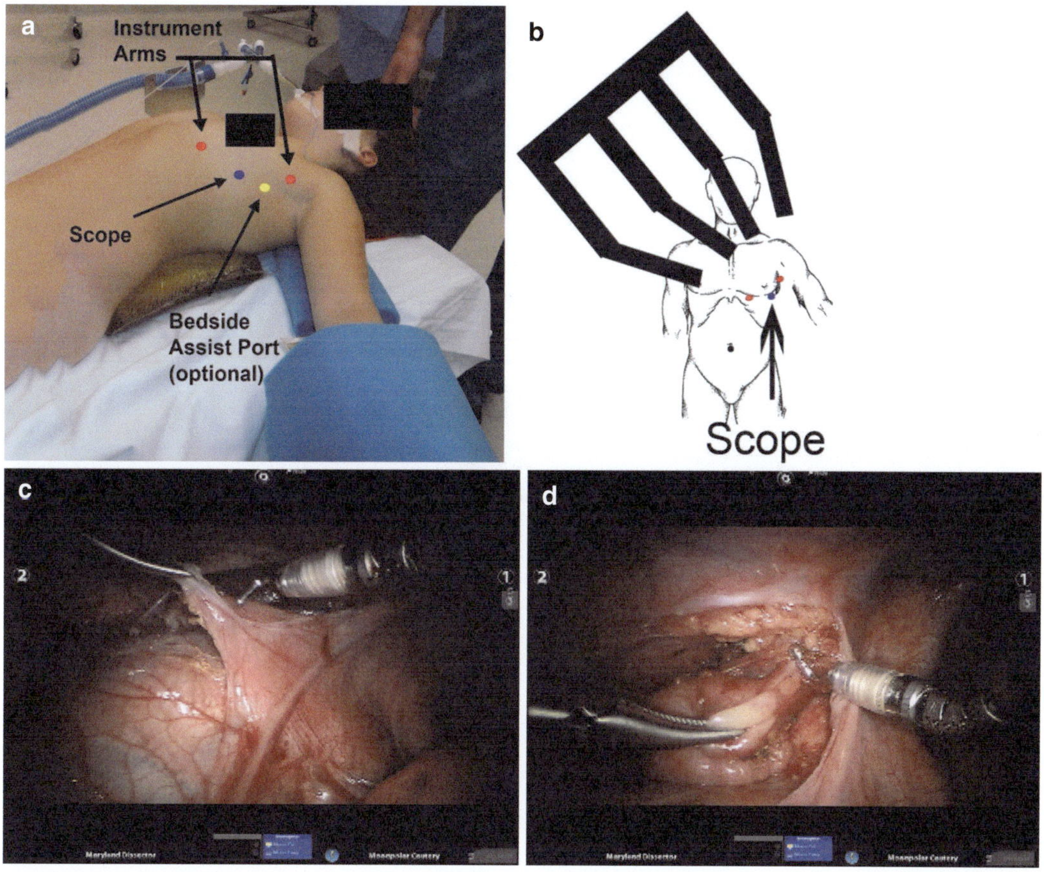

Fig. 6 Anterior mediastinum—thymectomy. (**a**) Patient positioning for a left-sided approach. (**b**) Robot cart location and port placement along inframammary line. (**c**) Starting the dissection, note the phrenic nerve and importance of staying 1 cm or more away from this structure at all times. (**d**) Following the thymic tissue up into the right neck is especially well suited to the articulating robotic instruments

3 Examples of Posterior Mediastinal Tumors

The neurogenic tumors such as ganglioneuroma, ganglioneuroblastoma, and neuroblastoma originate in the posterior mediastinum. Ganglioneuromas are benign, while neuroblastomas are malignant. Ganglioneuroblastomas are considered an intermediate between the neuroblastoma and ganglioneuroma with features of both, often with rests of potentially malignant elements nestled in more benign appearing tissue [6]. Resection is usually recommended. While ganglioneuromas were historically resected without hesitation in years past, recent questions whether these benign masses require resection have led some surgeons to watch these masses [7]. Others advocate for their resection whenever possible as the risk of complications may be small.

A mass suspicious for neuroblastoma often requires an initial biopsy for confirmation of the pathology and determination of critical features which will direct chemotherapy. A multidisciplinary team including an institutional tumor board should be involved to best determine the best therapeutic approach including when surgical intervention is warranted [8]. It should also be noted that some neuroblastomas have extension into the neural foramina causing compression of the spinal cord, and a neurosurgery consult would be required in those circum-

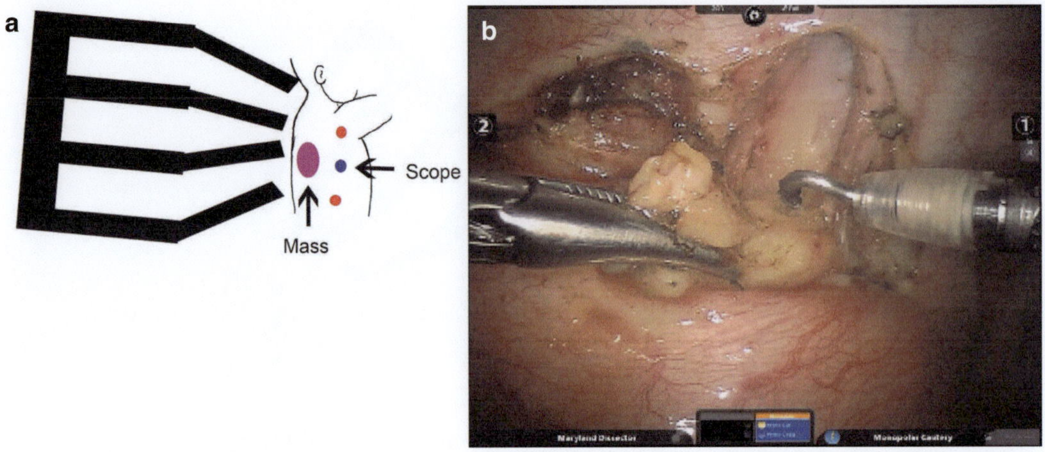

Fig. 7 Posterior mediastinum—ganglioneuroblastoma. (**a**) Robot cart location and port placement. (**b**) Resection of the mass along the posterior mediastinum

stances. Cord compromise often necessitates an immediate surgical intervention where the neurosurgeons handle the component within the spinal column including the vertebral foramina, while the pediatric surgeon may be asked to tackle at least a portion of the thoracic component. When the spinal cord is not involved, resection is often deferred as most neuroblastomas will respond well to chemotherapy, and resection is delayed until the mass has shrunk significantly. Principles of oncology surgery and highest chance for cure should always take precedence over any minimally plans. If a neuroblastoma is amenable to a MIS approach, the robot can certainly be used safely and effectively in neuroblastoma resection [5–8].

An otherwise healthy 8-year-old boy patient presented with a mild cough. A chest X-ray revealed a mass and further workup with CT demonstrated the solid right posterior mediastinal mass. No other disease was noted elsewhere. In this case, the mass is almost directly central in the right hemithorax at mid-level. The robot cart positioning and port are shown in Fig. 7a. Dissection was very straightforward using mainly hook electrocautery with only three ports required for this case. The 3-d vision of the robotic camera was particularly helpful demonstrating how these types of neural tumors invaginate between the vertebral bodies (Fig. 7b).

4 Other Anomalies: Bronchogenic and Esophageal Duplication Cysts

4.1 Bronchogenic Cyst

Before we conclude this chapter, we should also talk about mediastinal masses that are better thought of as congenital anomalies. The first, and one of the easier anomalies to resect robotically, is the bronchogenic cyst. These are usually the smallest masses we may encounter compared to the other mediastinal masses. These benign anomalies occur during fetal development, and many months or years may pass before a patient develops symptoms. They may present with fever or a mild persistent cough, or occasionally the anomaly creates a mass effect causing other symptoms as it impedes either the airway or nearby esophagus. Bronchogenic cysts are often first detected on chest X-ray, and a follow-up CT will demonstrate the fluid filled mass usually in the middle mediastinum. They are commonly, but not always, close to the bifurcation of the trachea. Sometimes there may be confusion or speculation over whether the anomaly is a bronchogenic cyst or a duplication cyst in which case an EGD may help delineate the two possibilities.

Bronchogenic cysts are ideally suited for robotic resection. They are usually relatively easy to resect due to their small size and tend to peel away from the nearby structures quite readily. In fact, some of the shortest robotic cases we've ever done in the chest or the abdomen have been bronchogenic cysts with surgeon console time frequently well below 15 minutes. The surgical planning for robot cart location is once again based on the exact location of the anomaly within the mediastinum following the same principles as outlined in the previous sections. We don't hesitate to drain large cysts if it will aid in an easier dissection. Figure 8 shows a bronchogenic cyst resecting undergoing robotic resection, and the console time for this particular case was 8 minutes.

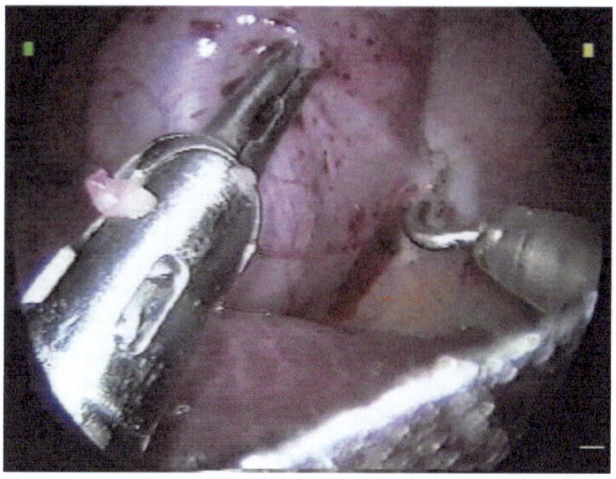

Fig. 8 Middle mediastinum—bronchogenic cyst: On the pleural surface and one of the easier mediastinal anomalies to resect robotically. This case took only 8 minutes of console time

4.2 Esophageal Duplication

Esophageal duplications may be small or quite extensive, and the surgical plan will depend on the size and location of the pathology. As the esophagus is slightly more to the left in the proximally and distally and slightly more to the right in the middle, the laterality of the approach will be influenced by its location proximal, middle, or distal on the esophagus.

A 16-year-old girl had dysphagia. A chest X-ray suggested a mediastinal mass, and MRI demonstrated an esophageal duplication in the proximal to mid-esophageal location (Fig. 9a). Following our positioning principles for this posterior and superior anomaly, a right chest approach with the cart in a posterior and superior location would be best (Fig. 9b). The patient is placed in a lateral decubitus position rolled slightly anteriorly to allow the lung to fall away anteriorly. Again we prefer to use hook electrocautery for the majority of the dissection (Fig. 9c). At some point, the esophageal duplication will need to be opened and drained of contents. It is important to only remove only the outer layer of the duplication and check the inner wall with concurrent endoscopy to be sure an esophageal perforation has not occurred. If a communication exists, it should be sutured with absorbable interrupted sutures, and a postoperative esophageal swallowing study is recommended before initiating feeds as EGD may miss small perforations. If a small perforation is noted, conservative management usually suffices and leaks generally seal spontaneously which can be confirmed with a repeat esophageal study a few days later.

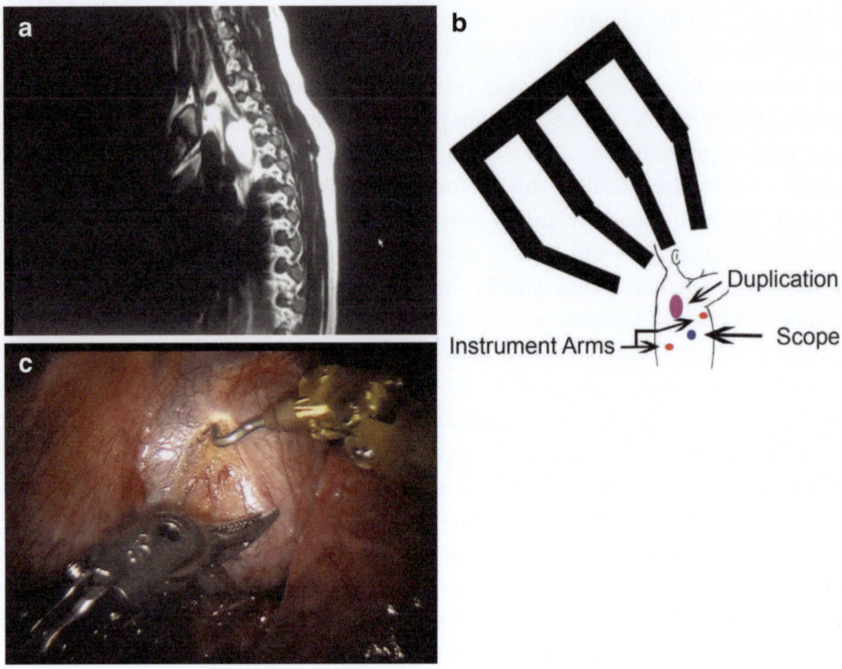

Fig. 9 Posterior mediastinum—esophageal duplication. (**a**) MRI demonstrating a superior esophageal duplication. (**b**) Robot cart and port location. (**c**) Resecting the esophageal duplication. Open and marsupialize the duplication. A concomitant EGD can assist in staying out of the true esophageal lumen. A contrast radiograph should be considered before reinitiating feeds

5 Conclusion

Mediastinal robotic surgery has many possible decision points, but it can all be simplified by knowing the type of mass of and the location of the mass. Following a stepwise algorithm for identification of the likely pathology based on patient symptoms coupled with the mass or anomaly's radiographic features and mass location will help dictate the direction of the operative plan. While the surgeon still needs to have a thorough knowledge of mediastinal anatomy, operative planning can be accomplished by following a few basic principles based on location of the mass and the likely pathology.

References

1. Carter BW, Benveniste MF, Madan R, et al. ITMIG classification of mediastinal compartments and multidisciplinary approach to mediastinal masses. Radiographics. 2017;37:413–36.
2. Simpson I, Campbell PE. Mediastinal masses in childhood: a review from a paediatric pathologist's point of view. Prog Pediatr Surg. 1991;27:92–126. https://doi.org/10.1007/978-3-642-87767-4_7.
3. Verma S, Kalra K, Rastogi S, Sidhu HS. Clinical approach to childhood mediastinal tumors and management. Mediastinum. 2020;4:21. https://doi.org/10.21037/med-19-82.
4. Pearson JK, Tan GM. Pediatric anterior mediastinal mass: a review article. 2015;19(3):248–54. https://doi.org/10.1177/1089253215578931. Epub 2015 Mar 26.
5. Kaba E, Cosgun T, Ayalp K, Toker A. Robotic thymectomy for myasthenia gravis. Ann Cardiothorac Surg. 2019;8(2):288–91. https://doi.org/10.21037/acs.2019.02.02.
6. Sreedher G, Tadros SS, Janitz E. Pediatric mediastinal masses. Pediatr Radiol. 2022;52(10):1935–47. https://doi.org/10.1007/s00247-022-05409-4. Epub 2022 Jun 8.
7. Wright CD. Mediastinal tumors and cysts in the pediatric population. Thorac Surg Clin. 2009;19:47–61.
8. Gun F, Erginel B, Unüvar A, Kebudi R, Salman T, Celik A. Mediastinal masses in children: experience with 120 cases. Pediatr Hematol Oncol. 2012;29(2):141–7. https://doi.org/10.3109/08880018.2011.646385.

Oncology

Tips and Tricks for Robotic Pediatric Oncology

Marie Bousquet, Pauline Lopez, Sarah Amar, Pauline Clermidi, Pierre Meignan, Quentin Ballouhey, Karim Braïk, Thomas Blanc, Mario Mendoza, Laurent Fourcade, and Hubert Lardy

1 General Concerns

In many countries, robotic surgery is becoming a common surgical approach in pediatric surgery[1, 2].

Probably due to the availability and costs of the platform, robotic surgeons prefer performing more reconstructive procedures than robotic removal procedures [3, 4].

M. Bousquet · S. Amar · P. Meignan · K. Braïk · H. Lardy (✉)
CHU Tours service de chirurgie pédiatrique, Tours, France
e-mail: marie.bousquet@chu-tours.fr; s.amar@chu-tours.fr; p.meignan@chu-tours.fr; k.braik@chu-tours.fr; hubert.lardy@univ-tours.fr

P. Lopez · Q. Ballouhey · L. Fourcade
CHU Limoges service de chirurgie pédiatrique, Limoges, France
e-mail: pauline.lopez@chu-limoges.fr; quentin.ballouhey@chu-limoges.fr; laurent.fourcade@chu-limoges.fr

P. Clermidi
Hôpital Robert Debré AP-HP Paris, Paris, France
e-mail: pauline.clermidi@aphp.fr

T. Blanc
Hôpital Necker AP-HP, Paris, France
e-mail: thomas.blanc@aphp.fr

M. Mendoza
Service de chirurgie pédiatrique Bellinzona, Bellinzona, Switzerland
e-mail: mario.mendozasagaon@eoc.ch

The best definition for robotic surgery is laparoscopic 3D tele-microsurgery.

- In fact, robotic surgery is a laparoscopic (or thoracoscopic) surgery.
- The term “robotic” is not entirely appropriate: It is more accurately described as telesurgery.
- The dissection is made in a small operating space with 3D vision and magnification as microsurgery [5, 6, 7].

This constitutes one of the key elements of minimally invasive surgery (MIS) programs in most pediatric centers, which also include laparoscopy, retroperitoneoscopy, thoracoscopy, video-assisted thoracotomy, and mini-open approaches [8, 9].

Minimally invasive surgery now integrates modern techniques such as robotic surgery, complementing the approaches mentioned above.

Surgeons aiming to establish a robotic program should follow general training principles similar to laparoscopy. These include structured training pathways, skill development using simulators, dry and wet lab sessions, and animal model training. Proctoring is highly recommended for novice surgeons to ensure a successful learning curve.

In certain strategies, combining different surgical approaches (e.g., robotics, laparoscopy, or open transumbilical procedures) can be advanta-

C. Esposito et al. (eds.), *Pediatric Robotic Assisted Surgery*,
https://doi.org/10.1007/978-3-031-99532-3_25

geous. For instance, in reconstructive surgery for choledochal cyst, excision may be performed robotically, while the "Roux en Y" intestinal loop is created via an umbilical incision [10, 12, 13].

Implementing a robotic program requires a multidisciplinary approach. Team learning and training pathways should be organized in collaboration with anesthesiologists and scrub nurses.

Communication is essential between the robotic surgeon (operating from the console) and the assistant (positioned beside the patient). The microphone volume should be adjusted appropriately, and the surgeon must communicate clearly. Additionally, effective communication with anesthesiologists is critical. Indeed, a good communication is the key of a successful procedure, whereas poor communication before or during the procedure can have severe consequences for the patient [14, 15].

Systematic video recording and storage of procedures are recommended for use in case of complications or for scientific and educational purposes. Particular attention must be given to obtaining patient consent and adhering to privacy laws.

The following advices could be useful for procedures with the Da Vinci Robotic platform.

2 Operating Room Setting

- *Preparation*: All equipment must be set up before patient enters the operating room (OR). Anticipation and early preparation are key (staff with surgeon(s), scrub nurses, and anesthetists). For routine procedures, the OR setup should be standardized. For rare procedures, staff discussions may be needed to reorganize the setup.
- *Team* installation: Assistant surgeon and scrub nurse installation must be the priority!
- *Room* requirements: Robotic surgery requires larger Ors than conventional setups. These should include multiple screens, strategic placement of the surgical lights, a console (potentially located outside the OR), and dedicated tables for robotic and conversion instruments.
- *Dual consoles*: Dual-console systems are highly beneficial for teaching and mentoring.
- *Anesthesia setup*: Anesthesiologists require a comfortable, well-organized workspace for patient conditioning.
- *Cart positioning*: Cart positioning should be coordinated with scrub nurses before surgery.
- *Camera setup*: A small table to support camera during preparation is useful.

3 Installation

Port placement and insertion: One port is used for the camera (0 or 30 degrees), two ports are used for robotic arms, and one or two additional ports are used for accessory instruments (5 mm). Strategies for accessory laparoscopic trocar placement (5 or 3 mm) depend on the type of procedure. This should be anticipated as much as possible. The number of accessory ports does not matter.

The first port for camera should be placed with open Hasson procedure.

The camera cable should be passed over the telescope before introducing the telescope into the trocar.

Sufficient space between ports is crucial to avoid arm collisions. For small children, we recommend maintaining a distance of 6 to 7.5 cm when using the Xi Da Vinci Platform.

The use of the fourth arm is rarely needed.

There are different methods for port placement:

- One-line placement (modern technique)
- Curved placement targeting the organ (traditional technique)
- SLIP (single-line inguinal placement) even for supra-mesocolic procedures
- Retroperitoneoscopy (subcostal approach)
- Thoracoscopy (midaxillary line or W port placement)
- Single-port robot (new SP Da Vinci platform)

For small children (< 12 Kg), particular care should be taken during installation. A thorough assessment of the setup is essential for these younger patients.

It is preferable to perform robotic procedures using a robotic operating bed that could be associated with the robot during the procedure. This allows safe adjustments to the patient's position during the procedure if needed.

The use of a vacuum shell mattress can be helpful, particularly for thoracoscopic procedures where lateral decubitus is required. In such cases, take care to position the child's arm properly to avoid collisions with the robotic arms

Patient positioning and fixation are key factors for ensuring a safe and successful robotic procedure.

4 Docking

There is different type of robot. Some models (e.g., Da Vinci) can be connected to the operating table (Trump Table), allowing the patient's position to be adjusted during the procedure once the robot is docked. If this feature is unavailable, the table must remain stationary once docking is complete.

Docking can be performed either by moving the patient to the robot or the robot to the patient.

Beginners should undergo specific training for docking.

In case of robotic instrument retrieval, the assistant must clutch the arm to prevent unintended movement.

During the robotic procedure, the assistant should maintain continuous control over the robotic arm movements to detect potential collisions with the patient's body.

We recommend creating a catalog of the various robotic setups and patient positions specific to each type of procedure.

5 Exposure

Transparietal suspension with sutures should be considered to optimize visualization (PUJ repair, vesical suspension for rectal or genital surgery, gallbladder suspension for hepatobiliary surgery, or round hepatic ligament).

Ensure that the robotic instruments always remain within the surgeon's field of vision.

At the console, the surgeon can use the clutch to reposition the manipulators (joysticks) if the ergonomics are suboptimal or in case of hand collisions.

Robotic ports can be suspended (2 or 3 cm higher) to elevate the abdominal wall. For small children, it is recommended to carefully adapt the robotic trocar tips to ensure proper fulcrum points and smooth robotic arm movements.

Air seal is not very useful for robotic surgery but can be used if surgical team has regular uses of this equipment. Special attention should be given to preventing of hypothermia particularly for young children. CO_2 leakage is the main cause of hypothermia and camera fogging. Keeping a thermos of warm saline solution on the instrument table can help warm the optic and prevent fogging. Another tip is to avoid attaching the insufflator tube to the optic trocar.

6 Hemostatic Devices and Robotic Instrumentation

Monopolar (green cable) and bipolar (blue cable) coagulations are the most frequently used energy sources. To avoid accidents, attach the cables to the robotic instrument before introducing the instrument into the trocar, and verify the energy intensity settings.

Ultrasonic coagulation or thermofusion devices can be used by the assistant with external instruments or via the robotic system. The same applies to clip applicators or staplers.

It is crucial to be familiar with all robotic instruments available in your hospital, especially when working within multidisciplinary teams.

7 Ligatures and Suturing

After tying a knot, ensure it is tightened under direct visual control, as there is no haptic feedback in robotic surgery.

8 Miscellaneous

Suction/aspiration If needed, increase the CO_2 flow rate to maintain a clear operative field.

Endobag Should be used for specimen retrieval.

Closure Close the trocar's site and skin incisions meticulously using absorbable sutures. Superficial fascia must be sutured for a better cosmetic outcome. Local anesthetics should be infiltrated into the port incisions to minimize postoperative pain and facilitate quicker recovery.

9 Conversion

In experienced hands, conversion is rarely necessary. However, in emergencies, either an open or a laparoscopic approach can be chosen. An instrument table for conversion should always be prepared before starting the robotic procedure.

References

1. Elbakry AA, Abdelhalim A, Al-Omar O. Tips and tricks for the extravesical robotic-assisted laparoscopic ureteral reimplantation for pediatric vesicoureteral reflux. J Pediatr Urol. 2023;19(6):816–7.
2. Esposito C, Yamataka A, Varlet F, Castagnetti M, Scalabre A, Fourcade L, Ballouhey Q, Nappo S, Escolino M. Current trends in 2021 in surgical management of vesico-ureteral reflux in pediatric patients: results of a multicenter international survey on 552 patients. Minerva Urol Nephrol. 2023;75(1):106–15.
3. Blanc T, Meignan P, Vinit N, Ballouhey Q, Pio L, Capito C, Harte C, Vatta F, Galmiche-Rolland L, Minard V, Orbach D, Berteloot L, Muller C, Kohaut J, Broch A, Braik K, Binet A, Heloury Y, Fourcade L, Lardy H, Sarnacki S. Robotic surgery in pediatric oncology: lessons learned from the first 100 tumors—a nationwide experience. Ann Surg Oncol. 2022;29(2):1315–26.
4. Spampinato G, Binet A, Fourcade L, Mendoza Sagaon M, Villemagne T, Braik K, Grosos C, Lardy H, Ballouhey Q. Comparison of the learning curve for robot-assisted laparoscopic pyeloplasty between senior and junior surgeons. J Laparoendosc Adv Surg Tech A. 2021;31(4):478–83.
5. Moncayo S, Compagnon R, Caire F, Grosos C, Bahans C, Ilhero P, Fourcade L, Ballouhey Q. Transition effects from laparocscopic to robotic surgery skills in small cavities. J Robot Surg. 2020;14(3):525–30.
6. Binet A, Fourcade L, Amar S, Alzahrani K, Cook AR, Braïk K, Cros J, Longis B, Villemagne T, Lardy H, Ballouhey Q. Robot-assisted laparoscopic fundoplications in pediatric surgery: experience review. Eur J Pediatr Surg. 2019;29(2):173–8.
7. Meignan P, Ballouhey Q, Lejeune J, Braik K, Longis B, Cook AR, Lardy H, Fourcade L, Binet A. Robotic-assisted laparoscopic surgery for pediatric tumors: a bicenter experience. J Robot Surg. 2018;12(3):501–8.
8. Binet A, Ballouhey Q, Chaussy Y, de Lambert G, Braïk K, Villemagne T, Becmeur F, Fourcade L, Lardy H. Current perspectives in robot-assisted surgery. Minerva Pediatr. 2018;70(3):308–14.
9. Ballouhey Q, Clermidi P, Cros J, Grosos C, Rosa-Arsène C, Bahans C, Caire F, Longis B, Compagnon R, Fourcade L. Comparison of 8- and 5-mm robotic instruments in small cavities: 5- or 8-mm robotic instruments for small cavities? Surg Endosc. 2018;32(2):1027–34.
10. Li B, Lindgren BW, Liu DB, Gong EM. Robot-assisted laparoscopic megaureter tapering with ureteral reimplantation: Tips and tricks. J Pediatr Urol. 2017;13(6):637–8.
11. Ballouhey Q, Dib N, Binet A, Carcauzon-Couvrat V, Clermidi P, Longis B, Lardy H, Languepin J, Cros J, Fourcade L. How robotic-assisted surgery can decrease the risk of mucosal tear during Heller myotomy procedure? J Robot Surg. 2017;11(2):255–8.
12. Muller CO, Blanc T, Peycelon M, El Ghoneimi A. Laparoscopic treatment of ureteropelvic junction obstruction in five pediatric cases of pelvic kidneys. J Pediatr Urol. 2015;11(6):353.e1–5.
13. Ballouhey Q, Villemagne T, Cros J, Szwarc C, Braik K, Longis B, Lardy H, Fourcade L. A comparison of robotic surgery in children weighing above and below 15.0 kg: size does not affect surgery success. Surg Endosc. 2015;29(9):2643–50.
14. Ballouhey Q, Villemagne T, Cros J, Vacquerie V, Bérenguer D, Braik K, Szwarc C, Longis B, Lardy H, Fourcade L. Assessment of paediatric thoracic robotic surgery. Interact Cardiovasc Thorac Surg. 2015;20(3):300–3.
15. de Lambert G, Fourcade L, Centi J, Fredon F, Braik K, Szwarc C, Longis B, Lardy H. How to successfully implement a robotic pediatric surgery program: lessons learned after 96 procedures. Surg Endosc. 2013;27(6):2137–44.

Robotic-Assisted Laparoscopic Surgery for Ovary-Sparing Mass Excision

Giuseppe Autorino, Ernesto Montaruli, and Mario Mendoza-Sagaon

1 Introduction

Abdominal masses are frequently found in pediatric female patients and often originate from the ovaries. Ovarian masses, comprising both non-neoplastic and neoplastic growths, can manifest across all age groups. The occurrence, clinical manifestation, and histological characteristics of such masses in children and adolescents differ significantly from those observed in adults, necessitating a specialized therapeutic approach. Ovarian masses in this population encompass a spectrum from simple functional cysts to malignant tumors. The prevalence of ovarian malignancy is reported to be between 3% and 8% among children and adolescents presenting with adnexal masses, representing 1–2% of all childhood cancers [1].

The most common type of ovarian masses in children is functional cyst especially in adolescents. Ovarian germ cell tumors (OGTs) represent approximately 70% of ovarian neoplasms in children and adolescents, among which the most common presentation is ovarian teratomas (OTs). In particular, OGTs generate directly from germ cells and account for 47.3% to 87.7% among all gynecological tumors, thus being the most common with very rare cases of malignancy [2].

While the prevalence of bilateral mature cystic teratomas is around 10%, conducting a biopsy on the contralateral ovary is a matter of debate. This procedure carries the risk of follicle damage, infection, hemorrhage, and potential adhesion formation. Numerous studies propose that examining the histology of a seemingly normal contralateral ovary results in identifying a teratoma in fewer than 1% of cases [3].

On the other hand, OTs consist of various histological categories of tumors, each containing tissues of germ cell (pluripotential) origin, whether mature or immature; the most common among this group of tumors, the mature cystic teratoma, typically contains tissue from all three embryological layers.

The majority of developed teratomas appear as cystic formations enclosed by a variable-thickness capsule and commonly filled with sebaceous fluid. In contrast, solid mature teratomas are infrequent. They may exhibit a concentrated projection within the cyst referred to as the Rokitansky nodule or dermoid plug, housing components such as hair, bone, dental structures, muscle, calcifications, and cartilage [1].

G. Autorino (✉)
Centre Universitaire Romand de Chirurgie Pédiatrique, Division of Pediatric Surgery of Lausanne, CHUV, Lausanne, Switzerland
e-mail: Giuseppe.Autorino@chuv.ch

E. Montaruli · M. Mendoza-Sagaon
Division of Pediatric Surgery, Ospedale Regionale di Bellinzona e Valli, Bellinzona, Switzerland
e-mail: Ernesto.Montaruli@eoc.ch; Mario.MendozaSagaon@eoc.ch

C. Esposito et al. (eds.), *Pediatric Robotic Assisted Surgery*,
https://doi.org/10.1007/978-3-031-99532-3_26

Another type of commonly benign tumor is the group of epithelial tumors, also known as cystadenomas. They represent around 15–20% of all pediatric ovarian tumors, being much more common among adult patients as they appear to be connected to hormonal stimulation. They can have different histological aspects (serous, mucinous, endometrioid, clear-cell, seromucinous, and Brenner tumors) and different grades of malignancy, although being mostly benign in children. Malignancy in these cases is associated with high level of CA-125 levels. Imaging varies a lot with the grade of malignancy: Imaging characteristics indicative of borderline or malignant tumors include larger size, complex structures, thick and irregular walls, septa thicker than 5 mm, and solid areas with necrosis [1].

Torsion represents the most frequent complication associated with ovarian tumors in children, occurring at an incidence ranging from 3% to 16%. Interestingly, findings from our study and others suggest that ovarian tumors undergoing torsion are typically benign [3]. One possible explanation for the lower incidence of torsion among malignant neoplasms is their capacity to induce inflammation, adhesions, local invasion, and consequently, adherence to surrounding structures. Solid ovarian masses in children have a higher likelihood of being malignant in comparison to either complex (solid and cystic) or simple cysts. When an ovarian lesion is suspected to be malignant, it is important to establish the staging performing a meticulous examination of the peritoneal surfaces, the underside of the diaphragm, the omentum, and the opposite ovary; in these cases, ovarian-sparing surgery is very rarely considered an option [3].

Due to the very low rate of malignancies registered in children and adolescents, patients with ovarian masses, when treated, generally have a favorable long-term prognosis. The preservation of gonadal function is crucial not only for maintaining fertility but also for the normal course of puberty. Moreover, abdominal scars can lead to psychological challenges and diminished self-confidence, particularly in young girls. Therefore, the approach to managing ovarian masses in children and adolescents should aim for a cure, emphasizing preservation of function and minimally invasive methods whenever possible, such as through laparoscopic ovary-sparing surgery [4].

As it happened for other types of technological advancements, the feasibility of robotic surgery has been firstly described by adult gynecologists with the possibility to perform, with a 3-D vision, better accurate movements and more precise dissection, allowing to execute minimally invasive detailed resection of adnexal masses [5].

When studying literature, the first examples of robotic surgery usage, among adult population, have been published in the early 2000s, with papers describing ovarian transpositions, myectomies, treatment of endometriosis, etc. During that period, however, instruments were still only available in 12 mm, and costs and disadvantages of the first models of the DaVinci system were still probably surpassing the advantages of using this technology for pediatric patients.

Progression in technology then brought both the miniaturization of the instruments down to 8 mm and the advancements of the new DaVinci system, making robotic-assisted surgery viable for pediatric patients; this way many centers followed up on the utility of this kind of technology, utilizing it more and more with a wider range of indications, among which ovarian surgery.

Another important development emerged with robotic surgery is the evolution of training: The availability of simulation programs and the presence of a second console seem to speed up the learning curve for every robotic-assisted procedure, but data specific for gynecological surgery has also been produced by adult surgeons. Teams with prior experience in standard laparoscopy might undergo a smoother transition to robotics, but the essential strategy for a secure adaptation to robotic surgery lies in gradually beginning with simpler cases [6–8].

The diagnostic work-up for these patients differs greatly based on the initial clinical presentation: Benign pathologies can be associated with adnexal torsion or be discovered incidentally.

In case of adnexal torsion, clinical presentation is the typical acute abdomen, with pain described as "never felt before," referred to the lower abdomen, associated with frequent episodes of vomiting. Blood tests typically don't show significant alterations in the early stages; thus, diagnosis is based on ultrasound with color Doppler. The prevalent sonographic observation is an echogenic mass in the pelvic region, accompanied by the absence of visualization of the ovary on the same side. The presence of fluid in the cul-de-sac typically appears as a late manifestation and is commonly linked to hemorrhagic ovarian tissue. The lack of blood flow detected through Doppler sonography indicates arterial occlusion and implies the nonviability of the organ. In case of uncertainty, which can emerge especially with constipated patients, an MRI to confirm diagnosis should be considered to eventually rule out more improbable causes. Even if not always diagnostic, tumoral markers should also be requested, to have a preoperative status of the lesion. Due to the urgent nature of this presentation, however, the robotic-assisted approach should not be considered [3, 9].

Should the mass be discovered incidentally, a second-level imaging is always important. The typical ultrasound presentation of a mature teratoma is a cystic mass featuring a hyperechoic Rokitansky nodule. This nodule originates from the cyst wall and extends into the cyst lumen, frequently leading to posterior acoustic shadowing.

CT scans have the ability to detect cystic lesions showing fat density, calcification along the cyst wall, Rokitansky nodules, hair tufts, and fat-fluid levels. This comprehensive imaging approach allows for a conclusive diagnosis in 98% of cases. Even though this method is diagnostic in most cases, it has a higher exposure to radiation, which should always be taken into consideration when choosing a diagnostic exam in children. Thus, MRI imaging, with the possibility to easily identifying the fatty tissue and fluid levels, is a very valid alternative to pose diagnosis with a good margin of certainty without the necessity of radiating young and fertile patients exposing one of the most sensitive tissues. Second-level imaging should also be capable to distinguish, at least with a certain grade of certainty, if a suspect of malignancy is present, thus helping the surgeon to determine the best approach for each patient [1].

2 Patient Positioning and Planning

Once diagnosis has been completed with tumor markers and imaging, surgical indication and planning must be discussed. It is important to stress that masses with a diameter equal or greater of 5 cm carry a high risk of causing an ovarian torsion; this parameter should thus always be taken into consideration when deciding on the urgency of the operation. Also, should malignancy be suspected, robotic-assisted minimally invasive surgery should probably not be taken into consideration due to the higher possibility of abdominal contamination.

However, since the majority of masses in girls don't have such features, robotic surgery could represent a valid alternative to perform a fine dissection requested to spare as much ovarian tissue as possible; this last point is of paramount importance, especially when treating pediatric patients, to reduce as much as possible the risk of infertility in the future [10].

Achieving success in robot-assisted surgery relies on four key factors. These encompass a thorough comprehension of the procedure, advanced surgical expertise and training, seamless teamwork, and, notably, precise patient positioning and strategic placement of robotic ports. The primary objectives of patient positioning and port placements include ensuring patient safety, preventing compression injuries, enabling optimal mobility of the robotic arms, and facilitating a seamless and efficient surgical process. This point gets more important with the reduction in size of the patients [8].

The patient is placed supine adjusting the table with small angle in the Trendelenburg position. This setup allows to get the intestinal loops far away from the pelvis and thus having a better view of the ovarian mass (Fig. 1). The Trendelenburg position also helps maintaining distance between the patient and the trocars, reducing the risk of traumatic/pression robotic

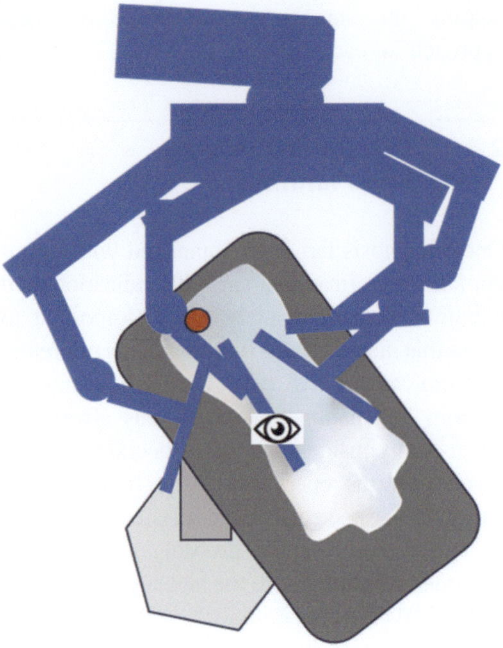

Fig. 1 Robot docking

arm injuries. To this regard, it is very important that the bedside surgeon is always careful about trocars moving during the operation, in order to warn the first operator should the possibility of traumatic injuries arise. It is important to be mindful that, if a Da Vinci compatible table is not available, positioning must be completed before the robot is completely docked, because the bed won't change position afterward without the necessity to redock the robot.

3 Incision and Port Placement

Pediatric surgeons have indeed adapted port positioning over the years, reducing distance and changing the setup to better fit smaller patients. The first incision is made at the umbilical level for the camera, two other 8 mm trocars are placed 7–8 cm apart each other when operating on big enough patients, on a straight transverse umbilical line; should the patient be smaller, distance can be reduced as low as 6 cm, and trocars can also be placed on a lightly curved line (Fig. 2). The use of all four robotic arms is advised, when possible, with the fourth arm placed contralaterally to the position of the mass to have more space available for maneuvers for retraction. The assistant's 5-mm trocar is usually placed ipsilaterally between the two other robotic arms.

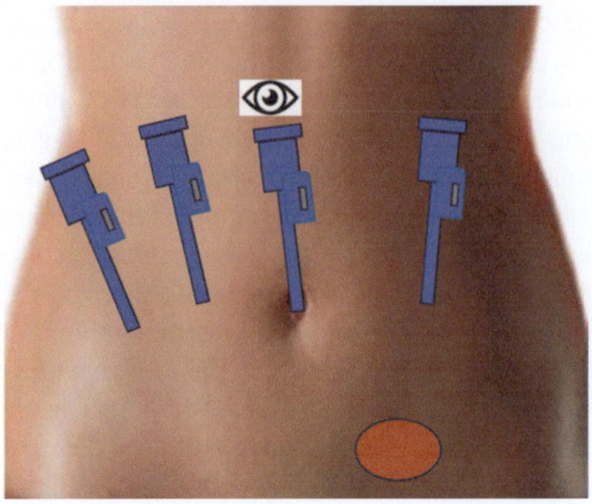

Fig. 2 Port placement

4 Robotic Positioning

The Da Vinci robot should be adjusted to pelvic setting and should be positioned contralaterally to the mass, so that the bedside surgeon can have more mobility when assisting the first operator.

5 Procedure Steps

When performing ovarian-sparing surgery, the dissection usually begins far away from the hilum and the fallopian tube (Fig. 3). Atraumatic graspers and monopolar coagulation (either with Maryland forceps or scissors) starting to slowly dissect the tumor until finding the correct plain of separation between the mass and the normal ovarian tissue (Fig. 4). When treating mature teratomas in particular, the plain of dissection can be easily identified; however, it is important to be careful not to create false planes of dissection; otherwise, there is a risk of rupturing the cystic part of the tumor. Sometimes rupture of normal follicles can mimic perforation of the cystic part. Once the plane of dissection is clearly visible,

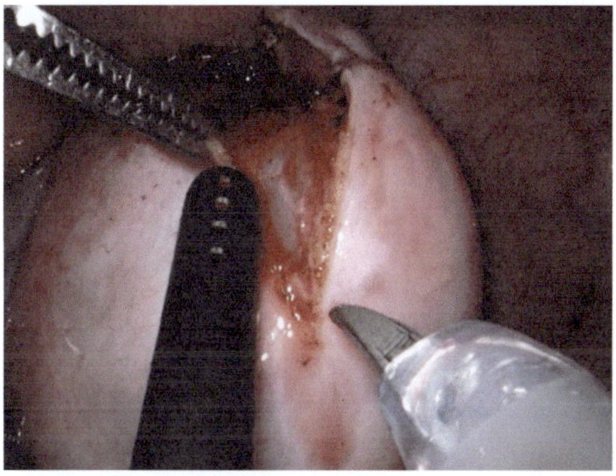

Fig. 3 Incision through the normal tissue up to the tumor

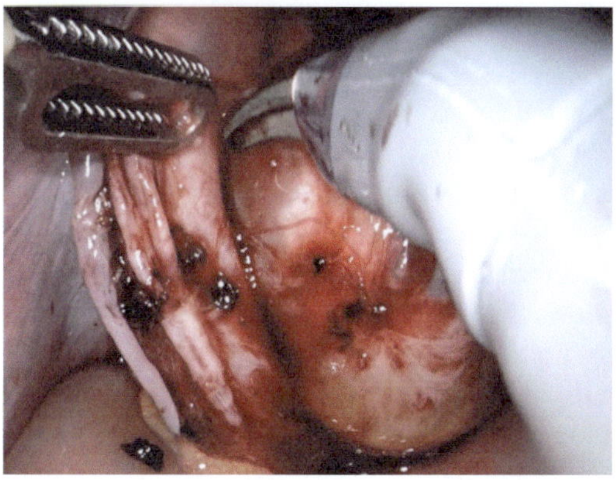

Fig. 4 Plane of dissection between tumor (inside) and normal ovary (outside)

slow and fine blunt dissection with low-intensity monopolar or bipolar energy can begin. The use of low energy, as far away from the ovarian tissue as possible, is very important to limit the damage to the good ovarian tissue. Once a good portion of the ovarian tissue has been peeled away from the mass, the fourth arm comes into play: the possibility to perform traction on both ends of the normal ovarian tissue allows the dissection to proceed smoothly without excessive force on the mass to reduce risk of rupture (Fig. 5). During this delicate part, laparoscopic aspiration should be always ready and the bedside surgeon vigilant to start aspiration right away in case of rupture, reducing at minimum the contamination of the abdominal cavity; should the cyst be open, intraoperative antibiotic prophylaxis should be considered. Once the mass is completely removed, it should be placed inside an endo-bag, whose dimension varies together with the maximum diameter of the mass; it is very important to use imaging as a reference to calculate the correct volume needed of the bag and always have different measures ready in case of discrepancies with pre-op images (Fig. 6). Some surgeons advise the introduction of an endo-bag (without the stick) to be placed underneath the compromised ovary before starting the dissection to decrease the risk of contamination in case of rupture of the mass (Fig. 7).

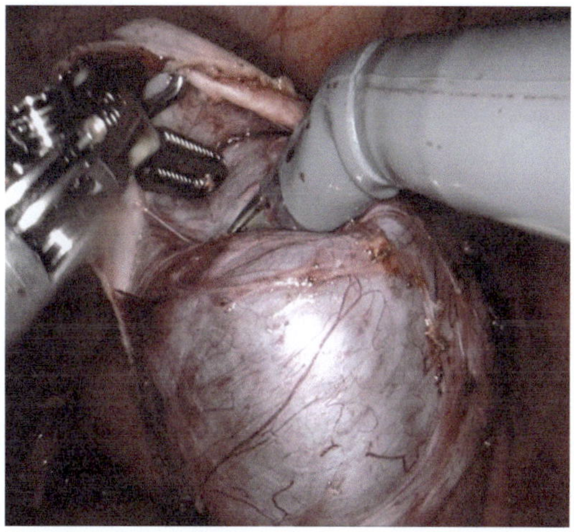

Fig. 5 Use of the fourth robotic arm to optimize traction

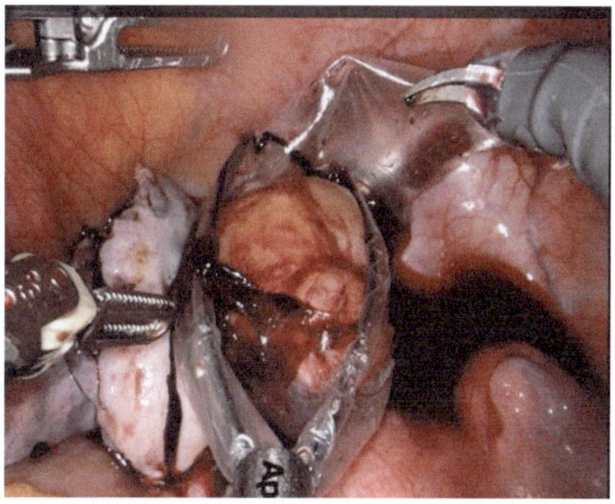

Fig. 6 Use of endo-bag for a safer extraction

Once the mass is inside the endo-bag without risk of contamination, we usually proceed to control hemostasis and suture the edges of the spared ovarian tissue with a 4-0 reabsorbed barbed

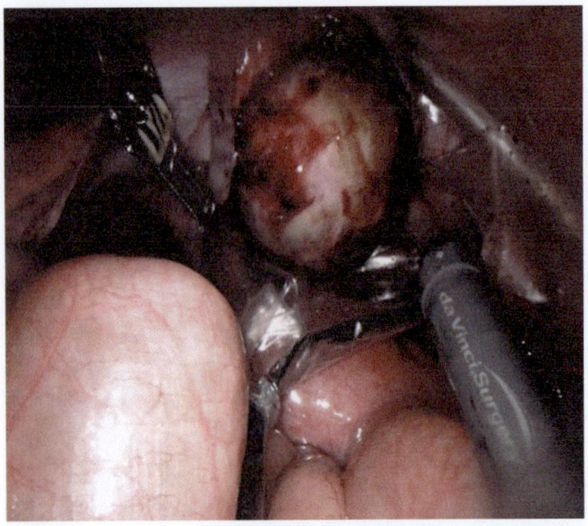

Fig. 7 Use of endo-bag to prevent spreading in case of rupture as much as possible

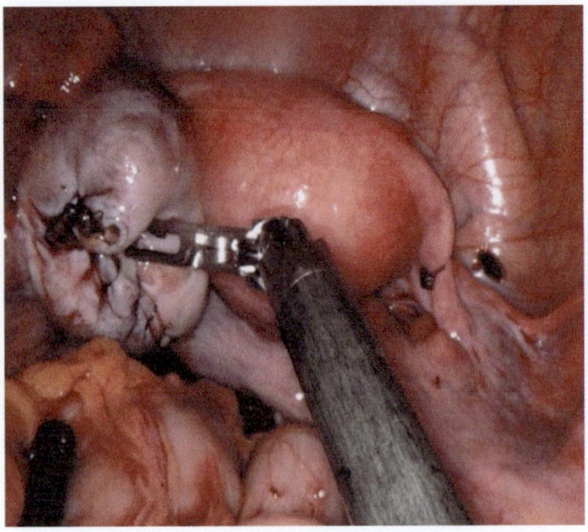

Fig. 9 Final aspect of the ovarian suture

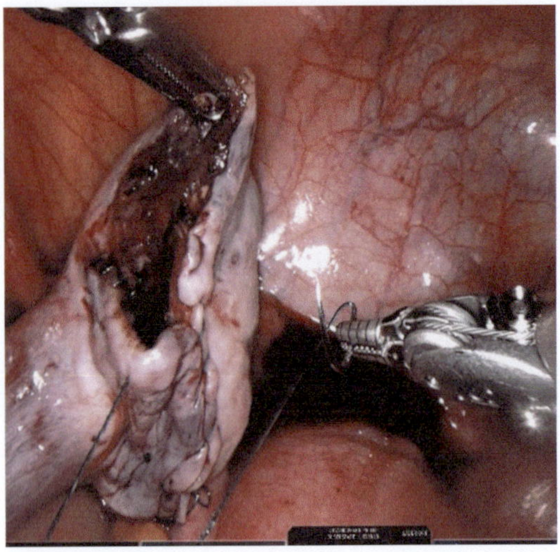

Fig. 8 Ovarian suture with a barbed string

suture (Figs. 8 and 9). This point is not clearly identified in literature; while it is not advisable to employ a lot of energy for electrical coagulation, an interesting prospective randomized study on adults has shown no reduction in ovarian reserve in women between suturing and bipolar coagulation after enucleation of ovarian cysts (endometrial cysts, in particular) [11].

There are multiple options for extraction. In case of big and mostly solid masses, a Pfannesteil incision appears to be the best way to completely remove the mass. In case a cystic part of the mass is present, however, the margins of the endo-bag can be extracted through the navel and under direct vision a controlled puncture of the mass allows for aspiration of the liquid inside. Once the liquid is aspirated, the fluid inside the syringe must be sent for cytological analysis, and the surgeon who performed the aspiration must change gloves in order to reduce the possibility of contamination by, albeit unlikely, possible malignant cells. At this point, the mass can be easily extracted through the navel.

6 Postoperative Period

Postoperative care, in case of no complications, is relatively straightforward. Patients usually only need pain control medication that can gradually be switched to oral administration with the reduction of the pain, usually after 24–48 h; this changes in case of Pfannenstiel incision, associated with higher level of pain. Once patient is discharged, routine follow-up ultrasound is scheduled 1 month after surgery. Eventually, a long-term follow-up at 6 and 12 months after surgery up is advised [12].

7 Tips and Tricks

- Exclude malignancy as much as possible.
- Be mindful of completing positioning before docking if a Da Vinci table is not available.
- The use of fourth robotic arm is highly advised.
- Give the bedside surgeon enough space to help properly.
- Once the plain of dissection is found, coagulate ovarian tissue as little as possible.
- For cystic lesions, safe puncture inside an endo-bag helps greatly with extraction.

Bibliography

1. Birbas E, Kanavos T, Gkrozou F, Skentou C, Daniilidis A, Vatopoulou A. Ovarian masses in children and adolescents: a review of the literature with emphasis on the diagnostic approach. Children (Basel). 2023;10(7):1114. https://doi.org/10.3390/children10071114. PMID: 37508611; PMCID: PMC10377960.
2. Vaysse C, Delsol M, Carfagna L, Bouali O, Combelles S, Lemasson F, Le Mandat A, Castex MP, Pasquet M, Moscovici J, Guitard J, Pienkowski C, Rubie H, Galinier P, Vaysse P. Ovarian germ cell tumors in children. Management, survival and ovarian prognosis. A report of 75 cases. J Pediatr Surg. 2010;45(7):1484–90. https://doi.org/10.1016/j.jpedsurg.2009.11.026. PMID: 20638529.
3. Kokoska ER, Keller MS, Weber TR. Acute ovarian torsion in children. Am J Surg. 2000;180(6):462–5. https://doi.org/10.1016/s0002-9610(00)00503-1. PMID: 11182398.
4. Tarca E, Trandafir LM, Cojocaru E, Costea CF, Rosu ST, Butnariu LI, Iordache AC, Munteanu V, Luca AC. Diagnosis difficulties and minimally invasive treatment for ovarian masses in adolescents. Int J Women's Health. 2022;14:1047–57. https://doi.org/10.2147/IJWH.S374444. PMID: 35971543; PMCID: PMC9375555.
5. Gala RB, Margulies R, Steinberg A, Murphy M, Lukban J, Jeppson P, Aschkenazi S, Olivera C, South M, Lowenstein L, Schaffer J, Balk EM, Sung V; Society of Gynecologic Surgeons Systematic Review Group. Systematic review of robotic surgery in gynecology: robotic techniques compared with laparoscopy and laparotomy. J Minim Invasive Gynecol. 2014;21(3):353–61. https://doi.org/10.1016/j.jmig.2013.11.010. Epub 2013 Dec 1. PMID: 24295923.
6. Marengo F, Larraín D, Babilonti L, Spinillo A. Learning experience using the double-console da Vinci surgical system in gynecology: a prospective cohort study in a University hospital. Arch Gynecol Obstet 2012;285(2):441–445. https://doi.org/10.1007/s00404-011-2005-8. Epub 2011 Jul 22. PMID: 21779771.
7. Hassan SO, Dudhia J, Syed LH, Patel K, Farshidpour M, Cunningham SC, Kowdley GC. Conventional laparoscopic vs robotic training: which is better for naive users? A randomized prospective crossover study. J Surg Educ 2015;72(4):592–9. https://doi.org/10.1016/j.jsurg.2014.12.008. Epub 2015 Feb 14. PMID: 25687957.
8. Chang C, Steinberg Z, Shah A, Gundeti MS. Patient positioning and port placement for robot-assisted surgery. J Endourol. 2014;28(6):631–638. https://doi.org/10.1089/end.2013.0733. Epub 2014 Apr 25. PMID: 24548088; PMCID: PMC4382714.
9. Joudi N, Adams Hillard PJ. Adnexal torsion in a pediatric population: Acute presentation with question of chronicity. Eur J Obstet Gynecol Reprod Biol. 2022;268:82–86. https://doi.org/10.1016/j.ejogrb.2021.11.435. Epub 2021 Dec 2. PMID: 34883338.
10. Nakib G, Calcaterra V, Scorletti F, Romano P, Goruppi I, Mencherini S, Avolio L, Pelizzo G. Robotic assisted surgery in pediatric gynecology: promising innovation in mini invasive surgical procedures. J Pediatr Adolesc Gynecol 2013;26(1):e5–7. https://doi.org/10.1016/j.jpag.2012.09.009 Epub 2012 Nov 15. PMID: 23158752.
11. Owczarek D, Malinowski A, Wilczyński M. Ovarian reserve evaluation after laparoscopic cyst enucleation, depending on applied haemostasis technique and with particular consideration of endometrial cysts. Menopause Rev/Przegląd Menopauzalny. 2018;17(1):22–7. https://doi.org/10.5114/pm.2018.74899.
12. Upasani A, Mariotto A, Eassa W, Subramaniam R. Robot-assisted reconstructive surgery of lower urinary tract in children: a narrative review on technical aspects and current literature. Transl Pediatr. 2023;12(8):1540–51. https://doi.org/10.21037/tp-22-533. Epub 2023 Aug 17. PMID: 37692545; PMCID: PMC10485640.

MIX
Papier aus verantwortungsvollen Quellen
Paper from responsible sources
FSC® C105338

If you have any concerns about our products,
you can contact us on
ProductSafety@springernature.com

In case Publisher is established outside the EU,
the EU authorized representative is:
Springer Nature Customer Service Center GmbH
Europaplatz 3, 69115 Heidelberg, Germany

Printed by Libri Plureos GmbH
in Hamburg, Germany